Choosing the Correct

Gary X. Wang • Mark A. Anderson
Lauren Uzdienski • Susanna I. Lee

Choosing the Correct Radiologic Test

Case-Based Teaching Files

Second Edition

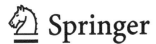

Gary X. Wang
Department of Radiology
Massachusetts General Hospital
Boston, MA
USA

Lauren Uzdienski
Independent Scholar
Boston, MA
USA

Mark A. Anderson
Department of Radiology
Massachusetts General Hospital
Boston, MA
USA

Susanna I. Lee
Department of Radiology
Massachusetts General Hospital
Boston, MA
USA

ISBN 978-3-030-65187-9   ISBN 978-3-030-65185-5   (eBook)
https://doi.org/10.1007/978-3-030-65185-5

This Springer imprint is published by the registered company Springer Nature Switzerland AG
The registered company address is: Gewerbestrasse 11, 6330 Cham, Switzerland

Preface

Few areas in medicine have undergone the dramatic expansion of technical capabilities experienced in diagnostic imaging or radiology over the past 50 years. As precision cross-sectional and molecular imaging has rendered older diagnostic tests obsolete, radiology has become one of the fastest expanding and rapidly changing components of healthcare, providing clinicians with powerful and precise tools to diagnose and treat illness. The ultimate beneficiaries have been patients, who enjoy earlier detection of and improved outcomes from disease.

Unfortunately, the training of healthcare providers has failed to keep pace with these rapid advances in radiologic imaging. Medical education, training, and recertification requirements for physicians, nurse practitioners, and physician assistants rarely include provisions to insure current knowledge on the utility and the risks and benefits of radiologic exams. Yet correct imaging utilization, when integrated into patient management algorithms, often expedites diagnosis, enables cost-effective treatment planning, and offers longitudinal monitoring of therapies for safety and efficacy.

This textbook is a guide to appropriate image ordering for the general healthcare provider. The chapters are organized by organ system or patient demographics and focus on commonly encountered clinical scenarios. These chapters cover breast, cardiac, thoracic, gastrointestinal, urologic, women's, pediatric, vascular, musculoskeletal, and neurologic imaging. The teaching is structured in a case-based multiple-choice quiz format. The practitioner is presented with a patient with a specific complaint, physical exam finding, or clinical need (e.g., cancer staging) and asked to choose a radiologic exam that is most likely to be appropriate. Once a choice has been made, the usefulness of each option is evaluated according to the American College of Radiology (ACR) Appropriateness Criteria as "usually," "may be," or "usually not" appropriate. In the answer key, an exam type is described as the "most" appropriate when it is both usually appropriate and preferred over all other answer choices. In some cases, when imaging is not indicated, "no ideal imaging exam" may be the correct answer. Each case is accompanied by an image from the correct radiologic exam choice, illustrating a possible diagnosis for the patient presented in the case, and a brief explanation of the answer. While the goal is to offer advice that is applicable internationally, some of the advanced technologies (e.g., magnetic resonance imaging, positron emission tomography) may not be available in limited resource settings.

Boston, MA, USA   Gary X. Wang
Boston, MA, USA   Mark A. Anderson
Boston, MA, USA   Lauren Uzdienski
Boston, MA, USA   Susanna I. Lee

Contents

1	**Introduction**.	1
	1.1 ACR Appropriateness Criteria	1
	1.2 Imaging Modalities	2
	1.2.1 X-ray and Fluoroscopy	2
	1.2.2 Ultrasound	4
	1.2.3 Computed Tomography	4
	1.2.4 Magnetic Resonance Imaging	5
	1.2.5 Nuclear Medicine Scan	6
	1.2.6 Interventional Procedures	6
	Bibliography	7
2	**Breast Imaging**	9
	2.1 Palpable Breast Lump	9
	2.2 Breast Pain	23
	2.3 Nipple Discharge	33
	2.4 Symptomatic Male Breast	41
	2.5 Imaging During Pregnancy and Lactation	47
	2.6 Breast Implant Evaluation	55
3	**Cardiac Imaging**	61
	3.1 Acute Chest Pain	61
	3.2 Chronic Chest Pain	65
	3.3 Coronary Artery Disease	69
	3.4 Infective Endocarditis	75
	3.5 Nonischemic Myocardial Disease	77
	3.6 Pulmonary Embolism.	85
	3.7 Shortness of Breath	91
4	**Thoracic Imaging**	97
	4.1 Blunt Chest Trauma	97
	4.2 Rib Fractures	101
	4.3 Hemoptysis	105
	4.4 Acute Respiratory Illness in an Immunocompetent Patient.	111
	4.5 Acute Respiratory Illness in an Immunocompromised Patient	127
	4.6 Chronic Dyspnea, Suspected Pulmonary Origin	135

4.7   Possible Tuberculosis.................................. 139
4.8   Occupational Lung Disease.............................. 143
4.9   Routine Chest Radiography.............................. 151
4.10 Solitary Pulmonary Nodule............................. 157
4.11 Bronchogenic Carcinoma Staging........................ 163

5   Gastrointestinal Imaging................................ 167
5.1   Blunt Abdominal Trauma................................ 167
5.2   Right Upper Quadrant Pain.............................. 173
5.3   Right Lower Quadrant Pain: Suspected Appendicitis........... 183
5.4   Left Lower Quadrant Pain: Suspected Diverticulitis........... 189
5.5   Acute Abdominal Pain and Fever or Suspected Abdominal
      Abscess... 191
5.6   Suspected Small Bowel Obstruction...................... 199
5.7   Jaundice... 203
5.8   Acute Pancreatitis................................... 209
5.9   Dysphagia... 217
5.10 Crohn's Disease..................................... 225
5.11 Liver Lesion Characterization.......................... 231
5.12 Colorectal Cancer Screening........................... 243
5.13 Colorectal Cancer Staging............................. 255

6   Urologic Imaging..................................... 259
6.1   Renal Trauma....................................... 259
6.2   Lower Urinary Tract Trauma............................ 265
6.3   Acute Onset Flank Pain or Suspected Urolithiasis........... 271
6.4   Acute Pyelonephritis................................. 277
6.5   Acute Onset Scrotal Pain.............................. 281
6.6   Hematuria.. 283
6.7   Hematospermia...................................... 289
6.8   Recurrent Lower Urinary Tract Infections in Women........... 293
6.9   Benign Prostatic Hyperplasia........................... 297
6.10 Renal Failure....................................... 299
6.11 Renal Transplant Dysfunction.......................... 303
6.12 Renovascular Hypertension............................ 305
6.13 Incidentally Discovered Adrenal Mass.................... 311
6.14 Indeterminate Renal Mass............................. 321
6.15 Prostate Cancer Detection, Staging, and Surveillance............ 325
      6.15.1 American Joint Committee on Cancer (AJCC)
              Prostate Cancer Staging......................... 325
      6.15.2 Prostate Cancer Risk Stratification................. 326
6.16 Renal Cell Carcinoma Staging.......................... 335
6.17 Invasive Bladder Cancer Staging........................ 337
6.18 Testicular Cancer Staging............................. 339
Bibliography... 340

7   Women's Imaging 341
   7.1   Abnormal Vaginal Bleeding. 341
   7.2   First-Trimester Bleeding 353
   7.3   Acute Pelvic Pain in the Reproductive Age Group 355
   7.4   Clinically Suspected Adnexal Mass. 363
   7.5   Infertility 369
   7.6   Pelvic Floor Dysfunction. 375
   7.7   Ovarian Cancer Screening 379
   7.8   Ovarian Cancer Pretreatment Imaging and Follow-Up 383
   7.9   Endometrial Cancer of the Uterus 387
   7.10 Staging of Invasive Cancer of the Cervix 395

8   Pediatric Imaging 401
   8.1   Head Trauma in a Child. 401
       8.1.1   Glasgow Coma Scale (GCS) 401
       8.1.2   Pediatric Emergency Care Network (PECARN)
               Clinical Criteria for Minor Head Trauma 402
   8.2   Seizures 411
   8.3   Headache 425
   8.4   Sinusitis 433
   8.5   Pneumonia in the Immunocompetent Child 437
   8.6   Vomiting in Infants. 445
   8.7   Suspected Appendicitis 453
   8.8   Urinary Tract Infection 463
   8.9   Hematuria. 471
   8.10 Developmental Dysplasia of the Hip 483
   8.11 Acutely Limping Child Up to Age 5 491
   8.12 Suspected Physical Abuse 497
   Bibliography 503

9   Vascular Imaging 505
   9.1   Penetrating Neck Injury. 505
   9.2   Suspected Pulmonary Arteriovenous Malformation 511
   9.3   Thoracic Aortic Aneurysm. 513
   9.4   Pulsatile Abdominal Mass 515
   9.5   Mesenteric Ischemia 517
   9.6   Suspected Upper Extremity Deep Vein Thrombosis 521
   9.7   Suspected Lower Extremity Deep Vein Thrombosis 523
   9.8   Sudden Onset of Cold, Painful Leg 525
   9.9   Vascular Claudication 527

10   Musculoskeletal Imaging 529
   10.1 Suspected Spine Trauma 529
       10.1.1   NEXUS Criteria. 529
       10.1.2   Canadian C-Spine Rules (CCR). 530

10.2 Traumatic Shoulder Pain 551
10.3 Acute Hand and Wrist Trauma. 567
10.4 Acute Hip Pain, Suspected Fracture 579
10.5 Acute Trauma to the Knee 583
10.6 Acute Trauma to the Ankle 595
      10.6.1 Ottawa Ankle Rules 595
10.7 Acute Trauma to the Foot 601
10.8 Stress (Fatigue or Insufficiency) Fracture 609
10.9 Osteoporosis and Bone Mineral Density 623
10.10 Atraumatic Shoulder Pain 631
10.11 Chronic Elbow Pain 645
10.12 Chronic Wrist Pain 661
10.13 Chronic Hip Pain 675
10.14 Chronic Knee Pain 685
10.15 Chronic Ankle Pain 689
10.16 Chronic Foot Pain 699
10.17 Chronic Back Pain: Suspected Sacroiliitis/Spondyloarthropathy . . 717
10.18 Chronic Extremity Joint Pain: Suspected Inflammatory Arthritis . . 723
10.19 Osteonecrosis of the Hip 731
10.20 Suspected Foot Osteomyelitis in Patients with Diabetes Mellitus. . 735
10.21 Suspected Osteomyelitis, Septic Arthritis, or Soft Tissue Infection
      (Excluding Spine and Diabetic Foot). 741
10.22 Soft Tissue Masses. 751
10.23 Primary Bone Tumors 757
10.24 Imaging After Shoulder Arthroplasty. 769
10.25 Imaging After Total Hip Arthroplasty 775
10.26 Imaging After Total Knee Arthroplasty 781
Bibliography 789

11 Neurologic Imaging. 791
11.1 Head Trauma 791
      11.1.1 Glasgow Coma Scale (GCS) 791
      11.1.2 New Orleans Criteria (NOC) 792
      11.1.3 Canadian CT Head Rule (CCHR) 793
      11.1.4 National Emergency X-Radiography Utilization Study
              (NEXUS-II) 794
11.2 Cerebrovascular Disease 811
11.3 Acute Mental Status Change, Delirium, and New-Onset
      Psychosis 833
11.4 Seizures and Epilepsy 839
11.5 Headache 847
11.6 Dementia 859
11.7 Movement Disorders and Neurodegenerative Diseases. 869

11.8   Ataxia... 879
11.9   Orbits, Vision, and Visual Loss 883
11.10 Hearing Loss and Vertigo................................ 897
11.11 Tinnitus 909
11.12 Sinonasal Disease...................................... 915
11.13 Thyroid Disease 921
11.14 Neck Mass and Adenopathy.............................. 929
11.15 Low Back Pain.. 935
Bibliography 947

1.1 ACR Appropriateness Criteria

The ACR Appropriateness Criteria (American College of Radiology n.d.-a) are practice guidelines for healthcare providers on how to best use imaging in caring for patients with common clinical problems. For each clinical scenario, possible radiology exam choices are evaluated as "usually," "may be," or "usually not" appropriate as defined in Table 1.1. They have been devised by a series of expert panels comprised of radiologists and treating physicians, with each panel devoted to a specific medical specialty or organ system (e.g., pediatric imaging, neurologic imaging). When available, recommendations for exam ordering are derived from clinical research results published in the peer-reviewed literature. However, in the absence of relevant evidence, recommendations are drawn as a consensus expert opinion of the panel members. The guidelines are freely available online and are kept current, with updates every 2–3 years.

Table 1.1 Exam appropriateness rankings

Appropriateness ranking	Definition
Usually appropriate	Imaging is indicated, and the exam choice is likely to benefit the patient The most preferable exam choice in this category is described as the "most appropriate" in the answer key
May be appropriate	Imaging is indicated, and the exam choice is second line to another more likely to benefit the patient Imaging may be indicated, and the exam choice may benefit the patient
Usually not appropriate	Imaging is indicated, but the exam choice is unlikely to benefit the patient Imaging is probably not indicated, and the exam choice is unlikely to benefit the patient
No ideal imaging exam	Imaging is not indicated

G. X. Wang et al., *Choosing the Correct Radiologic Test*,
https://doi.org/10.1007/978-3-030-65185-5_1

While comprehensive, the Appropriateness Criteria is far from exhaustive. On many clinical issues where no or little research evidence or expert consensus is available (e.g., posttreatment surveillance, chronic pain), the Appropriateness Criteria, as well as this textbook, is silent. Finally, for many scenarios, the underlying assumption is that the referring practitioner has evaluated the patient and determined that a radiologic exam may be indicated. Only rarely do the guidelines speak to the question, "Should imaging be undertaken at all?" Few cases that address this query define specific clinical criteria (i.e., patient complaints or physical exam findings) that should be present before imaging has been shown useful.

1.2   Imaging Modalities

Radiologic exams are generally classified by the imaging modality. These include X-ray plain film (also called radiography) and fluoroscopy, ultrasound (US), computed tomography (CT), magnetic resonance imaging (MRI), nuclear medicine scan (also called scintigraphy) and positron emission tomography (PET), and image-guided interventional procedures. As diagnostic tests, each carry known advantages and disadvantages. The language of radiology, like that for all other medical specialties, is replete with acronyms. Those commonly used in this textbook have been defined in Table 1.2.

1.2.1   X-ray and Fluoroscopy

X-ray plain film (also called radiography) is the oldest and most widely available radiologic modality. Evaluation of many body parts (e.g., chest, abdomen, extremities) is possible at the bedside at many sites. Images of reasonable diagnostic quality can be obtained even in patients who cannot cooperate with breath-holding instructions as acquisition times are on the order of seconds. Extremely high resolution allows for optimal evaluation of bone and lung. Exams deliver 0.001–1 mSv of ionizing radiation, well below the average annual radiation dose of 3 mSv from background radiation (RadiologyInfo.org n.d.).

With fluoroscopy, the patient is evaluated in real time with X-ray. Thus, movement such as that of bowel, diaphragm, or the joints can be assessed. Enteric contrast, either barium-based (non-water soluble) or iodine-based (water soluble), is administered orally (e.g., X-ray swallow exam) or rectally (e.g., X-ray contrast enema) for the visualization of the esophagus, stomach, and small bowel or the colon, respectively. X-ray fluoroscopy confers higher radiation doses than plain film with effective doses of 6–8 mSv for abdominal exams (RadiologyInfo.org n.d.). Because exams require that the patient be able to follow swallowing, positioning, and breath-holding instructions, it cannot be used effectively to evaluate the critically ill or debilitated patients.

Table 1.2 List of acronyms

ACR	American College of Radiology
AJCC	American Joint Committee on Cancer
β-HCG	β-Human chorionic gonadotropin
CCHR	Canadian CT head rule
CCR	Canadian C-spine rules
CT	Computed tomography
CTA	Computed tomography angiogram
DMSA	Dimercaptosuccinic acid
DTPA	Diethylenetriaminepentaacetic acid
ERCP	Endoscopic retrograde cholangiopancreatogram
F-18	Fluorine-18
FAST	Focused assessment with sonography for trauma
FDG	Fluorodeoxyglucose
FIGO	International Federation of Gynecology and Obstetrics
Ga-67	Gallium-67
GCS	Glasgow coma scale
HMPAO	Hexamethylpropyleneamine oxime
HU	Hounsfield units
I-123	Iodine-123
In-111	Indium-111
MAA	Macroaggregated albumin
MAG3	Mercaptoacetyltriglycine
MDP	Methylene diphosphonate
mGy	Milli-Gray
MIBG	Metaiodobenzylguanidine
MIP	Maximum intensity projection
MRA	Magnetic resonance angiogram
MRCP	Magnetic resonance cholangiopancreatogram
MRI	Magnetic resonance imaging
mSv	Milli-Sievert
NEXUS	National emergency X-radiography utilization study
NOC	New Orleans criteria
PECARN	Pediatric emergency care network
PET	Positron emission tomography
PSA	Prostate-specific antigen
SPECT	Single-photon emission computerized tomography
Tc-99m	Metastable technetium-99m
US	Ultrasound
V/Q	Ventilation-perfusion
Xe-133	Xenon-133

1.2.2 Ultrasound

Ultrasound (US) is a modality that is widely available and can be performed at the bedside for critically ill patients. It also has the advantage that no ionizing radiation is involved. No biologic effects have been documented from diagnostic US exams, even in the fetus, despite widespread use over several decades. With Doppler, the theoretical risks to a fetus from heat and cavitation are a consideration; hence, it is used judiciously, minimizing the exposure time and acoustic output. Intravenous contrast is an option available for specific indications (e.g., liver or renal mass characterization) but is not administered in the routine diagnostic US exam.

US as an imaging tool is hampered by its inability to penetrate through many tissues (e.g., typically <10 cm in soft tissue, 0 cm through air or bone). Also, the width of the image is limited by the transducer which is typically <15 cm. This limited field of view means US is not useful as a comprehensive search tool for the whole body or even a body part. In essence, you find what you are looking for where you are looking for it, but rarely anything more. Image acquisition protocols are not standardized, and most practices do not acquire volumetric cine images of the target body part, meaning that test results rely on real-time operator assessment. Consequently, it is challenging to test the reported diagnostic accuracies for reproducibility or inter-reader agreement. In this sense, US is more analogous to an extension of the physical exam rather than a diagnostic test.

1.2.3 Computed Tomography

Computed tomography (CT) is widely available in both outpatient and inpatient settings. Exams are well tolerated, as imaging a given body part typically requires <15 s on most scanners. Thus, even in a patient who is unresponsive or unable to cooperate with breathing instructions, CT has a high likelihood of yielding diagnostic quality images. Imaging involves an X-ray beam capable of penetrating through most tissue types (metallic implants being the notable exception) and yields large field-of-view images for complete assessment of the entire body. Bone, soft tissue, fluid, fat, and air are all imaged with high resolution and reproducibility. Intravenous contrast is iodine based and is administered to evaluate vessels and to improve soft tissue contrast of the solid and hollow viscera, renal collecting systems, and neoplasms.

Ionizing radiation exposure is the most significant drawback of CT. While effective doses administered by a diagnostic CT exam (1–20 mSv in adult) have not been directly shown to pose a health risk, extrapolation from higher levels estimate, for instance, an added fatal cancer risk of approximately 1:1000 in an adult undergoing an abdomen CT exam (RadiologyInfo.org n.d.; National Research Council 2006). While this may seem negligible in the context of the general lifetime risk of 1:5 for fatal cancer, this risk is thought to be additive with each exam. The risk is also likely to be higher in the pediatric population and in the fetus.

Intravenous iodinated contrast is associated with a 3% incidence of allergic reaction, the vast majority of which are mild (e.g., itching, hives) and self-limited (American College of Radiology n.d.-b). However, 0.004–0.04% incidence of severe reactions (e.g., laryngeal edema, hypotension) requiring hospitalization has been reported. In patients with end stage renal disease (i.e., estimated glomerular filtration rate [eGFR] less than 30 mL/min/1.73 m^2), transient acute kidney injury (AKI) also represents a potential complication. The pre-disposing risk factors that should trigger a measurement of renal function before iodinated contrast administration is a history of kidney disease (e.g., chronic kidney disease, AKI, kidney surgery, or albuminuria) or diabetes.

1.2.4 Magnetic Resonance Imaging

Magnetic resonance imaging (MRI) affords the best soft tissue contrast of any of the radiologic modalities and involves no ionizing radiation. Brain and spinal cord, bone marrow, joints, muscles, and abdominopelvic solid organs (e.g., liver, kidneys, uterus, prostate) are all optimally depicted with MRI. The electromagnetic field, which is the basis for scanning, allows for multiplanar imaging with a large field of view. Application of multiple electromagnetic pulse sequences (e.g., T1-, T2-, proton density-weighted) enables differentiation of a large variety of soft tissues. For some indications, intravenous contrast that is gadolinium based is administered to better evaluate the vessels, solid viscera, and neoplasms. However, even in a patient who cannot receive intravenous contrast, specific flow-sensitive pulse sequences can be used to evaluate the blood vessels.

Disadvantages of MRI include limited access to the scanner itself or the radiologist expertise to implement and interpret the exams in some practice settings. Most exams entail that the patient lie still in an enclosed scanner for up to 20–40 min, although wider bore or "open" scanners if available can be used for some indications. For pediatric patients who are too young to cooperate or lie still sedation may be necessary. In critically ill patients, monitoring and supportive-care equipment that are usually incompatible with high field strength magnets would be a contraindication to scanning. Even in conscious patients, concerns such as claustrophobia or inability to lie still or cooperate with breath-holding procedures can hinder successful image acquisition.

Intravenous gadolinium contrast is associated with a much lower incidence (0.07%) of allergic reactions than iodinated contrast (3%) (American College of Radiology n.d.-b). Incidence of severe reactions requiring hospitalization is reported as <0.005%. However, gadolinium contrast administration in patients with renal failure has been associated with nephrogenic systemic fibrosis (NSF), a syndrome resulting in progressive fibrosis of the skin, joints, eyes, and organs, which is uniformly fatal. While the newer macrocyclic class of gadolinium agents now in use have not been associated with NSF, gadolinium is still considered relatively contraindicated in patients with end stage renal disease (i.e., eGFR less than 30 mL/min/1.73 m^2).

1.2.5   Nuclear Medicine Scan

Nuclear medicine scanning and positron emission tomography (PET) employs the physiologic and biochemical processes in the body to image-specific organs and their functions. Radiopharmaceuticals are administered, most often intravenously, but for some exams by other means such as inhalation (^{133}Xe into lung) or by catheter (^{99}Tc-pertechnetate into bladder). Their uptake and/or excretion by various tissues are then imaged by computer-aided detectors that can acquire and present the information in planar (e.g., anteroposterior, lateral) or tomographic (e.g., single-photon emission computerized tomography [SPECT], PET) format.

Because a physiologically active radiotracer is used, many nuclear medicine scans have the distinct advantage of being able to provide functional as well as anatomic information. Examples include cardiac myocardial perfusion (^{99}Tc-sestamibi), bone turnover (^{99}Tc-MDP), lung ventilation (^{133}Xe) and perfusion (^{99}Tc-MAA), and glucose metabolism (^{18}FDG). These are each tailored to answer a defined diagnostic question. Effective radiation doses range from 1 to 20 mSv and, hence, are comparable to a CT exam (RadiologyInfo.org n.d.). Because the imaging source is emitted from the body, rather than being external, whole-body evaluation is possible.

The major disadvantage of a nuclear medicine exam is poor spatial resolution, which for some exams has been mitigated by fusing the nuclear medicine images with concurrently acquired anatomic images (e.g., PET-CT). Availability of many exam types is often limited because a radiopharmacy and, for specific isotopes, a cyclotron, must be nearby to deliver isotopes with half-lives on the order of several minutes to days. Finally, image acquisition requires table times of 30 min to several hours rendering many exams unsuitable for the uncooperative or critically ill patient.

1.2.6   Interventional Procedures

Image-guided interventional procedures in diagnostic radiology typically use fluoroscopy, US, or CT to introduce a catheter or a needle into a particular anatomic space, such as a blood vessel (angiogram), a joint space (arthrogram), the spinal canal (myelogram), or a hollow viscera (e.g., cystogram, hysterosonogram). Contrast material is then introduced, thereby allowing for high-contrast visualization of the opacified lumen. Biopsies comprise the other general category of diagnostic radiologic interventions. Here an aspiration and/or cutting needle is introduced into the lesion or organ of interest under imaging guidance to obtain samples for histology, culture, or other laboratory studies.

Most image-guided interventions are performed as same-day outpatient procedures. Procedures on superficial targets (e.g., skin, breast) or joints can be performed on cooperative patients without sedation. Angiograms and deep tissue biopsies, however, usually require conscious sedation for which the patient will need to fast before and be monitored after the procedures. Major complications requiring hospitalization are very rare (Society of Interventional Radiology Standards of Practice

Committee 2003). Minor complications include bleeding (usually self-limited), localized infection, and allergic reaction to administered contrast.

Bibliography

American College of Radiology. ACR Appropriateness Criteria. n.d.-a. Available at https://acsearch.acr.org/list. Accessed 20 Mar 2020.

American College of Radiology committee on drugs and contrast media. ACR manual on contrast media, version 10.2. n.d.-b. Available at https://www.acr.org/-/media/ACR/Files/Clinical-Resources/Contrast_Media.pdf. Accessed 20 Mar 2020.

National Research Council committee to assess health risks from exposure to low levels of ionizing radiation. Health risks from exposure to low levels of ionizing radiation: BEIR VII phase 2. Washington, DC: National Academies Press; 2006.

RadiologyInfo.org. Radiation dose in X-ray and CT exams. n.d.. Available at https://www.radiologyinfo.org/en/info.cfm?pg=safety-xray. Accessed 20 Mar 2020.

Society of Interventional Radiology Standards of Practice Committee. Quality improvement guidelines for image-guided percutaneous biopsy in adults. J Vasc Interv Radiol. 2003;14:S227–30.

Breast Imaging

2

2.1 Palpable Breast Lump

A 54-year-old woman with a palpable breast lump.

a. Mammography diagnostic
b. US breast
c. MRI breast without and with contrast
d. FDG-PET breast
e. No ideal imaging exam

© The Author(s), under exclusive license to Springer Nature
Switzerland AG 2021
G. X. Wang et al., *Choosing the Correct Radiologic Test*,
https://doi.org/10.1007/978-3-030-65185-5_2

A woman 40 years of age or older, initial evaluation.

a. *Mammography diagnostic* is the most appropriate.
b. US breast may be appropriate as the initial imaging exam if the patient has had a mammogram within the past 6 months.
c. MRI breast without and with contrast is usually not appropriate.
d. FDG-PET breast is usually not appropriate.

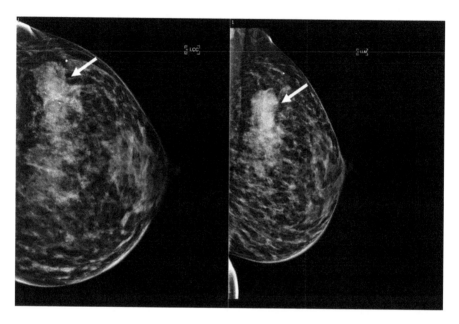

Fig. 2.1 Breast cancer. Diagnostic mammography craniocaudal (left) and mediolateral (right) views of the left breast show an irregular mass at the site of a palpable lump (arrows). Core needle biopsy of the mass revealed invasive ductal carcinoma

Solution

Diagnostic mammography is the primary exam for initial imaging assessment of a palpable lump and is performed under the direct supervision of a radiologist. A small radio-opaque marker is placed on the skin overlying the lump to identify its position. If a clearly benign correlate is identified, then mammography alone may be enough. Otherwise, additional imaging with another modality is indicated.

A 54-year-old woman with a palpable breast lump. Mammography shows a finding suspicious for malignancy.

a. US breast
b. MRI breast without and with contrast
c. FDG-PET breast
d. Image-guided fine needle aspiration breast
e. No ideal imaging exam

A woman 40 years of age or older, mammography finding suspicious for malignancy.

a. *US breast* is the most appropriate.
b. MRI breast without and with contrast is usually not appropriate.
c. FDG-PET breast is usually not appropriate.
d. Image-guided fine needle aspiration breast is usually not appropriate.

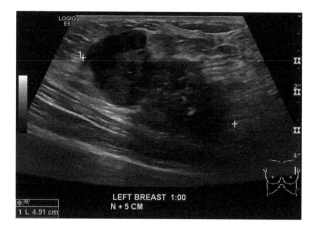

Fig. 2.2 Breast cancer. Breast US shows a 4.9 cm irregularly shaped mass (calipers). Core needle biopsy diagnosed invasive ductal carcinoma

Solution

US may help characterize a suspicious mammographic finding and identify additional lesions not evident on mammography. If a US correlate to the mammographic finding is identified, then biopsy can be performed under sonographic guidance. US-guided biopsy may be better tolerated by some patients than mammographic-guided biopsy and allows biopsy of areas difficult to access mammographically.

A 57-year-old woman with a palpable breast lump. Mammography is negative.

a. US breast
b. MRI breast without and with contrast
c. FDG-PET breast
d. Image-guided core biopsy breast
e. No ideal imaging exam

A woman 40 years of age or older, mammography is negative.

a. *US breast* is the most appropriate.
b. MRI breast without and with contrast is usually not appropriate.
c. FDG-PET breast is usually not appropriate.
d. Image-guided core biopsy breast is usually not appropriate.

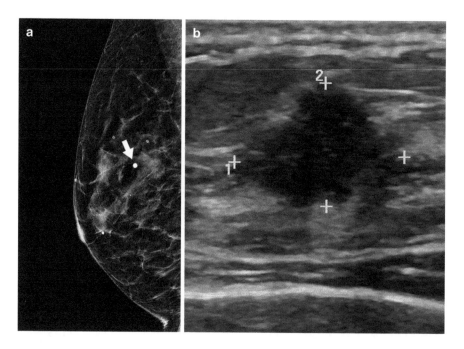

Fig. 2.3 Breast cancer. Diagnostic mammography mediolateral view of the right breast (**a**) shows scattered fibroglandular tissue without focal abnormality at the site of a palpable lump indicated by a radio-opaque marker (arrow). Breast US (**b**) found an irregularly shaped mass (calipers) that was obscured by surrounding breast tissue on mammogram. Core needle biopsy diagnosed invasive ductal carcinoma

Solution
US allows direct correlation of the palpable lump with imaging findings. When both mammography and US are negative or benign in the evaluation of a palpable breast lump, the negative predictive value excluding malignancy is very high, over 97%.

A 29-year-old woman with a palpable breast lump.

a. Mammography diagnostic
b. US breast
c. MRI breast without and with contrast
d. Image-guided fine needle aspiration breast
e. No ideal imaging exam

A woman younger than 30 years of age, initial evaluation.

a. Mammography diagnostic is usually not appropriate.
b. *US breast* is the most appropriate.
c. MRI breast with contrast is usually not appropriate.
d. Image-guided fine needle aspiration breast is usually not appropriate.

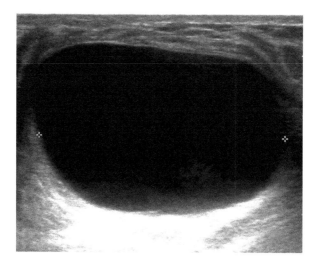

Fig. 2.4 Breast cyst. Breast US shows a simple cyst (calipers) corresponding to the palpable lump

Solution
US is the preferred exam because it avoids ionizing radiation and because of the low incidence of breast cancer in women age <30 years. In addition, most benign lesions in young women are not visualized on mammography.

A 22-year-old woman with a palpable breast lump. US shows a probably benign finding.

a. Mammography diagnostic
b. US breast follow-up in 6–12 months
c. MRI breast without and with contrast
d. Image-guided core biopsy breast
e. No ideal imaging exam

A woman younger than 30 years of age, US findings probably benign.

a. Mammography diagnostic is usually not appropriate.
b. *US breast follow-up in 6–12 months* is the most appropriate.
c. MRI breast without and with contrast is usually not appropriate.
d. Image-guided core biopsy breast is usually not appropriate.

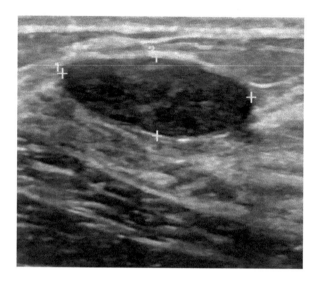

Fig. 2.5 Fibroadenoma. Breast US shows an oval circumscribed hypoechoic mass oriented parallel to the chest wall, corresponding to the palpable lump. This was stable on 2 years of US follow-up, consistent with a benign lesion, and presumptively diagnosed as a fibroadenoma

Solution

For women aged <30 years, US follow-up is an appropriate alternative to biopsy for palpable solid masses with benign US features if the clinical evaluation also suggests a benign etiology. Benign US features include an oval or round shape, well-defined margin, homogenous echogenicity, orientation parallel to chest wall, and lack of posterior acoustic shadowing. Follow-up is usually at 6–12 months intervals for 2–3 years.

A 28-year-old woman with a palpable breast mass. US is negative.

a. Mammography diagnostic
b. US breast short-interval follow-up
c. MRI breast without and with contrast
d. FDG-PET breast
e. No ideal imaging exam

A woman younger than 30 years of age, US negative.

a. Mammography diagnostic is usually not appropriate.
b. US breast short-interval follow-up is usually not appropriate.
c. MRI breast without and with contrast is usually not appropriate.
d. FDG-PET breast is usually not appropriate.
e. *No ideal imaging exam* is the correct answer.

Solution
Mammography following a negative US is usually not appropriate in women aged <30 years unless clinical findings are highly suspicious for malignancy.

A 34-year-old woman with a palpable breast mass.

a. Mammography diagnostic
b. US breast
c. MRI breast without and with contrast
d. FDG-PET breast
e. No ideal imaging exam

Woman 30–39 years of age, initial evaluation.

a. *Mammography diagnostic* and choice (b) are equally the most appropriate.
b. *US breast* and choice (a) are equally the most appropriate.
c. MRI breast without and with contrast is usually not appropriate.
d. FDG-PET breast is usually not appropriate.

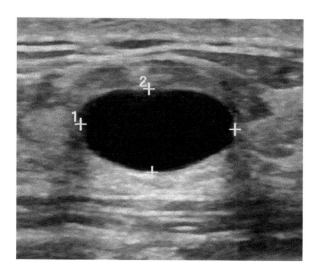

Fig. 2.6 Breast cyst. Breast US shows a simple cyst (calipers) corresponding to the palpable mass

Solution

US is an appropriate alternative to mammography as the initial imaging study given the relatively low risk of breast cancer in women aged 30–39 years, if clinical presentation does not suggest malignancy and breast cancer risk factors are not present. If either of these features are present, then mammography is recommended.

2.2 **Breast Pain**

A 43-year-old woman with diffuse left breast pain that waxes and wanes with her menstrual cycle.

a. Mammography diagnostic
b. US breast
c. MRI breast without and with contrast
d. FDG-PET breast
e. No ideal imaging exam

Cyclical breast pain, unilateral or bilateral

a. Mammography diagnostic is usually not appropriate.
b. US breast is usually not appropriate.
c. MRI breast without and with contrast is usually not appropriate.
d. FDG-PET breast is usually not appropriate.
e. *No ideal imaging exam* is the correct answer.

Solution
Cyclical breast pain is diffuse unilateral or bilateral pain and/or tenderness that waxes and wanes with the menstrual cycle. This is more common than noncyclical pain and is most likely hormonal in origin. Since this scenario is not associated with an increased likelihood of breast cancer, imaging is not indicated.

A 26-year-old woman with focal right breast pain that does not wax or wane with her menstrual cycle.

a. Mammography diagnostic
b. US breast
c. FDG-PET breast
d. MRI breast without and with contrast
e. No ideal imaging exam

A woman younger than 30 years of age with noncyclical focal breast pain, unilateral or bilateral

a. Mammography diagnostic is usually not appropriate.
b. US breast may be appropriate.
c. FDG-PET breast is usually not appropriate.
d. MRI breast without and with contrast is usually not appropriate.
e. *No ideal imaging exam* is the correct answer.

Solution

Noncyclical focal breast pain is most likely inflammatory in nature and tends to be more focal than cyclical breast pain. Imaging is not routinely indicated given the low risk of malignancy with this clinical scenario. However, US may be used to help provide reassurance.

A 34-year-old woman with focal left breast pain that does not wax or wane with her menstrual cycle.

a. Mammography diagnostic
b. US breast
c. FDG-PET breast
d. MRI breast without and with contrast
e. No ideal imaging exam

A woman 30 years of age or older with noncyclical focal breast pain, unilateral or bilateral.

a. Mammography diagnostic may be appropriate.
b. US breast may be appropriate.
c. FDG-PET breast is usually not appropriate.
d. MRI breast without and with contrast is usually not appropriate.
e. *No ideal imaging exam* is the correct answer.

Solution

Noncyclical focal breast pain is most likely inflammatory in nature and tends to be more focal than cyclical breast pain. Imaging is not routinely indicated given the low risk of malignancy with this clinical scenario. However, mammography and US may be used to help rule out cancer as the cause of pain and to provide reassurance. Mammography should also be offered to patients who would normally qualify for a mammogram based on risk factors and the date of the last mammogram.

A 38-year-old woman with diffuse bilateral breast pain that does not wax or wane with her menstrual cycle.

a. Mammography diagnostic
b. US breast
c. MRI breast without and with contrast
d. FDG-PET breast
e. No ideal imaging exam

A woman younger than 40 years of age with noncyclical diffuse breast pain, unilateral or bilateral.

a. Mammography diagnostic is usually not appropriate.
b. US breast is usually not appropriate.
c. MRI breast without and with contrast is usually not appropriate.
d. FDG-PET breast is usually not appropriate.
e. *No ideal imaging exam* is the correct answer.

Solution
Diffuse breast pain is one that involves more than 25% of the breast and axillary tissue. In women aged <40 years presenting with diffuse breast pain, imaging is typically unnecessary due to the low likelihood of finding cancer or a specific cause for pain.

A 45-year-old woman with diffuse right breast pain that does not wax or wane with her menstrual cycle.

a. Mammography diagnostic
b. US breast
c. MRI breast without and with contrast
d. FDG-PET breast
e. No ideal imaging exam

A woman 40 years of age or older with noncyclical diffuse breast pain, unilateral or bilateral.

a. Mammography diagnostic may be appropriate.
b. US breast is usually not appropriate.
c. MRI breast without and with contrast is usually not appropriate
d. FDG-PET breast is usually not appropriate
e. *No ideal imaging exam* is the correct answer.

Solution

Diffuse breast pain is one that involves more than 25% of the breast and axillary tissue. Imaging evaluation of diffuse breast pain is usually unnecessary due to the low likelihood of finding cancer or a specific cause for pain. However, mammography should be offered to patients who would normally qualify for a mammogram based on risk factors and the date of the last mammogram.

2.3   Nipple Discharge

A 35-year-old woman with non-spontaneous discharge of yellow-colored fluid from both nipples.

a. Mammography diagnostic
b. US breast
c. MRI breast without and with contrast
d. Ductography
e. No ideal imaging exam

Woman of any age without pathologic features.

a. Mammography diagnostic is usually not appropriate.
b. US breast is usually not appropriate.
c. MRI breast without and with contrast is usually not appropriate.
d. Ductography is usually not appropriate.
e. *No ideal imaging exam* is the correct answer.

Solution

Features of pathologic nipple discharge include unilaterality, discharge from a single duct orifice, spontaneous, and serous or bloody in color. If none of these features are present, then the discharge may be considered physiologic. If the history and physical examination indicate physiologic discharge and routine screening mammography is up to date, then no imaging is needed.

A 42-year-old woman with spontaneous discharge of bloody fluid from one nipple.

a. Mammography diagnostic
b. US breast
c. MRI breast without and with contrast
d. Ductography
e. No ideal imaging exam

A man or woman 30 years of age or older with pathologic features.

a. *Mammography diagnostic* and choice (b) are equally the most appropriate. These exams are complementary.
b. *US breast* and choice (a) are equally the most appropriate. For women 30–39 years of age, US can be the initial exam. For older women and for men, mammography is the preferred initial exam.
c. MRI breast without and with contrast is usually not appropriate as the initial study but can be considered when other approaches have failed to identify a cause.
d. Ductography is usually not appropriate.

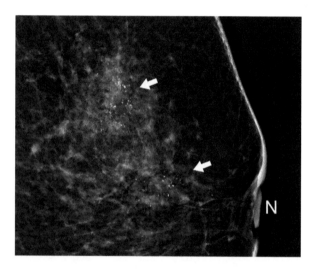

Fig. 2.7 Breast cancer. Diagnostic mammography mediolateral magnification view of the left breast shows calcifications (arrows) that extend to the subareolar region. Core needle biopsy diagnosed ductal carcinoma in situ and invasive ductal carcinoma. *N* nipple

Solution
Causes of pathologic nipple discharge include intraductal papilloma (the most common cause) and, less commonly, malignancy such as ductal carcinoma in situ and invasive carcinoma. Mammography and US in this scenario should include dedicated evaluation of the subareolar region.

A 27-year-old woman with spontaneous discharge of serous fluid from both nipples.

a. Mammography diagnostic
b. US breast
c. MRI breast without and with contrast
d. Ductography
e. No ideal imaging exam

A woman younger than 30 years of age with pathologic features.

a. Mammography diagnostic may be appropriate if initial US shows a suspicious finding, or if the patient has a genetic mutation predisposing to breast cancer.
b. *US breast* is the most appropriate.
c. MRI breast without and with contrast is usually not appropriate.
d. Ductography is usually not appropriate.

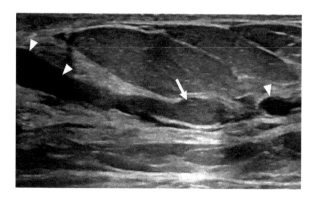

Fig. 2.8 Papilloma. Breast US of the subareolar region of the right breast shows a mass (arrow) within a dilated duct (arrowheads). Core needle biopsy diagnosed papilloma

Solution
Due to low cancer incidence in women younger than 30 years, initial imaging evaluation is performed with US to avoid ionizing radiation.

A 26-year-old man with spontaneous bloody discharge from one nipple.

a. Mammography diagnostic
b. US breast
c. MRI breast without and with contrast
d. Ductography
e. No ideal imaging exam

A man younger than 30 years of age with pathologic features.

a. *Mammography diagnostic* is the most appropriate.
b. *US breast* is usually appropriate, but there is a better choice here. It may be used as the initial imaging study when the patient is younger than 25 years of age.
c. MRI breast without and with contrast is usually not appropriate.
d. Ductography is usually not appropriate.

Solution
There is a high incidence of malignancy among men with pathologic nipple discharge. Therefore, imaging evaluation is indicated in this scenario. For men 25 years of age and older, mammography is recommended as the initial imaging exam, and US is complementary. For those younger than 25 years of age, US may be used as the initial exam.

2.4 Symptomatic Male Breast

A 22-year-old man with a palpable breast lump. Clinical findings are indeterminate for gynecomastia.

a. Mammography diagnostic
b. US breast
c. MRI breast without contrast
d. MRI breast without and with contrast
e. No ideal imaging exam

A man, younger than 25 years of age, indeterminate palpable breast lump.

a. Mammography diagnostic may be appropriate if US demonstrates suspicious features or is inconclusive. Benign processes such as gynecomastia and oil cysts can have a suspicious appearance on US but can typically be diagnosed as benign on mammography.
b. *US breast* is the most appropriate.
c. MRI breast without contrast is usually not appropriate.
d. MRI breast without and with contrast is usually not appropriate.

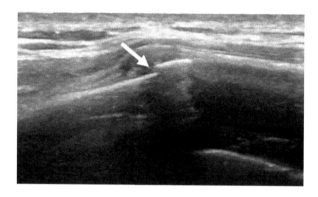

Fig. 2.9 Rib fracture. Breast US shows abrupt discontinuity of the cortex of the right second rib (arrow) consistent with a fracture at the site of a palpable lump. This male patient had a recent history of mild trauma to the chest

Solution
Most men with breast symptoms can be diagnosed based on clinical evaluation without imaging. Gynecomastia often presents as a soft, rubbery, or firm mass directly under the nipple, can be unilateral or bilateral, and is more likely to be painful than cancer, especially if symptoms have been present for <6 months. If clinical findings are indeterminate, US may be useful as the initial imaging exam in men age <25 years.

A 33-year-old man with a palpable breast lump. Clinical findings are indeterminate for gynecomastia.

a. Mammography diagnostic
b. US breast
c. MRI breast without contrast
d. MRI breast without and with contrast
e. No ideal imaging exam

A man 25 years of age or older, indeterminate palpable breast lump.

a. *Mammography diagnostic* is the most appropriate.
b. US breast may be appropriate.
c. MRI breast without contrast is usually not appropriate.
d. MRI breast without and with contrast is usually not appropriate.

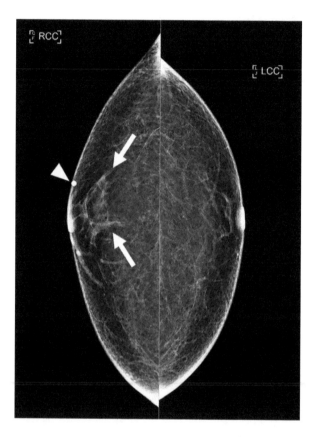

Fig. 2.10 Gynecomastia. Diagnostic mammography craniocaudal views of the right (RCC) and left (LCC) breasts show right subareolar densities (long arrows) consistent with gynecomastia, at the site of the palpable lump indicated by a radio-opaque marker (arrowhead)

Solution
Mammography is highly sensitive and specific for malignancy in a man with a palpable breast lump. If mammography shows gynecomastia or another cause to explain the symptoms, then US is typically unnecessary. US can complement mammography if the mammogram is indeterminate, suspicious, or does not demonstrate a cause for the palpable finding.

A 47-year-old man with a palpable breast lump and nipple retraction.

a. Mammography diagnostic
b. US breast
c. MRI breast without contrast
d. MRI breast without and with contrast
e. No ideal imaging exam

Palpable breast lump with clinical suspicion for malignancy.

a. *Mammography diagnostic* is the most appropriate.
b. US breast is usually appropriate, but there is a better choice here.
c. MRI breast without contrast is usually not appropriate.
d. MRI breast without and with contrast is usually not appropriate.

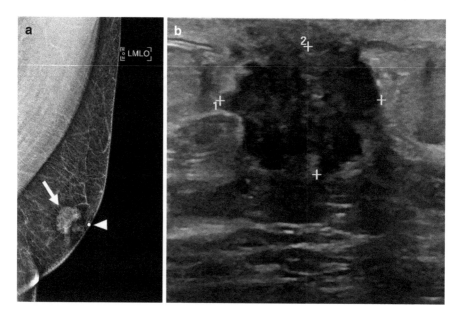

Fig. 2.11 Breast cancer. Diagnostic mammography (**a**) mediolateral oblique view of the left breast shows a subareolar mass (arrow) and nipple retraction at the site of the palpable lump marked by a radio-opaque marker (arrowhead). Breast US (**b**) shows a corresponding irregular mass (calipers). Core needle biopsy diagnosed invasive ductal carcinoma

Solution
Mammography is performed in men presenting with signs and symptoms suggesting cancer. Male breast cancer typically presents differently from gynecomastia, usually as a unilateral, painless, hard subareolar lump eccentric to the nipple. Other findings include skin or nipple retraction, discharge, and axillary lymphadenopathy.

2.5 Imaging During Pregnancy and Lactation

A 41-year-old woman is currently breastfeeding. She asks about breast cancer screening.

a. Mammography screening
b. US breast
c. MRI breast without contrast
d. MRI breast without and with contrast
e. No ideal imaging exam

Breast cancer screening during lactation.

a. *Mammography screening* is the most appropriate.
b. US breast may be appropriate.
c. MRI breast without contrast is usually not appropriate.
d. MRI breast without and with contrast is usually not appropriate.

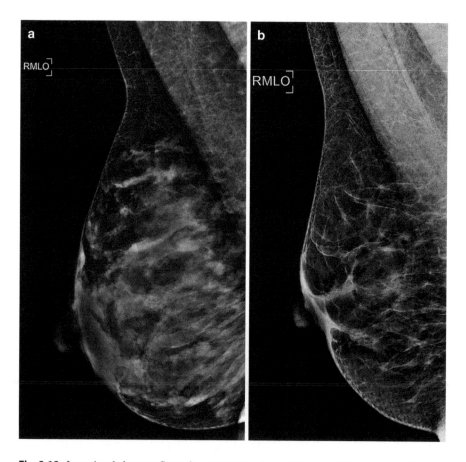

Fig. 2.12 Lactational changes. Screening mammography mediolateral oblique views of the right breast of the same woman imaged when she was breastfeeding (**a**) and 4 years after she had stopped breastfeeding (**b**) show increased breast density during lactation

Solution

Mammography is not contraindicated during lactation. However, mammographic breast density increases during lactation due to distention of lobules with milk. Breastfeeding or pumping prior to imaging is encouraged to minimize breast density and optimize sensitivity of screening mammography.

A 43-year-old woman is currently pregnant. She asks about breast cancer screening.

a. Mammography screening
b. US breast
c. MRI breast without contrast
d. MRI breast without and with contrast
e. No ideal imaging exam

Breast cancer screening during pregnancy.

a. *Mammography screening* is the most appropriate.
b. US breast may be appropriate.
c. MRI breast without contrast is usually not appropriate.
d. MRI breast without and with contrast is usually not appropriate.

Solution

Mammography can be safely performed during pregnancy without endangering the fetus. The fetal radiation dose from a standard four-view screening mammogram is <0.03 mGy. No teratogenic effects have been demonstrated below 50 mGy. Use of lead shielding for pregnant patients is recommended.

A 32-year-old pregnant woman with a palpable breast lump.

a. Mammography diagnostic
b. US breast
c. MRI breast without contrast
d. MRI breast without and with contrast
e. No ideal imaging exam

A pregnant woman with palpable breast lump.

a. Mammography diagnostic may be appropriate as an adjunct to US and can evaluate for additional findings such as calcifications and architectural distortion.
b. *US breast* is the most appropriate.
c. MRI breast without contrast is usually not appropriate.
d. MRI breast without and with contrast is usually not appropriate.

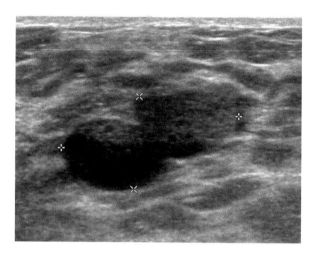

Fig. 2.13 Galactocele in a pregnant patient. Breast US shows a cyst with complex fluid (calipers)
at the site of a palpable lump. Milky fluid was aspirated under US guidance, consistent with a
galactocele

Solution

US is highly sensitive for pregnancy-associated breast cancer, defined as breast cancer diagnosed during pregnancy, throughout the first postpartum year, or during
lactation. Though this usually presents as a palpable mass, most masses in pregnant
and breastfeeding women are benign, such as fibroadenomas, hamartomas, lactating
adenomas, and galactoceles, with the latter two being unique to pregnancy and
lactation.

A 28-year-old pregnant woman with spontaneous discharge of bloody fluid from one nipple.

a. Mammography diagnostic
b. US breast
c. MRI breast without contrast
d. MRI breast without and with contrast
e. No ideal imaging exam

A pregnant woman, with nipple discharge that has pathologic features.

a. *Mammography diagnostic* and choice (b) are equally the most appropriate. The two exams are complementary.
b. *US breast* and choice (a) are equally the most appropriate. The two exams are complementary.
c. MRI breast without contrast is usually not appropriate.
d. MRI breast without and with contrast is usually not appropriate.

Solution

US is the first-line imaging exam and is used to evaluate the retroareolar location for a papilloma or other mass. Mammography is complementary to US and is performed with retroareolar magnification views to look for calcifications which can be occult on US. Persistent unilateral bloody discharge may be caused by infection, papilloma, or less commonly, breast cancer. More commonly, proliferative epithelial changes and increased breast vascularity may result in physiologic bloody nipple discharge during pregnancy or early lactation. This is usually self-limited.

2.6   Breast Implant Evaluation

A 29-year-old woman, clinical examination equivocal for saline breast implant rupture.

a. Mammography diagnostic
b. US breast
c. MRI breast without contrast
d. MRI breast without and with contrast
e. No ideal imaging exam

A woman younger than 30 years of age, clinical examination equivocal for saline breast implant rupture.

a. Mammography diagnostic is usually not appropriate.
b. *US breast* is the most appropriate.
c. MRI breast without contrast is usually not appropriate.
d. MRI breast without and with contrast is usually not appropriate.

Solution

Typically, saline breast implant rupture is clinically evident as the saline is resorbed by the body over a period of days, and the patient experiences a change in breast size and shape. In younger women with equivocal clinical findings, US is the recommended initial study and can visualize the collapsed implant shell.

A 36-year-old woman, clinical examination equivocal for saline breast implant rupture.

a. Mammography diagnostic
b. US breast
c. MRI breast without contrast
d. MRI breast without and with contrast
e. No ideal imaging exam

A woman, 30 years of age or older, clinical examination equivocal for saline breast implant rupture.

a. *Mammography diagnostic* and choice (b) are equally the most appropriate for women 30–39 years of age. Mammography is the preferred initial exam for women 40 years of age or older.
b. *US breast* and choice (a) are equally the most appropriate for women 30–39 years of age. For older women, mammography is the preferred initial exam. US is used for problem-solving after mammography and for those unable to undergo mammography.
c. MRI breast without contrast is usually not appropriate.
d. MRI breast without and with contrast is usually not appropriate.

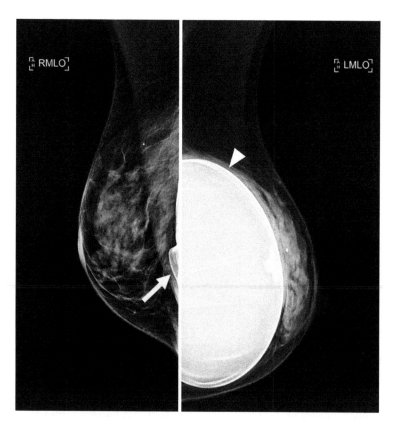

Fig. 2.14 Ruptured saline implant. Diagnostic mammography mediolateral oblique views of the right (RMLO) and left (LMLO) breasts show a ruptured right (arrow) and intact left (arrowhead) saline implants

Solution
On mammography, visualization of the collapsed implant shell is diagnostic for saline implant rupture.

A 42-year-old woman suspected with complication from silicone breast implant.

a. Mammography diagnostic
b. US breast
c. MRI breast without contrast
d. MRI breast without and with contrast
e. No ideal imaging exam

A woman, 30 years of age or older, suspected complication from silicone breast implant.

a. *Mammography diagnostic* and choice (c) are equally the most appropriate.
b. US breast may be appropriate for women aged 40 years or older and is equally as appropriate as choices (a) and (c) for younger women.
c. *MRI breast without contrast* and choice (a) are equally the most appropriate.
d. MRI breast without and with contrast is usually not appropriate.

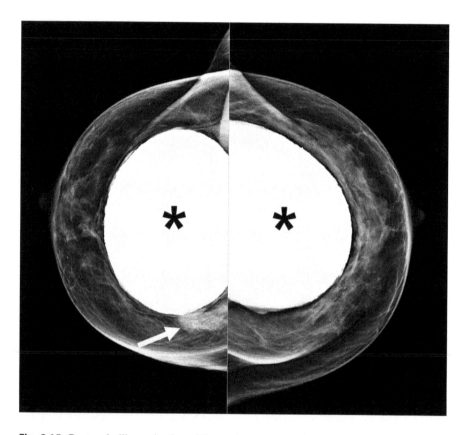

Fig. 2.15 Ruptured silicone implant. Diagnostic mammography craniocaudal views of both breasts show bilateral silicone implants (stars) and high-density material outside the right breast implant capsule (arrow) consistent with silicone from extracapsular rupture. Subsequent breast MRI confirmed intra- and extracapsular implant rupture on the right

Solution
MRI without contrast is the gold standard for silicone implant evaluation and reliably identifies both intracapsular (the more common type) and extracapsular ruptures. Mammography can identify extracapsular rupture, which presents as high-density material outside the implant shell. However, this exam does not reliably diagnose intracapsular rupture.

Cardiac Imaging

3

3.1 Acute Chest Pain

A 25-year-old man with acute chest pain with low probability of coronary artery disease.

a. X-ray chest
b. CTA coronary arteries
c. CTA chest (noncoronary)
d. Radionuclide myocardial scan with stress perfusion
e. No ideal imaging exam

G. X. Wang et al., *Choosing the Correct Radiologic Test*,
https://doi.org/10.1007/978-3-030-65185-5_3

Low probability of coronary artery disease. Initial imaging study.

a. *X-ray chest* is the most appropriate.
b. CTA coronary arteries is usually appropriate, but there is a better choice here.
c. CTA chest (noncoronary) is usually appropriate, but there is a better choice here.
d. Radionuclide myocardial scan with stress perfusion may be appropriate.

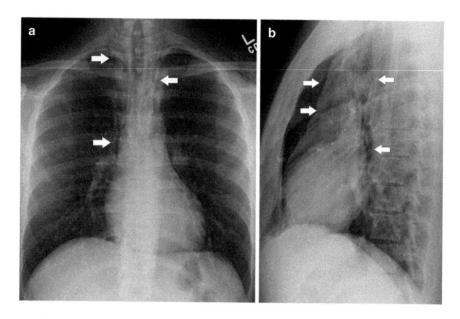

Fig. 3.1 Pneumomediastinum. Chest X-ray posteroanterior (**a**) and lateral (**b**) views show linear lucencies (arrows) indicating mediastinal air

Solution
Chest x-ray identifies sources of nonspecific chest pain such as pneumothorax, pneumomediastinum, fractured ribs, infections, and malignancies. Depending on the clinical presentation, CTA coronary arteries and CTA chest can also be appropriate. For low-risk patients, CTA of the coronary arteries has high negative predictive value for significant coronary artery disease.

A 54-year-old man with acute chest pain. Aortic dissection is suspected.

a. US echocardiography transesophageal
b. CTA chest and abdomen
c. MRA chest and abdomen without contrast
d. MRA chest and abdomen without and with contrast
e. No ideal imaging exam

Suspected aortic dissection.

a. US echocardiography transesophageal is usually appropriate, but there is a better choice here.
b. *CTA chest and abdomen* is the most appropriate.
c. MRA chest and abdomen without contrast is usually appropriate, but there is a better choice here.
d. MRA chest and abdomen without and with contrast is usually appropriate, but there is a better choice here.

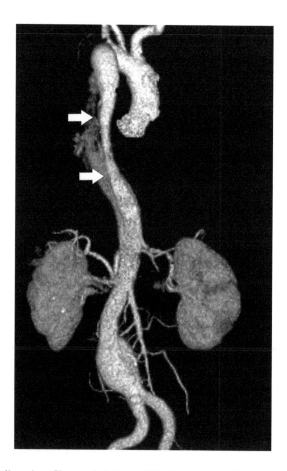

Fig. 3.2 Aortic dissection. Chest and abdomen CTA 3D reconstruction image of the thoracoabdominal aorta shows a dissection flap (arrows) separating the true and false lumens

Solution
For suspected aortic dissection, CTA chest and abdomen is the definitive imaging study. MRA without and with contrast is an alternative for patients with a contraindication to iodinated contrast. As contrast-enhanced imaging is preferred to confirm aortic dissection, MRA without contrast is reserved only for cases when both iodinated and gadolinium-based contrast agents are contraindicated.

3.2   Chronic Chest Pain

A 70-year-old man with chronic chest pain and high probability of coronary artery disease.

a. CT coronary calcium without contrast
b. CTA coronary arteries
c. MRI heart with vasodilator stress perfusion without and with contrast
d. Radionuclide myocardial scan with stress perfusion
e. Coronary angiography

High probability of coronary artery disease.

a. CT coronary calcium without contrast is usually not appropriate.
b. CTA coronary arteries is usually appropriate, but there is a better choice here.
c. *MRI heart with vasodilator stress perfusion without and with contrast* and choices (d) and (e) are equally the most appropriate.
d. *Radionuclide myocardial scan with stress perfusion* and choices (c) and (e) are equally the most appropriate.
e. *Coronary angiography* and choices (c) and (d) are equally the most appropriate.

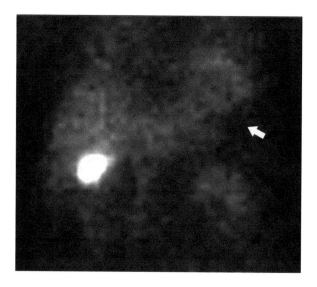

Fig. 3.3 Cardiac ischemia. Radionuclide myocardial scan with stress perfusion planar frontal image shows decreased tracer uptake in the left ventricular inferolateral wall (arrow). Note high levels of tracer excretion into the gallbladder

Solution

Coronary angiography is the gold standard for evaluating coronary artery disease and allows immediate intervention but is an invasive procedure with associated risks. MRI and radionuclide stress perfusion imaging are first-line noninvasive options for identifying ischemia and indirectly assessing coronary artery disease.

A 74-year-old woman presents with chronic chest pain with low to intermediate probability of coronary artery disease.

a. X-ray chest
b. CTA coronary arteries
c. CTA chest (noncoronary)
d. Radionuclide myocardial scan with stress perfusion
e. No ideal imaging exam

Low to intermediate probability of coronary artery disease.

a. *X-ray chest* is the most appropriate.
b. CTA coronary arteries is usually appropriate, but there is a better choice here.
c. CTA chest (noncoronary) is usually appropriate, but there is a better choice here.
d. Radionuclide myocardial scan with stress perfusion is usually appropriate, but there is a better choice here.

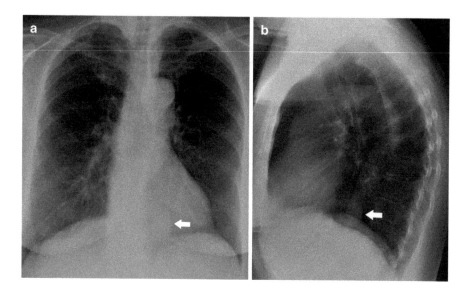

Fig. 3.4 Hiatal hernia. Chest X-ray posteroanterior (**a**) and lateral (**b**) views show a soft tissue density (arrows) superior to the esophageal hiatus

Solution
Chest X-ray as the initial imaging study can help identify causes of chronic noncardiac chest pain, which is most commonly related to gastroesophageal reflux or other esophageal diseases.

3.3   Coronary Artery Disease

A 65-year-old asymptomatic man at high risk for coronary artery disease.

a. CT coronary calcium without contrast
b. MRI heart function and morphology without and with contrast
c. MRI heart with stress perfusion without and with contrast
d. Radionuclide myocardial scan with stress perfusion
e. No ideal imaging exam

Evaluation of disease burden: asymptomatic high-risk individuals.

a. CT coronary calcium without contrast is usually not appropriate.
b. MRI heart function and morphology without and with contrast is usually not appropriate.
c. MRI heart with stress perfusion without and with contrast may be appropriate.
d. Radionuclide myocardial scan with stress perfusion may be appropriate.
e. *No ideal imaging exam.*

Solution
There is no ideal imaging exam to help guide preventive interventions for atherosclerotic cardiovascular disease among asymptomatic high-risk individuals. Certain groups of patients such as those with diabetes may benefit from use of cardiac stress imaging and coronary artery CTA to detect subclinical coronary atherosclerosis and thus help guide early intervention.

A 65-year-old asymptomatic woman at intermediate risk for coronary artery disease.

a. CT coronary calcium without contrast
b. Radionuclide myocardial scan with stress perfusion
c. MRI heart with stress perfusion without and with contrast
d. MRI heart function and morphology without and with contrast
e. No ideal imaging exam

Evaluation of disease burden: asymptomatic intermediate-risk individuals.

a. *CT coronary calcium without contrast* is the most appropriate.
b. Radionuclide myocardial scan with stress perfusion is usually not appropriate.
c. MRI heart with stress perfusion without and with contrast is usually not appropriate.
d. MRI heart function and morphology without and with contrast is usually not appropriate.

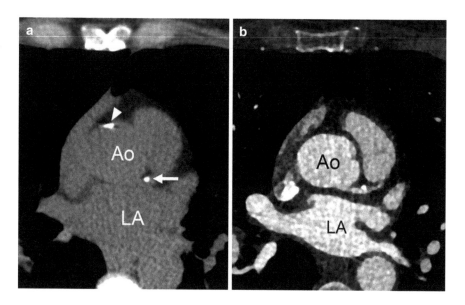

Fig. 3.5 Coronary artery calcium score. Cardiac CT without contrast (**a**) performed for coronary artery calcium scoring (CACS) shows calcified plaque in the left main coronary artery (arrow). Calcification along the aorta (arrowhead) is not used for CACS. Though scoring is performed without contrast, cardiac CT with contrast (**b**) of the same patient is shown to better demonstrate anatomy. *Ao* aorta, *LA* left atrium

Solution

CACS is recommended for coronary artery disease risk stratification in intermediate-risk patients. It correlates strongly with future mortality and cardiovascular events.

A 55-year-old asymptomatic man at low risk for coronary artery disease.

a. CT coronary calcium without contrast
b. Radionuclide myocardial scan with stress perfusion
c. MRI heart with stress perfusion without and with contrast
d. MRI heart function and morphology without and with contrast
e. No ideal imaging exam

Evaluation of disease burden in asymptomatic low-risk individuals.

a. CT coronary calcium without contrast is usually not appropriate.
b. Radionuclide myocardial scan with stress perfusion is usually not appropriate.
c. MRI heart with perfusion without and with contrast is usually not appropriate.
d. MRI heart function and morphology without and with contrast is usually not appropriate.
e. *No ideal imaging exam*

Solution

In low-risk patients, imaging is usually not appropriate. However, coronary artery calcium score determination may be useful for some low-risk patients with a strong family history of premature coronary artery disease.

3.4   Infective Endocarditis

A 36-year-old man suspected with infective endocarditis.

a. US echocardiography transthoracic resting
b. CT chest without contrast
c. CT chest with contrast
d. CT heart function and morphology with contrast
e. No ideal imaging exam

Suspected infective endocarditis.

a. *US echocardiography transthoracic resting* is the most appropriate.
b. CT chest without contrast is usually not appropriate.
c. CT chest with contrast may be appropriate.
d. CT heart function and morphology with contrast may be appropriate.

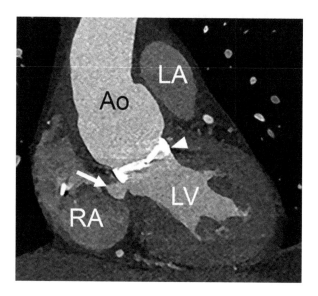

Fig. 3.6 Paravalvular pseudoaneurysm. Cardiac CT with contrast coronal reconstruction image shows a paravalvular pseudoaneurysm (arrow) in a patient with infectious endocarditis and a metallic aortic valve (arrowhead). Subsequent surgery found infection along the suture lines of the valve with a tract underneath that extended toward the right atrium. *Ao* aorta, *LA* left atrium, *LV* left ventricle, *RA* right atrium

Solution
Transthoracic echocardiography is the standard of care for confirming infective endocarditis, as it can demonstrate valvular vegetation and regurgitation and paravalvular abscess. CT heart function and morphology is most useful in cases of suspected paravalvular infections and for the evaluation of prosthetic heart valves. CT chest can help evaluate for related pulmonary findings such as septic infarcts.

3.5   Nonischemic Myocardial Disease

A 25-year-old woman with subacute chest pain and recent history of fever and fatigue. Viral myocarditis is suspected.

a. US echocardiography transthoracic resting
b. CTA chest
c. CT heart function and morphology with contrast
d. MRI heart function and morphology without and with contrast
e. FDG-PET/CT heart

Suspected acute or subacute myocardial disease.

a. *US echocardiography transthoracic resting* and choice (d) are equally the most appropriate.
b. CTA chest is usually not appropriate.
c. CT heart function and morphology with contrast is usually not appropriate.
d. *MRI heart function and morphology without and with contrast* and choice (a) are equally the most appropriate.
e. FDG-PET/CT heart is usually not appropriate.

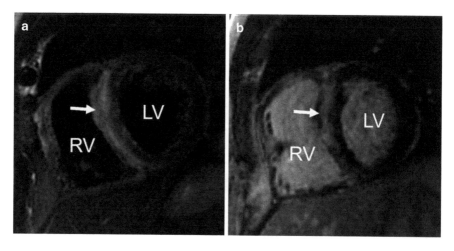

Fig. 3.7 Acute viral myocarditis. Cardiac MRI short-axis T2-weighted (**a**) and post-contrast (**b**) images show myocardial edema co-localizing with late gadolinium enhancement (arrows) along the basal interventricular septum between the left (LV) and right (RV) ventricles

Solution
In patients with myocarditis, both echocardiography and cardiac MRI can show global or regional wall motion abnormalities. Cardiac MRI provides additional information by demonstrating myocardial edema and characteristic patterns of myocardial enhancement.

A 19-year-old man with shortness of breath and palpitations. Arrhythmogenic right ventricular cardiomyopathy is suspected.

a. US echocardiography transthoracic resting
b. CT heart function and morphology with contrast
c. MRI heart function and morphology without and with contrast
d. FDG-PET/CT heart
e. No ideal imaging exam

Suspected arrhythmogenic right ventricular cardiomyopathy.

a. US echocardiography transthoracic resting is usually appropriate, but there is a better choice here.
b. CT heart function and morphology with contrast may be appropriate. CT is an alternative if the patient has a contraindication to MRI.
c. *MRI heart function and morphology without and with contrast* is the most appropriate.
d. FDG-PET/CT heart is usually not appropriate.

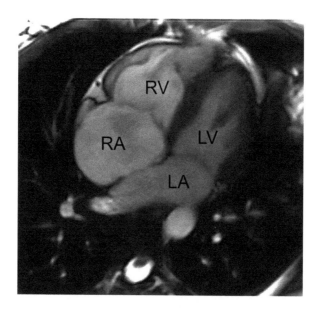

Fig. 3.8 Arrhythmogenic right ventricular cardiomyopathy. Cardiac MRI four-chamber view bright blood gradient echo image shows a dilated right ventricle (RV). Additional cine images showed depressed right ventricular resting systolic function and regional dyssynchrony at the right ventricular apex. *LA* left atrium, *LV* left ventricle, *RA* right atrium

Solution
Right ventricle dilation and dysfunction are hallmarks of arrhythmogenic right ventricular cardiomyopathy and are well-demonstrated by cardiac MRI. This study can also evaluate for the fibrofatty infiltration of the myocardium seen in this disease.

A 20-year-old professional athlete with a recent history of syncope. Hypertrophic obstructive cardiomyopathy is suspected.

a. US echocardiography transthoracic resting
b. CTA chest
c. CT heart function and morphology with contrast
d. MRI heart function and morphology without and with contrast
e. No ideal imaging exam

Suspected hypertrophic obstructive cardiomyopathy.

a. *US echocardiography transthoracic resting* and choice (d) are equally the most appropriate.
b. CTA chest is usually not appropriate.
c. CT heart function and morphology with contrast is usually not appropriate.
d. *MRI heart function and morphology without and with contrast* and choice (a) are equally the most appropriate.

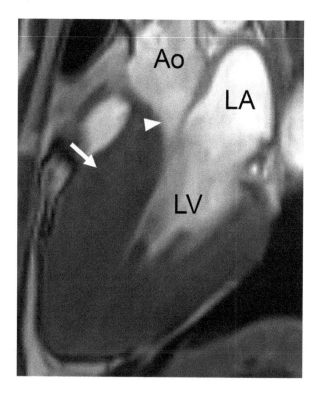

Fig. 3.9 Hypertrophic obstructive cardiomyopathy. Cardiac MRI three-chamber view bright blood gradient echo image shows a thickened interventricular septum (arrow) and narrowed left ventricular outflow tract (arrowhead). *Ao* aorta, *LA* left atrium, *LV* left ventricle

Solution
Both echocardiography and cardiac MRI can evaluate left ventricle outflow obstruction and systolic anterior motion of the mitral valve, characteristic features of hypertrophic obstructive cardiomyopathy.

A 45-year-old woman with known pulmonary sarcoidosis and new complete heart block. Cardiac sarcoidosis is suspected.

a. US echocardiography transthoracic resting
b. CT heart function and morphology with contrast
c. MRI heart function and morphology without and with contrast
d. FDG-PET/CT heart
e. No ideal imaging exam

Suspected myocardial infiltrative disease.

a. US echocardiography transthoracic resting is usually appropriate, but there is a better choice here.
b. CT heart function and morphology with contrast may be appropriate.
c. *MRI heart function and morphology without and with contrast* is the most appropriate. For sarcoidosis, choice (d) is equally as appropriate.
d. *FDG-PET/CT heart* and choice (c) are equally the most appropriate for sarcoidosis. For other types of infiltrative disease, this exam is also usually appropriate, but MRI is preferred.

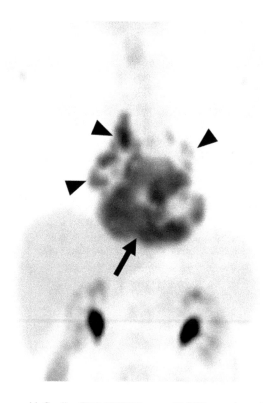

Fig. 3.10 Cardiac sarcoid. Cardiac FDG-PET/CT coronal MIP image shows hypermetabolic ventricular myocardium (arrow) as well as mediastinal and hilar lymph nodes (arrowheads). This study is performed using patient preparation to suppress normal myocardial FDG metabolism

Solution
Due to the low yield and invasiveness of endomyocardial biopsy, imaging is often used for suspected myocardial infiltrative disease. Amyloidosis and sarcoidosis are most common and show typical enhancement patterns on MRI. For sarcoidosis, FDG-PET/CT shows sites of active disease and can be as good as MRI for initial diagnosis and superior for follow-up.

3.6   Pulmonary Embolism

A 35-year-old man with shortness of breath. There is an intermediate pretest probability of pulmonary embolism with a negative D-dimer.

a. X-ray chest
b. US duplex Doppler lower extremity
c. CT chest without and with contrast
d. CTA chest
e. CTA chest with CT angiography lower extremities

Suspected pulmonary embolism, with low pretest probability or intermediate probability with negative D-dimer.

a. *X-ray chest* is the most appropriate.
b. US duplex Doppler lower extremity is usually not appropriate.
c. CT chest without and with contrast is usually not appropriate.
d. CTA chest may be appropriate.
e. CTA chest with CT angiography lower extremities is usually not appropriate.

Solution

In these clinical scenarios, pulmonary embolism may be safely excluded without imaging. Chest X-ray is the most appropriate initial imaging exam to evaluate for alternative explanations for the acute symptoms, such as pneumonia or a large pleural effusion.

A 57-year-old man with acute pleuritic chest pain and shortness of breath. There is a high pretest probability of pulmonary embolism.

a. US duplex Doppler lower extremity
b. CTA chest
c. Tc-99m ventilation perfusion lung scan
d. Pulmonary angiography with right heart catheterization
e. No ideal imaging exam

Suspected pulmonary embolism, with intermediate pretest probability and positive D-dimer or high probability.

a. US duplex Doppler lower extremity is usually appropriate, but there is a better choice here.
b. *CTA chest* is the most appropriate and should be optimized to evaluate the pulmonary arteries.
c. Tc-99m ventilation perfusion lung scan is usually appropriate and may be an alternative to CTA. Use if chest X-ray is negative and CTA is contraindicated or nondiagnostic.
d. Pulmonary angiography with right heart catheterization is usually not appropriate. This is usually reserved for cases where catheter-directed thrombectomy or thrombolysis is clinically indicated.

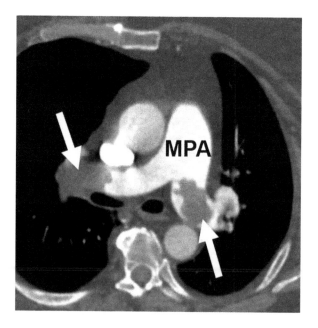

Fig. 3.11 Pulmonary embolus. Chest CTA shows thrombus in the left and right pulmonary arteries (arrows). *MPA* main pulmonary artery

Solution

CTA chest is highly accurate for pulmonary embolism and can also identify signs of right ventricular dysfunction.

A 28-year-old pregnant woman with chest pain and shortness of breast. Pulmonary embolism is suspected.

a. X-ray chest
b. US duplex Doppler lower extremity
c. CTA chest
d. MRA chest
e. Tc-99m ventilation perfusion lung scan

Pregnant patient, pulmonary embolism suspected.

a. *X-ray chest* is the most appropriate.
b. US duplex Doppler lower extremity is usually appropriate, but there is a better choice here.
c. CTA chest is usually appropriate, but there is a better choice here. This study should be optimized to evaluate the pulmonary arteries.
d. MRA chest is usually not appropriate.
e. Tc-99m ventilation perfusion lung scan is usually appropriate, but there is a better choice here.

Solution
In pregnancy, minimizing ionizing radiation is a priority. Chest X-ray is the most appropriate initial exam as it may show other causes for the acute symptoms. Lower extremity duplex US is recommended when there are also signs and symptoms of lower extremity deep venous thrombosis. Although CTA for suspected pulmonary embolism can be performed in pregnant patients, it is most appropriate only when chest X-ray and, where indicated, lower extremity duplex US are non-diagnostic. Choice of CTA versus ventilation perfusion scan remains a matter of debate.

3.7   Shortness of Breath

A 47-year-old man with dyspnea due to suspected heart failure. Cardiac ischemia has been excluded.

a. X-ray chest
b. US echocardiography transthoracic resting
c. CT heart function and morphology with contrast
d. MRI heart function and morphology without and with contrast
e. No ideal imaging exam

Suspected heart failure, ischemia has been excluded.

a. *X-ray chest* and choices (b) and (d) are equally the most appropriate.
b. *US echocardiography transthoracic resting* and choices (a) and (d) are equally the most appropriate.
c. CT heart function and morphology with contrast may be appropriate. This is primarily used for coronary artery evaluation.
d. *MRI heart function and morphology without and with contrast* and choices (a) and (b) are equally the most appropriate.

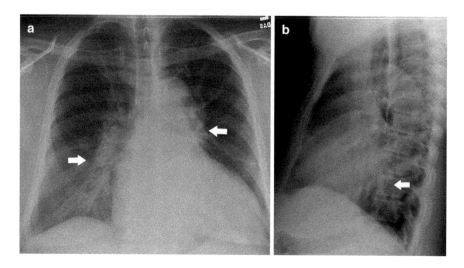

Fig. 3.12 Heart failure. Chest X-ray posteroanterior (**a**) and lateral (**b**) views show bilaterally enlarged pulmonary vessels (arrows) and cardiac enlargement

Solution
Chest X-ray findings include upper lung zone flow redistribution, alveolar or interstitial edema, bilateral pleural effusions, and cardiac enlargement. Transthoracic echocardiography demonstrates abnormalities of the myocardium, heart valves, and pericardium. Cardiac MRI can characterize most causes of heart failure by imaging cardiac function, myocardial edema, and myocardial scarring.

A 41-year-old woman with shortness of breath. Valvular heart disease is suspected.

a. X-ray chest
b. US echocardiography transthoracic resting
c. CT heart function and morphology with contrast
d. MRI heart function and morphology without and with contrast
e. No ideal imaging exam

Suspected valvular heart disease.

a. *X-ray chest* and choice (b) are equally the most appropriate.
b. *US echocardiography transthoracic resting* and choice (a) are equally the most appropriate.
c. CT heart function and morphology with contrast may be appropriate.
d. MRI heart function and morphology without and with contrast is usually appropriate, but there is a better choice here.

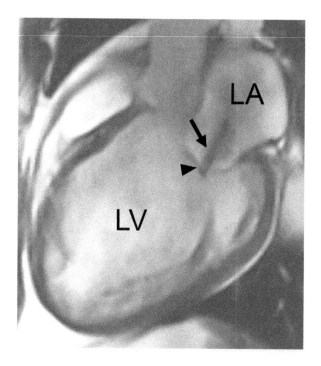

Fig. 3.13 Mitral valve regurgitation. Cardiac MRI three-chamber view bright blood gradient echo image shows a regurgitant jet of blood (arrow) passing from the left ventricle (LV) into the left atrium (LA) through the mitral valve (arrowhead)

Solution
Cardiac echocardiography with Doppler is the primary imaging study for the evaluation of valvular heart disease. It accurately assesses the presence and severity of valve obstruction or regurgitation and comprehensively evaluates valve morphology. Cardiac MRI provides additional information on cardiac anatomy, measures blood flow and pressure gradients across valves, and complements echocardiography findings.

A 55-year-old man with shortness of breath. Pericardial disease is suspected.

a. X-ray chest
b. US echocardiography transthoracic resting
c. CT chest without contrast
d. CT heart function and morphology with contrast
e. MRI heart function and morphology without and with contrast

Suspected pericardial disease.

a. *X-ray chest* and choices (b) and (e) are equally the most appropriate.
b. *US echocardiography transthoracic resting* and choices (a) and (e) are equally the most appropriate.
c. CT chest without contrast is usually appropriate, but there is a better choice here.
d. CT heart function and morphology with contrast is usually appropriate, but there is a better choice here.
e. *MRI heart function and morphology without and with contrast* and choices (a) and (b) are equally the most appropriate.

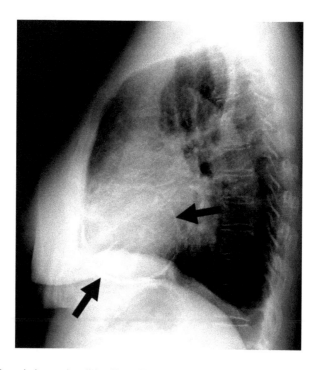

Fig. 3.14 Constrictive pericarditis. Chest X-ray lateral view shows pericardial calcifications (arrows) circumferentially around the heart

Solution
Pericardial disease is usually diagnosed by transthoracic cardiac echocardiography but may be seen on chest X-ray. MRI can also provide the diagnosis and help differentiate constrictive pericardial disease from restrictive cardiomyopathy. CT improves assessment of pericardial calcifications and of associated extracardiac disease.

Thoracic Imaging

4

4.1   Blunt Chest Trauma

A 28-year-old man involved in a high-speed motor vehicle accident

a. X-ray chest
b. US chest
c. CTA chest
d. MRI chest without and with contrast
e. No ideal imaging exam

High-energy mechanism. First-line evaluation.

a. *X-ray chest* and choice (c) are equally the most appropriate.
b. US chest may be appropriate.
c. *CTA chest* and choice (a) are equally the most appropriate.
d. MRI chest without and with IV contrast is usually not appropriate.

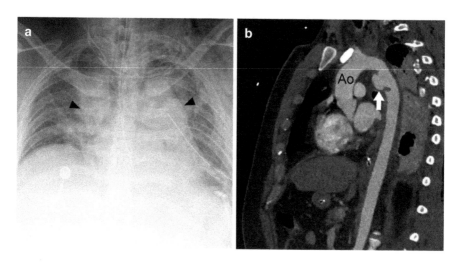

Fig. 4.1 Aortic injury. Chest X-ray anteroposterior view (**a**) shows widening of the mediastinum (arrowheads). Subsequent chest CTA sagittal oblique reconstruction image (**b**) shows a traumatic pseudoaneurysm (arrow) at the isthmus of the thoracic aorta (Ao)

Solution
Chest X-ray and CTA are complementary in blunt trauma evaluation. Chest X-ray can quickly assess for major injuries and detect misplacement of lines and tubes, but its quality may be limited if the patient cannot co-operate. Chest CTA is the gold standard in thoracic trauma evaluation, but the necessary technology and resources are less readily available than a chest X-ray.

A 37-year-old man involved in a low speed motor vehicle accident. He is alert. Physical examination and chest X-ray are normal.

a. US chest
b. CT chest with contrast
c. CTA chest
d. MRI chest without and with contrast
e. No ideal imaging exam

No high-energy mechanism. Normal mental status, physical examination, and anteroposterior chest radiograph.

a. US chest is usually not appropriate.
b. CT chest with contrast may be appropriate.
c. CTA chest may be appropriate.
d. MRI chest without and with contrast may be appropriate.
e. *No ideal imaging exam* is the correct answer.

Solution

In the absence of a high-energy mechanism for trauma with findings that indicate a low probability of significant thoracic injury (normal mental status, clinical examination and chest radiograph), further imaging is usually not indicated. In these patients, chest CT with contrast or CTA may be considered on a case-specific basis.

4.2   **Rib Fractures**

A 60-year-old man involved in minor blunt trauma with suspected rib fractures.

a. X-ray chest
b. X-ray chest with rib views
c. CT chest without contrast
d. CT chest with contrast
e. No ideal imaging exam

Suspected rib fractures from minor blunt trauma.

a. *X-ray chest* is the most appropriate. Posteroanterior, not an anteroposterior, view needed.
b. X-ray chest with rib views may be appropriate.
c. CT chest without contrast is usually not appropriate.
d. CT chest with contrast is usually not appropriate.

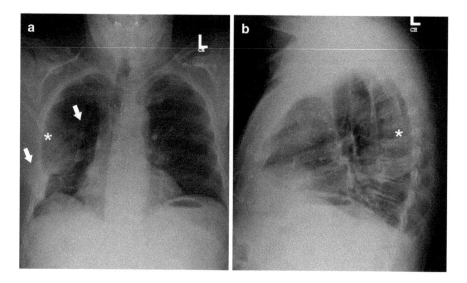

Fig. 4.2 Rib fracture. Chest X-ray posteroanterior (**a**) and lateral (**b**) views show multiple rib fractures (arrows) and a lung contusion (star)

Solution
Chest X-ray with a posteroanterior view is the initial diagnostic test for the detection of rib fractures. While chest X-ray offers limited sensitivity and may miss up to 50% of rib fractures, additional rib views rarely add information that would alter patient management or outcome. Also, chest X-ray can detect complications such as pneumothorax, hemothorax, flail chest, or contusion.

A 37-year-old woman with metastatic breast cancer with suspected pathologic rib fracture. Initial evaluation.

a. X-ray chest
b. X-ray chest with rib views
c. CT chest without contrast
d. Tc-99m bone scan whole body
e. FDG-PET/CT skull base to mid-thigh

Adult, with suspected pathologic rib fracture. Initial evaluation.

a. *X-ray chest* is the most appropriate.
b. X-ray chest with rib views may be appropriate.
c. CT chest without contrast is usually appropriate, but there is a better choice here.
d. Tc-99m bone scan ribs are usually appropriate, but there is a better choice here.
e. FDG-PET/CT skull base to mid-thigh may be appropriate.

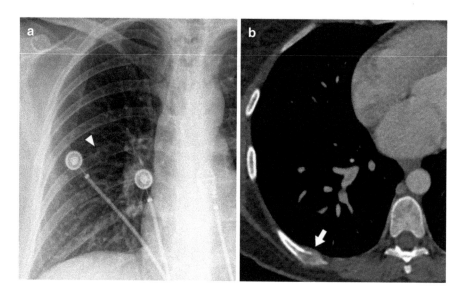

Fig. 4.3 Pathologic rib fracture. Chest X-ray anteroposterior view (**a**) shows a fracture along the right posterior 7th rib (arrowhead). Chest CT with contrast (**b**) shows a soft tissue mass associated with the pathologic fracture (arrow) in this patient with metastatic breast cancer

Solution

Chest X-ray may be sufficient to diagnose a pathologic fracture, though further imaging with chest CT, bone scan, or FDG-PET/CT may be necessary.

4.3 Hemoptysis

A 63-year-old woman with a 40 pack-year smoking history reports hemoptysis. Chest X-ray is unrevealing.

a. CT chest without contrast
b. CTA chest
c. Angiography pulmonary
d. Angiography bronchial without or with embolization
e. No ideal imaging exam

Hemoptysis of ≥30 cc or two risk factors (i.e., age >40 years and >30 pack-year smoking history).

a. CT chest without contrast may be appropriate. Consider if iodinated contrast is contraindicated.
b. *CTA chest* is the most appropriate.
c. Angiography pulmonary is usually not appropriate.
d. Angiography bronchial without or with embolization may be appropriate. Consider for patients with a known pre-procedure diagnosis and a high risk of recurrent hemorrhage.

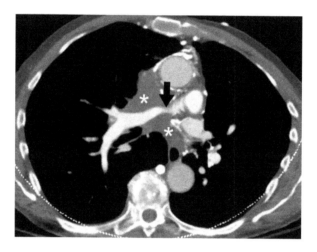

Fig. 4.4 Lung cancer. Chest CTA shows a centrally located mass (stars) that encases and narrows the right pulmonary artery (arrow) in this 68-year-old smoker who presented with hemoptysis

Solution
All patients with hemoptysis should be initially imaged with chest X-ray. For the population described in this scenario, chest CTA is recommended if radiography is inconclusive or negative. CTA can identify the cause of bleeding (most commonly bronchitis, bronchiectasis, and malignancy) and has comparable accuracy as bronchoscopy for localizing the bleeding site.

A 54-year-old woman with recurrent hemoptysis of <15 cc and a 15 pack-year smoking history.

a. X-ray chest
b. CT chest without contrast
c. CTA chest
d. Angiography pulmonary
e. No ideal imaging exam

Persistent or recurrent hemoptysis of <30 cc and one risk factor (i.e., age >40 years or >30 pack-year smoking history).

a. *X-ray chest* is the most appropriate.
b. CT chest without contrast may be appropriate. Consider if iodinated contrast is contraindicated.
c. CTA chest is usually appropriate, but there is a better choice here.
d. Angiography pulmonary is usually not appropriate.

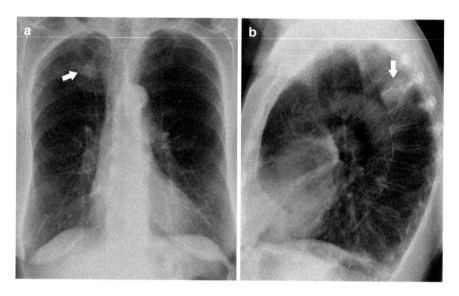

Fig. 4.5 Lung cancer. Chest X-ray posteroanterior (**a**) and lateral (**b**) views shows a 3 cm mass (arrows) in the right upper lobe. Hyperinflated lungs reflect underlying emphysema

Solution
Imaging evaluation of all patients with hemoptysis should begin with chest radiography, which may identify the etiology.

A 28-year-old woman with massive hemoptysis and no findings of cardiopulmonary compromise. Chest X-ray has been performed.

a. CT chest without contrast
b. CTA chest
c. Angiography pulmonary
d. Angiography bronchial without or with embolization
e. No ideal imaging exam

Massive hemoptysis without cardiopulmonary compromise.

a. CT chest without contrast may be appropriate.
b. *CTA chest* and choice (d) are equally the most appropriate.
c. Angiography pulmonary may be appropriate.
d. *Angiography bronchial without or with embolization* and choice (b) are equally the most appropriate.

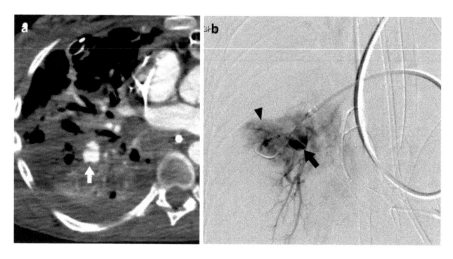

Fig. 4.6 Pulmonary artery pseudoaneurysm. Chest CTA (**a**) and subsequent pulmonary angiography (**b**) show a pulmonary artery pseudoaneurysm (arrow) with active extravasation (arrowhead) in this patient with hemoptysis and septic emboli. This was embolized during the angiography procedure

Solution
The source of hemoptysis is more commonly from systemic rather than pulmonary arteries. CTA can rapidly and accurately identify the cause of hemoptysis and localize the site of bleeding. Angiography is usually reserved for embolization to control acute hemorrhage.

4.4   Acute Respiratory Illness in an Immunocompetent Patient

A 51-year-old woman with new onset cough, sputum production, and dyspnea.

a. X-ray chest
b. CT chest without contrast
c. CT chest with contrast
d. CT chest without and with contrast
e. No ideal imaging exam

A patient older than 40 years of age.

a. *X-ray chest* is the most appropriate.
b. CT chest without contrast may be appropriate.
c. CT chest with contrast is usually not appropriate.
d. CT chest without and with contrast is usually not appropriate.

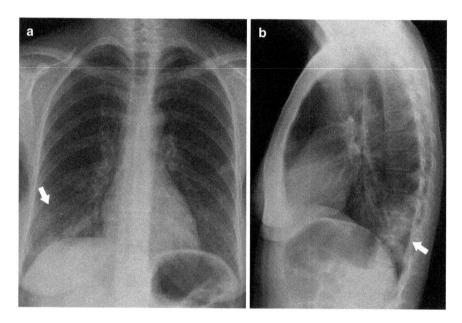

Fig. 4.7 Pneumonia. Chest X-ray posteroanterior (**a**) and lateral (**b**) views show air space consolidation (arrows) in the right lower lobe

Solution
Chest radiography for acute respiratory illness is recommended for immunocompetent patients if one or more of the following are present: age >40 years, dementia, a positive physical exam, hemoptysis, hypoxemia, leukocytosis, comorbidities (e.g., coronary artery disease, congestive heart failure), or drug-induced acute respiratory failure.

A 74-year-old man with a history of dementia, now with cough, sputum production, and dyspnea.

a. X-ray chest
b. CT chest without contrast
c. CT chest with contrast
d. CT chest without and with contrast
e. No ideal imaging exam

A patient of any age with dementia.

a. *X-ray chest* is the most appropriate.
b. CT chest without contrast may be appropriate. Exam may be indicated in patients with a negative chest X-ray where delayed diagnosis would result in morbidity.
c. CT chest with contrast is usually not appropriate.
d. CT chest without and with contrast is usually not appropriate.

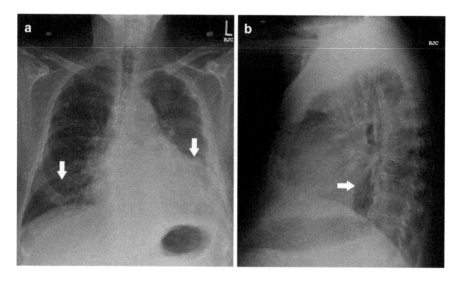

Fig. 4.8 Aspiration pneumonia. Chest X-ray posteroanterior (**a**) and lateral (**b**) views show pneumonia (arrows) bilaterally in the lower lobes

Solution
Chest radiography is recommended for acute respiratory illness in immunocompetent patients of all ages with dementia due to the high incidence of pneumonia in this population.

A 32-year-old man with cough, sputum production, and dyspnea. He has no other signs or symptoms for pneumonia and is otherwise healthy.

a. X-ray chest
b. CT chest without contrast
c. CT chest with contrast
d. Ga-67 scan lung
e. No ideal imaging exam

A patient younger than 40 years of age with a negative physical exam and no other signs, symptoms, or risk factors for pneumonia

a. X-ray chest may be appropriate.
b. CT chest without contrast is usually not appropriate.
c. CT chest with contrast is usually not appropriate.
d. Ga-67 scan lung is usually not appropriate.
e. *No ideal imaging exam* is the correct answer.

Solution

Imaging is not usually indicated for acute respiratory illness in this population.

A 25-year-old man with cough, sputum production, and dyspnea. Exam reveals unilateral decrease in breath sounds.

a. X-ray chest
b. CT chest without contrast
c. CT chest with contrast
d. Ga-67 scan lung
e. No ideal imaging exam

A patient younger than 40 years of age with a positive physical exam.

a. *X-ray chest* is the most appropriate.
b. CT chest without contrast may be appropriate.
c. CT chest with contrast is usually not appropriate.
d. Ga-67 scan lung is usually not appropriate.

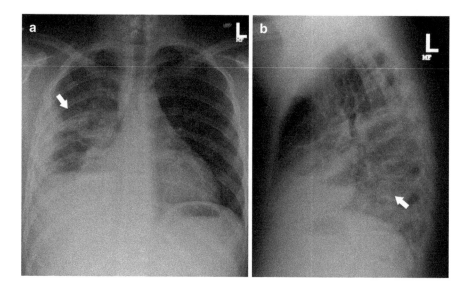

Fig. 4.9 Pneumonia. Chest X-ray posteroanterior (**a**) and lateral (**b**) views show air space opacity (arrows) in the right lower lobe

Solution

Chest radiography is recommended for adult patients presenting with an acute respiratory illness and clinical findings suggesting pneumonia.

A 32-year-old man with a history of asthma now with dyspnea. He has no other signs or symptoms.

a. X-ray chest
b. CT chest without contrast
c. CT chest with contrast
d. Tc-99m DTPA scan lung
e. No ideal imaging exam

Acute asthma, uncomplicated.

a. X-ray chest may be appropriate.
b. CT chest without contrast is usually not appropriate.
c. CT chest with contrast is usually not appropriate.
d. Tc-99m DTPA scan lung is usually not appropriate.
e. *No ideal imaging exam* is the correct answer.

Solution
In patients presenting with acute asthma and no signs or symptoms of complications, imaging is usually not indicated. However, imaging may be indicated in cases of suspected pneumonia or pneumothorax, or if one or more of the following are present: leukocytosis, chest pain, pulmonary edema, or a history of coronary artery disease or congestive heart failure.

A 37-year-old woman with a history of asthma, now with dyspnea, cough, and sputum. Acute asthma with pneumonia is suspected.

a. X-ray chest
b. CT chest without contrast
c. CT chest with contrast
d. Tc-99m DTPA scan lung
e. No ideal imaging exam

Acute asthma and suspected pneumonia or pneumothorax.

a. *X-ray chest* is the most appropriate.
b. CT chest without contrast is usually not appropriate.
c. CT chest with contrast is usually not appropriate.
d. Tc-99m DTPA scan lung is usually not appropriate.

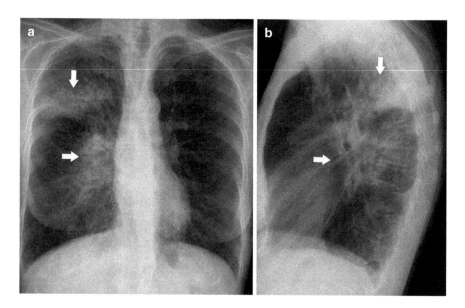

Fig. 4.10 Pneumonia. Chest X-ray posteroanterior (**a**) and lateral (**b**) views show multifocal air space opacities (arrows) in the right lung. Hyperinflated lungs and flattened diaphragms reflect acute asthma

Solution
Chest radiography is warranted in the evaluation of patients with acute asthma suspected with complications (e.g., pneumonia or pneumothorax).

A 62-year-old man with a history of chronic obstructive pulmonary disease (COPD) now with dyspnea. He has no other signs or symptoms and has no history of heart disease.

a. X-ray chest
b. CT chest without contrast
c. Ga-67 scan lung
d. Tc-99m DTPA scan lung
e. No ideal imaging exam

Acute exacerbation of COPD without leukocytosis, fever, or chest pain. No history of coronary artery disease or congestive heart failure.

a. X-ray chest may be appropriate.
b. CT chest without contrast is usually not appropriate.
c. Ga-67 scan lung is usually not appropriate.
d. Tc-99m DTPA scan lung is usually not appropriate.
e. *No ideal imaging exam* is the correct answer.

Solution
Imaging is usually not indicated in patients with COPD exacerbations as the findings are unlikely to alter clinical management. However, chest radiography should be considered if worsening dyspnea is accompanied by leukocytosis, chest pain, or edema or if there is a history of coronary artery disease or congestive heart failure.

A 65-year-old woman with a history of chronic obstructive pulmonary disease (COPD) now with dyspnea. She has a history of congestive heart failure.

a. X-ray chest
b. CT chest without contrast
c. CT chest with contrast
d. CT chest without and with contrast
e. No ideal imaging exam

Acute exacerbation of COPD with one or more of the following: chest pain, leukocytosis, edema, history of coronary artery disease, or congestive heart failure.

a. *X-ray chest* is the most appropriate.
b. CT chest without contrast may be appropriate.
c. CT chest with contrast is usually not appropriate.
d. CT chest without and with contrast is usually not appropriate.

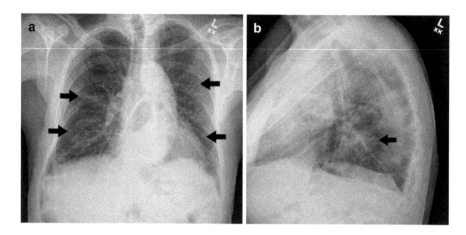

Fig. 4.11 Pulmonary edema and COPD. Chest X-ray posteroanterior (**a**) and lateral (**b**) views show increased bilateral interstitial opacities (arrows) consistent with pulmonary edema. Hyperinflated lungs and flattened diaphragms reflect underlying COPD

Solution
Chest radiography is indicated in patients with exacerbations of COPD when accompanied by leukocytosis, chest pain, or edema or if there is a history of coronary artery disease or congestive heart failure.

4.5   Acute Respiratory Illness in an Immunocompromised Patient

A 40-year-old neutropenic man with cough, sputum production, and dyspnea.

a. X-ray chest
b. CT chest without contrast
c. Ga-67 scan lung
d. Tc-99m DTPA scan lung
e. No ideal imaging exam

Cough, dyspnea, chest pain, or fever.

a. *X-ray chest* is the most appropriate.
b. CT chest without contrast is usually not appropriate.
c. Ga-67 scan lung is usually not appropriate.
d. Tc-99m DTPA scan lung is usually not appropriate.

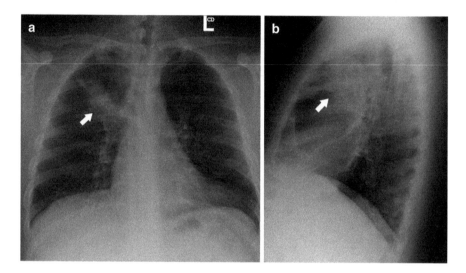

Fig. 4.12 Pneumonia. Chest X-ray posteroanterior (**a**) and lateral (**b**) views show air space opacity (arrows) in the right upper lobe

Solution

Chest radiography is the preferred initial imaging exam to evaluate immunocompromised patients presenting with cough, chest pain, dyspnea, or fever. The exam can demonstrate the presence and extent of pulmonary infection.

A 48-year-old man, HIV positive, with cough, sputum production, and dyspnea. Chest X-ray is negative.

a. CT chest without contrast
b. MRI chest without contrast
c. Ga-67 scan lung
d. Tc-99m DTPA scan lung
e. No ideal imaging exam

Negative, equivocal, or nonspecific chest radiograph.

a. *CT chest without contrast* is the most appropriate.
b. MRI chest without contrast is usually not appropriate.
c. Ga-67 scan lung is usually not appropriate. Consider if *Pneumocystis jirovecii* pneumonia is suspected.
d. Tc-99m DTPA scan lung is usually not appropriate. Consider if *Pneumocystis jirovecii* pneumonia is suspected.

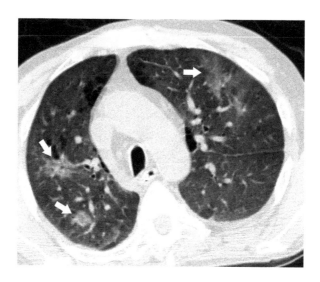

Fig. 4.13 *Pneumocystis jirovecii* pneumonia. Chest CT without contrast through the upper thorax shows multifocal bilateral ground glass opacities (arrows) in this patient with AIDS

Solution

In the immunocompromised patient, lack of an adequate inflammatory response to pulmonary infection may result in equivocal or negative chest radiography, despite high clinical suspicion for pulmonary disease. In this setting, chest CT is indicated.

A 34-year-old man, HIV positive, with cough, sputum production, and dyspnea. Chest X-ray shows diffuse confluent opacities.

a. CT chest without contrast
b. Ga-67 scan lung
c. Tc-99m DTPA scan lung
d. Transthoracic needle biopsy
e. No ideal imaging exam

Positive chest radiograph with multiple, diffuse, or confluent opacities.

a. *CT chest without contrast* is the most appropriate.
b. Ga-67 scan lung is usually not appropriate. Consider if *Pneumocystis jirovecii* pneumonia is suspected.
c. Tc-99m DTPA scan lung is usually not appropriate. Consider if *Pneumocystis jirovecii* pneumonia is suspected.
d. Transthoracic needle biopsy may be appropriate. Consider if an opportunistic infection is suspected.

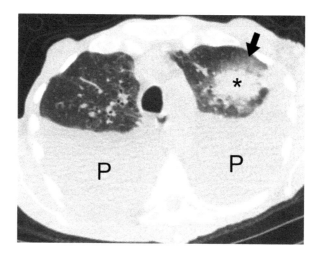

Fig. 4.14 Angio-invasive aspergillosis. Chest CT without contrast through the upper thorax shows a solid mass (star) with a surrounding halo of ground glass opacity representing hemorrhage (arrow). Large bilateral pleural effusions (P) are also present

Solution

Chest CT is indicated in immunocompromised patients with abnormal findings on initial chest X-ray. Patterns of disease seen on CT can help predict the underlying causative organisms and help guide transthoracic or transbronchial biopsy.

A 46-year-old man, HIV positive, with dyspnea. Chest X-ray shows lymphadenopathy suspected to be of noninfectious origin.

a. CT chest without contrast
b. Ga-67 scan lung
c. Tc-99m DTPA scan lung
d. Transthoracic needle biopsy
e. No ideal imaging exam

Positive chest radiograph, noninfectious disease suspected.

a. *CT chest without contrast* is the most appropriate.
b. Ga-67 scan lung is usually not appropriate.
c. Tc-99m DTPA scan lung is usually not appropriate.
d. Transthoracic needle biopsy may be appropriate. Consider if malignancy is suspected.

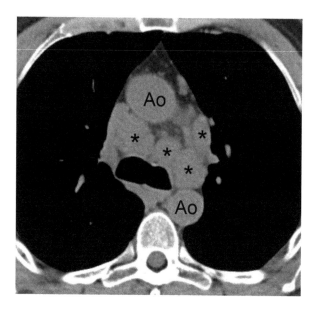

Fig. 4.15 Lymphoma. Chest CT without contrast through the mid thorax shows mediastinal lymphadenopathy (stars) in this patient with human immunodeficiency virus. Biopsy revealed classical Hodgkin lymphoma. *Ao* aorta

Solution
Chest CT can demonstrate and characterize findings not seen with radiography and help confirm suspected noninfectious diagnoses.

4.6   Chronic Dyspnea, Suspected Pulmonary Origin

A 58-year-old woman with chronic dyspnea suspected to be of pulmonary origin.

a. X-ray chest
b. CT chest with contrast
c. MRI chest without contrast
d. Tc-99m V/Q scan lung
e. No ideal imaging exam

Any age.

a. *X-ray chest* is the most appropriate.
b. CT chest with contrast is usually not appropriate.
c. MRI chest without contrast is usually not appropriate.
d. Tc-99m V/Q scan lung is usually not appropriate.

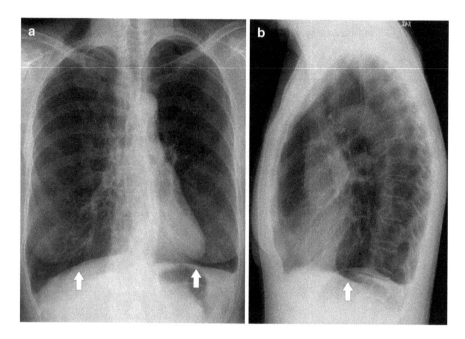

Fig. 4.16 Emphysema. Chest X-ray posteroanterior (**a**) and lateral (**b**) views show hyperinflated lungs and flattened diaphragm (arrows)

Solution

Chest radiography is the preferred initial imaging exam in patients with chronic dyspnea. Additional imaging may be necessary if the exam is negative. Of note, a negative chest X-ray does not exclude diffuse pulmonary disease.

A 65-year-old man with chronic dyspnea. Chest X-ray is nondiagnostic.

a. CT chest without contrast
b. CT chest with contrast
c. MRI chest without contrast
d. Tc-99m V/Q scan lung
e. No ideal imaging exam

Any age. Nondiagnostic clinical evaluation, chest X-ray, and laboratory tests.

a. *CT chest without contrast* is the most appropriate.
b. CT chest with contrast may be appropriate.
c. MRI chest without contrast is usually not appropriate.
d. Tc-99m V/Q scan lung is usually not appropriate.

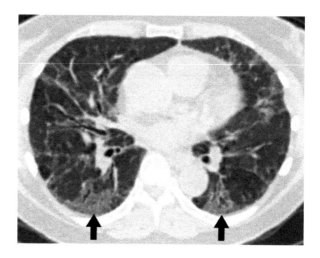

Fig. 4.17 Pulmonary fibrosis. Chest CT without contrast shows lower lobe-predominant peripheral reticulation, ground glass opacities (arrows), and bronchiolectasis, consistent with fibrotic interstitial lung disease

Solution

Chest CT performed with thin-section, high-resolution technique (i.e., high-resolution chest CT) is the preferred imaging exam for evaluating patients with suspected diffuse lung disease. Expiratory phase imaging helps assess for air trapping and tracheobronchomalacia. Intravenous contrast is rarely needed but may be helpful if mediastinal or hilar adenopathy or fibrosing mediastinitis is suspected.

4.7   **Possible Tuberculosis**

A 45-year-old man with suspected active tuberculosis.

a. X-ray chest
b. CT chest without contrast
c. MRI chest without contrast
d. FDG-PET/CT chest
e. No ideal imaging exam

Suspect active tuberculosis.

a. *X-ray chest* is the most appropriate.
b. CT chest without contrast is usually appropriate, but there is a better choice here. It is recommended if X-ray is equivocal.
c. MRI chest without contrast is usually not appropriate.
d. FDG-PET/CT chest is usually not appropriate.

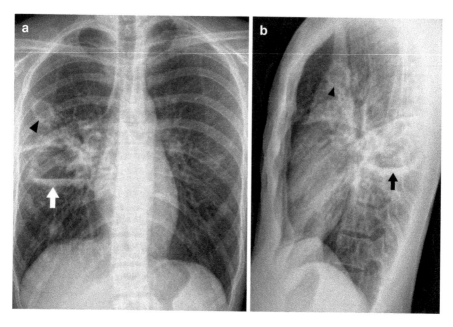

Fig. 4.18 Active tuberculosis. Chest X-ray posteroanterior (**a**) and lateral (**b**) views show a cavity in the right upper lobe (arrowhead) and the superior segment of the right lower lobe with an air-fluid level (arrows)

Solution
Chest radiography combined with clinical evaluation is sensitive but not specific for latent and active tuberculosis. In the appropriate clinical setting, upper-lobe or superior-segment lower-lobe fibro-cavitary disease on radiographs is sufficient to warrant respiratory isolation and sputum culture for definitive diagnosis. In immunocompromised patients (e.g., AIDS patients with low CD4 counts), chest X-ray may be normal.

A 41-year-old man with positive purified protein derivative (PPD) test. Prior PPD status is unknown. He is otherwise asymptomatic.

a. X-ray chest
b. CT chest without contrast
c. CT chest with contrast
d. FDG-PET/CT chest
e. No ideal imaging exam

Positive PPD or interferon-gamma release assay. Known to be newly positive or prior status is unknown. No clinical symptoms.

a. *X-ray chest* is the most appropriate.
b. CT chest without contrast is usually not appropriate.
c. CT chest with contrast may be appropriate. Consider if chest X-ray is equivocal and if results would inform treatment planning (e.g., transplantation, biologic agents for rheumatologic disease).
d. FDG-PET/CT chest is usually not appropriate.

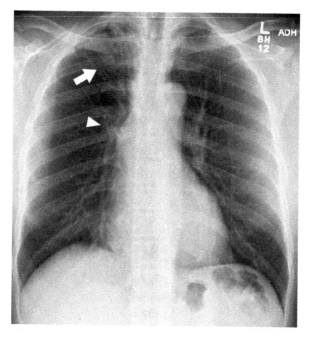

Fig. 4.19 Prior tuberculosis. Chest X-ray posteroanterior view shows scarring at the apex of the right lung (arrow) with superior retraction of the hilum (arrowhead), consistent with sequelae of prior tuberculosis

Solution
The purpose of performing chest radiography following a positive PPD is to distinguish latent from active TB. However, in the absence of clinical symptoms, the yield of radiographs for active TB is low.

4.8   Occupational Lung Disease

A 78-year-old man with history of silica exposure. Silicosis is suspected.

a. X-ray chest
b. CT chest without contrast
c. MRI chest without contrast
d. FDG-PET/CT chest
e. No ideal imaging exam

Silica exposure with suspected silicosis.

a. *X-ray chest* and choice (b) are equally the most appropriate. These two exams are complementary.
b. *CT chest without contrast* and choice (a) are equally the most appropriate. These two exams are complementary.
c. MRI chest without contrast is usually not appropriate.
d. FDG-PET/CT chest is usually not appropriate.

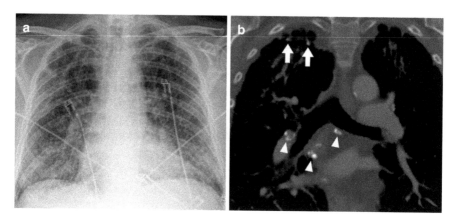

Fig. 4.20 Silicosis. Chest X-ray anteroposterior view (**a**) shows bilateral interstitial opacities. Chest CT coronal reconstruction image (**b**) shows calcified lung nodules (arrows) and mediastinal and right hilar lymph nodes (arrowheads), consistent with silicosis. This patient had occupational exposure to silica as a sandblaster

Solution
For suspected silicosis, chest radiography and CT without contrast are complementary. High-resolution chest CT demonstrates greater sensitivity for the detection of nodules and of complications of silicosis including bulla, pleural thickening, and progressive massive fibrosis.

A 63-year-old man with a history of coal dust exposure. Pneumoconiosis is suspected.

a. X-ray chest
b. CT chest without contrast
c. MRI chest without contrast
d. FDG-PET/CT chest
e. No ideal imaging exam

Coal dust exposure with suspected pneumoconiosis.

a. *X-ray chest* and choice (b) are equally the most appropriate. These two exams are complementary.
b. *CT chest without contrast* and choice (a) are equally the most appropriate. These two exams are complementary.
c. MRI chest without contrast is usually not appropriate.
d. FDG-PET/CT chest is usually not appropriate.

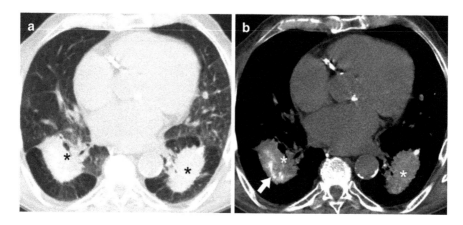

Fig. 4.21 Coal worker's pneumoconiosis. Chest CT without contrast in lung (**a**) and soft tissue (**b**) windows show mass-like conglomerates (stars) in both lungs with calcifications (arrow), consistent with pneumoconiosis with progressive massive fibrosis

Solution

For suspected pneumoconiosis, chest radiography and CT without contrast are complementary. Chest CT demonstrates greater sensitivity for detection of nodules and of complications such as pleural thickening and progressive massive fibrosis.

A 71-year-old man with a history of asbestos exposure. Interstitial lung disease is suspected.

a. X-ray chest
b. CT chest without contrast
c. MRI chest without contrast
d. FDG-PET/CT chest
e. No ideal imaging exam

Asbestos exposure with suspected interstitial lung disease.

a. *X-ray chest* and choice (b) are equally the most appropriate. These two exams are complementary.
b. *CT chest without contrast* and choice (a) are equally the most appropriate. These two exams are complementary.
c. MRI chest without contrast is usually not appropriate.
d. FDG-PET/CT chest is usually not appropriate.

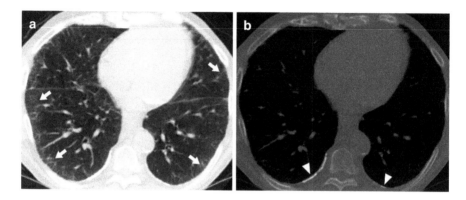

Fig. 4.22 Asbestosis. Chest CT without contrast in lung (**a**) and bone (**b**) windows show bilateral peripheral reticular opacities (arrows) and pleural calcifications (arrowheads), consistent with pulmonary and pleural fibrosis from asbestos exposure

Solution
Chest radiography and CT without contrast are complementary, and both should be performed. While radiography is the main method of screening for asbestos-related interstitial lung disease, CT is more sensitive for detection of lung abnormalities and complications related to asbestos exposure.

A 67-year-old man with history of asbestos exposure. Mesothelioma is suspected.

a. X-ray chest
b. CT chest with contrast
c. MRI chest without and with contrast
d. FDG-PET/CT chest
e. No ideal imaging exam

Asbestos exposure with suspected mesothelioma.

a. *X-ray chest* and choice (b) are equally the most appropriate. These two exams are complementary.
b. *CT chest with contrast* and choice (a) are equally the most appropriate. These two exams are complementary.
c. MRI chest without and with contrast may be appropriate.
d. FDG-PET/CT chest may be appropriate.

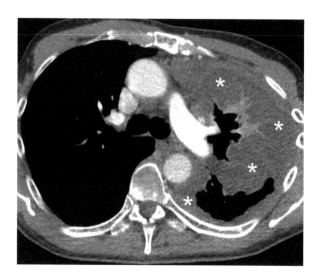

Fig. 4.23 Mesothelioma. Chest CT with contrast shows confluent pleural-based masses in the left hemithorax (stars)

Solution
When mesothelioma is suspected, chest radiography and CT with contrast are complementary and both should be performed. FDG-PET/CT may be useful for defining mediastinal and distal metastatic disease and for identifying potential biopsy sites.

4.9 Routine Chest Radiography

A 58-year-old man admitted for elective surgery. He is asymptomatic with no active diagnoses.

a. X-ray chest
b. CT chest without contrast
c. CTA coronary arteries
d. Tc-99m SPECT MPI
e. No ideal imaging exam

No clinical concern on the basis of history or physical examination.

a. X-ray chest is usually not appropriate.
b. CT chest without contrast is usually not appropriate.
c. CTA coronary arteries is usually not appropriate.
d. Tc-99m SPECT MPI is usually not appropriate.
e. *No ideal imaging exam* is the correct answer.

Solution
Routine imaging upon hospital admission, including chest radiography, is not recommended in the absence of clinical concerns. Screening chest X-ray rarely adds clinically significant information that would not have been predicted by a reliable history and physical examination.

A 43-year-old man admitted for elective surgery. Exam is positive for acute cardio-pulmonary findings.

a. X-ray chest
b. CT chest without contrast
c. CTA coronary arteries
d. Tc-99m SPECT MPI
e. No ideal imaging exam

Suspicion of acute or potentially unstable chronic cardiopulmonary disease by history or physical examination.

a. *X-ray chest* is the most appropriate.
b. CT chest without contrast is usually not appropriate.
c. CTA coronary arteries is usually not appropriate.
d. Tc-99m SPECT MPI is usually not appropriate.

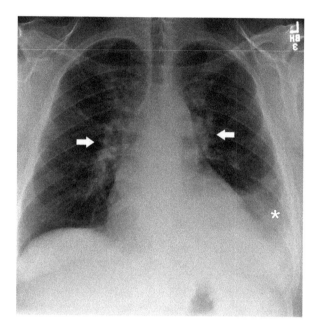

Fig. 4.24 Pulmonary edema. Chest X-ray posteroanterior view shows cardiomegaly, bilateral hilar prominence (arrows) and left pleural effusion (star)

Solution

In hospitalized or pre-intervention patients suspected to have acute or potentially unstable chronic cardiopulmonary disease, chest radiography is the most appropriate imaging exam. The decision to perform this exam is made based on whether the results could potentially influence care.

A 78-year-old man admitted for elective surgery.

a. X-ray chest
b. CT chest without contrast
c. CTA coronary arteries
d. Tc-99m SPECT MPI
e. No ideal imaging exam

Increased patient- or procedure-related risk (e.g., age >70 years, unreliable history or physical examination, high-risk surgery).

a. *X-ray chest* is the most appropriate.
b. CT chest without contrast is usually not appropriate.
c. CTA coronary arteries is usually not appropriate.
d. Tc-99m SPECT MPI is usually not appropriate.

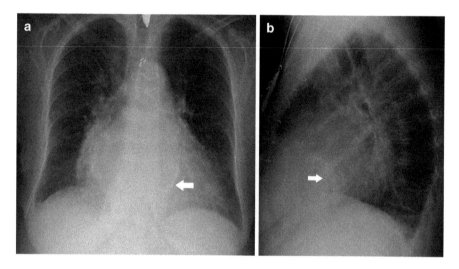

Fig. 4.25 Cardiomegaly. Chest X-ray posteroanterior (**a**) and lateral (**b**) views reveal an enlarged heart and a prosthetic mitral valve (arrows)

Solution
In the preoperative setting, chest radiography may provide added value in patients of advanced age (i.e., age >70 years), those with risk factors such as history of cardiopulmonary disease or unreliable clinical evaluation, and those undergoing a high-risk procedure. However, the ability of preoperative chest X-ray to predict postoperative pulmonary complications is low.

4.10   Solitary Pulmonary Nodule

A 62-year-old woman with 1.5 cm nodule seen on chest X-ray.

a. CT chest without contrast
b. CT chest with contrast
c. FDG-PET/CT skull base to mid-thigh
d. Transthoracic needle biopsy
e. No ideal imaging exam

Nodule ≥1 cm.

a. *CT chest without contrast* and choices (c) and (d) are equally the most appropriate.
b. CT chest with contrast may be appropriate.
c. *FDG-PET/CT skull base to mid-thigh* and choices (a) and (d) are equally the most appropriate.
d. *Transthoracic needle biopsy* and choices (a) and (c) are equally the most appropriate.

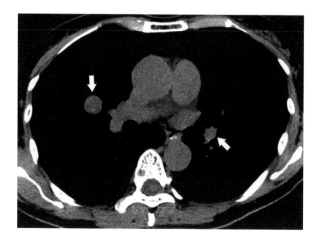

Fig. 4.26 Pulmonary hamartomas. Chest CT without contrast shows soft tissue density nodules (arrows) with punctate foci of high-density calcifications, one in each lung. There are consistent with hamartomas

Solution
Chest CT without contrast can characterize nodules as benign on appearance (e.g., calcification patterns) or after follow-up (e.g., solid nodule unchanged for ≥2 years). FDG-PET/CT and transthoracic needle biopsy are alternative methods to characterize lung nodules but are usually only used after a chest CT has been performed.

A 55-year-old woman with 0.8 cm nodule seen chest X-ray. There is low clinical suspicion for cancer.

a. CT chest without contrast
b. CT chest without contrast in 3–6 months
c. FDG-PET/CT whole body
d. Transthoracic needle biopsy
e. No ideal imaging exam

Nodule <1 cm, low clinical suspicion for cancer.

a. CT chest without contrast is usually appropriate, but there is a better choice here.
b. *CT chest without contrast in 3–6 months* is the most appropriate.
c. FDG-PET/CT whole body is usually not appropriate.
d. Transthoracic needle biopsy is usually not appropriate.

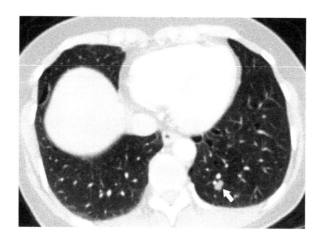

Fig. 4.27 Benign pulmonary nodule. Chest CT shows a 0.8 cm solid pulmonary nodule in the left lower lobe (arrow), which has remained stable in size over 2 years and is, therefore, considered benign

Solution

In patients with nodules <1 cm in size and no risk factors for cancer, it is appropriate to follow the nodules on CT to assess for interval change. Preferred follow-up interval varies with local institutional practice and choice of society guideline. For a solid nodule, stability in size for 2 years is sufficient to establish it as benign. Ground glass attenuation nodules may require longer follow-up as they can represent bronchoalveolar carcinoma, which demonstrate an indolent growth pattern.

A 50-year-old woman with 0.8 cm nodule seen on chest X-ray. There is high clinical suspicion for cancer.

a. CT chest without contrast
b. CT chest without contrast in 3–6 months
c. FDG-PET/CT whole body
d. Transthoracic needle biopsy
e. No ideal imaging exam

Nodule <1 cm, moderate to high clinical suspicion for cancer.

a. *CT chest without contrast* is the most appropriate.
b. CT chest without contrast in 3–6 months may be appropriate.
c. FDG-PET/CT whole body is usually not appropriate.
d. Transthoracic needle biopsy may be appropriate.

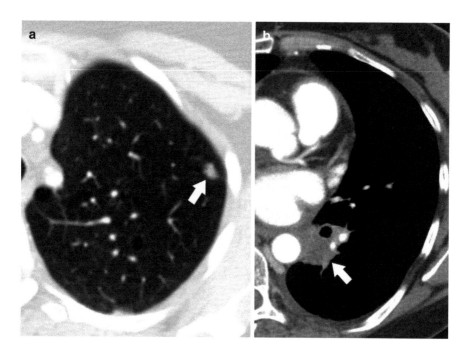

Fig. 4.28 Lung cancer. Chest CT with contrast in lung window (**a**) shows a spiculated subcentimeter left upper lobe pulmonary nodule (arrow) and in soft tissue window (**b**) shows adenopathy (arrow)

Solution

In a patient with risk factors for cancer and a subcentimeter nodule on chest radiography, CT without contrast is used to characterize the nodule and triage the patient to follow-up or biopsy. Transthoracic needle biopsy can help provide a definitive pathologic diagnosis. FDG-PET/CT is usually not appropriate as it often cannot characterize nodules <1 cm.

4.11   Bronchogenic Carcinoma Staging

An 84-year-old man newly diagnosed with non-small-cell lung carcinoma.

a. CT chest with or without contrast
b. CT abdomen with contrast
c. MRI head without and with contrast
d. FDG-PET/CT skull base to mid-thigh
e. No ideal imaging exam

Non-small-cell lung carcinoma.

a. *CT chest with or without contrast* and choice (d) are equally the most appropriate.
b. CT abdomen with contrast may be appropriate.
c. MRI head without and with contrast is usually appropriate, but there is a better choice here.
d. *FDG-PET/CT skull base to mid-thigh* and choice (a) are equally the most appropriate.

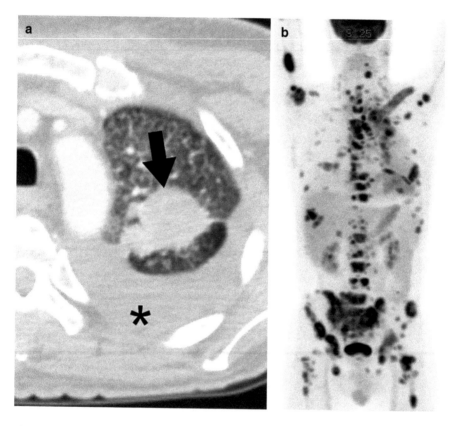

Fig. 4.29 Metastatic non-small-cell lung cancer. Chest CT with contrast (**a**) shows a left lung mass (arrow) and pleural effusion (star). FDG-PET/CT coronal MIP image (**b**) shows widespread metastases

Solution

In patients with non-small-cell lung cancer, chest CT includes imaging through the adrenal. Use of contrast varies with institutional preference. FDG-PET/CT, if used, is performed with the chest CT. Head MRI is appropriate when there is mediastinal adenopathy, neurological symptoms, or if the tumor is an adenocarcinoma measuring ≥3 cm.

A 64-year-old woman newly diagnosed with small-cell lung carcinoma.

a. CT chest and abdomen without contrast
b. CT chest and abdomen with contrast
c. MRI head without and with contrast
d. FDG-PET/CT skull base to mid-thigh
e. No ideal imaging exam

Small-cell lung carcinoma.

a. CT chest and abdomen without contrast may be appropriate.
b. *CT chest and abdomen with contrast* and choice (c) are equally the most appropriate.
c. *MRI head without and with contrast* and choice (b) are equally the most appropriate.
d. FDG-PET/CT skull base to mid-thigh is usually appropriate, but there is a better choice here. Use if diagnostic chest CT has not been performed.

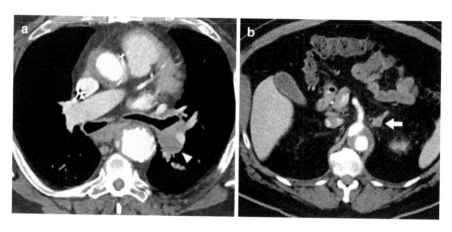

Fig. 4.30 Small-cell lung cancer. Chest (**a**) and abdomen (**b**) CT with contrast show a left parahilar mass (arrowhead) that abuts the airways and vessels and a left adrenal metastasis (arrow)

Solution
In patients with small-cell lung cancer, chest CT evaluates the extent of disease and relationship to mediastinal vessels. Abdominal CT with contrast and head MRI with contrast is also recommended due to the high incidence of metastases to the adrenal glands, liver, and brain.

Gastrointestinal Imaging

5

5.1 Blunt Abdominal Trauma

A 21-year-old man with blunt abdominal trauma. He is hemodynamically unstable.

a. US chest, abdomen, and pelvis for fluid
b. US abdomen and pelvis for organs
c. CT chest, abdomen, and pelvis with contrast
d. Angiography abdomen and pelvis
e. No ideal imaging exam

An unstable patient.

a. *US chest, abdomen, and pelvis for fluid* is the most appropriate. This exam (i.e., FAST scan) is complementary to X-ray chest and X-ray abdomen and pelvis. All three should be performed if clinically feasible.
b. US abdomen and pelvis for organs is usually not appropriate.
c. CT chest, abdomen, and pelvis is usually not appropriate for unstable patients.
d. Angiography abdomen and pelvis may be appropriate. This exam may be appropriate if site of active hemorrhage is known.

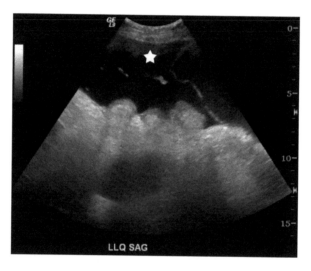

Fig. 5.1 Free abdominal fluid. Abdomen US shows complex free fluid (star), likely blood

Solution

Hemodynamically unstable patients presenting with blunt abdominal trauma should be evaluated with US of the chest, abdomen, and pelvis for fluid (i.e., FAST scan). A positive result can be used to support a decision to operate immediately.

A 22-year-old man with blunt abdominal trauma. He is hemodynamically stable.

a. X-ray abdomen and pelvis
b. US chest, abdomen, and pelvis for fluid
c. CT abdomen and pelvis with contrast
d. Angiography abdomen and pelvis
e. No ideal imaging exam

A stable patient.

a. X-ray abdomen and pelvis may be appropriate. Exam may be useful to initially evaluate for free intraperitoneal air and for pelvic or vertebral fractures.
b. US chest, abdomen, and pelvis for fluid may be appropriate.
c. *CT abdomen and pelvis with contrast* is the most appropriate. Exam can be tailored to evaluate for arterial, visceral, and skeletal injuries in the same sitting.
d. Angiography abdomen and pelvis may be appropriate.

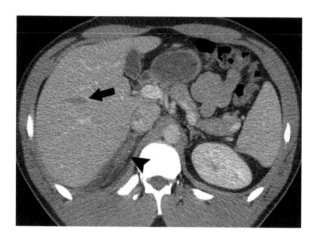

Fig. 5.2 Liver laceration. Abdomen CT with contrast shows a liver laceration (arrow) and soft tissue density posterior to the liver (arrowhead) consistent with a hematoma

Solution

CT with contrast should be performed in hemodynamically stable patients following blunt abdominal trauma. The need for urgent surgery versus a period of close observation can be assessed as CT identifies hemorrhage or injury to intra-abdominal organs (e.g., bowel, liver, spleen, or kidneys).

A 23-year-old man with blunt abdominal trauma. He is hemodynamically stable but has gross hematuria.

a. X-ray abdomen and pelvis
b. X-ray cystography
c. CT abdomen and pelvis with contrast
d. CT pelvis with bladder contrast (CT cystography)
e. No ideal imaging exam

Hematuria.

a. X-ray abdomen and pelvis may be appropriate. Exam may be useful to initially evaluate for free intraperitoneal air and for pelvic or vertebral fractures.
b. X-ray cystography may be appropriate. CT cystography is preferred.
c. *CT abdomen and pelvis with contrast* is the most appropriate. CT cystography should immediately follow in patients with known acute pelvic fractures or penetrating injury to the pelvis.
d. CT pelvis with bladder contrast (CT cystography) may be appropriate. Perform immediately after CT abdomen and pelvis.

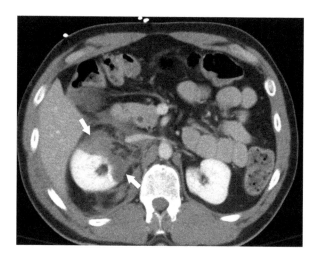

Fig. 5.3 Renal injury. Abdomen CT with contrast shows right renal contusions (arrows) and a hematoma around the kidney

Solution

CT abdomen and pelvis with contrast evaluates for injury to the kidneys and the renal collecting systems. CT cystography with intravesicular contrast should also be performed in cases of suspected bladder rupture and is preferred to X-ray cystography.

5.2   Right Upper Quadrant Pain

A 36-year-old woman with right upper quadrant pain, fever, and leukocytosis. Physical exam reveals a positive Murphy's sign.

a. US abdomen
b. CT abdomen with contrast
c. MRI abdomen without and with contrast
d. Cholescintigraphy
e. No ideal imaging exam

Fever, elevated white blood cell count, and positive Murphy sign.

a. *US abdomen* is the most appropriate.
b. CT abdomen with contrast may be appropriate.
c. MRI abdomen without and with contrast may be appropriate
d. Cholescintigraphy may be appropriate. This would follow an US exam indeterminate for acute cholecystitis.

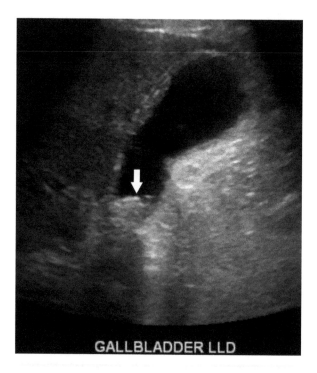

GALLBLADDER LLD

Fig. 5.4 Acute cholecystitis. Abdomen US shows stone lodged at the neck of the gallbladder (arrow). A sonographic Murphy's sign was also elicited

Solution

US is the initial imaging for suspected acute cholecystitis, with cholescintigraphy reserved for those cases where US is indeterminate. While cholescintigraphy is slightly more sensitive, US is more readily available, involves shorter exam times, and detects gallstones. CT or MRI may be helpful in equivocal cases to evaluate for other diagnoses.

An 82-year-old man with right upper quadrant pain, fever, and leukocytosis. US shows no gallstones. Acalculous cholecystitis is suspected.

a. US abdomen
b. CT abdomen with contrast
c. MRI abdomen without and with contrast
d. Cholescintigraphy
e. No ideal imaging exam

Suspected acalculous cholecystitis.

a. *US abdomen* is the most appropriate. If exam findings suggest acalculous cholecystitis, proceed with percutaneous cholecystostomy under US guidance.
b. CT abdomen with contrast may be appropriate.
c. MRI abdomen without and with contrast may be appropriate.
d. Cholescintigraphy may be appropriate.

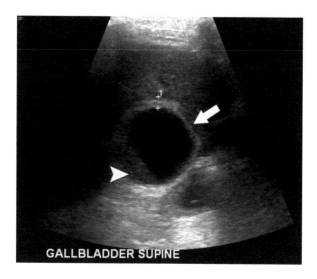

GALLBLADDER SUPINE

Fig. 5.5 Acalculous cholecystitis. Abdomen US shows a distended gallbladder (arrow) with a
thick wall (calipers) and biliary sludge (arrowhead). A sonographic Murphy's sign was elicited

Solution

US abdomen is the most appropriate initial exam for suspected acalculous cholecystitis. Although US and cholescintigraphy is used to evaluate for acalculous cholecystitis, diagnostic accuracies are limited as the gallbladder often appears abnormal
in these critically ill patients even when it is not inflamed. Percutaneous cholecystostomy may be both diagnostic and therapeutic in patients with acalculous
cholecystitis.

A 46-year-old woman with right upper quadrant pain. She has no fever or leukocytosis.

a. US abdomen
b. CT abdomen with contrast
c. MRI abdomen without and with contrast
d. Cholescintigraphy
e. No ideal imaging exam

No fever, normal white blood cell count.

a. *US abdomen* is the most appropriate. Exam would evaluate for gallstones and
   bile duct obstruction.
b. CT abdomen may be appropriate.
c. MRI abdomen without and with contrast may be appropriate.
d. Cholescintigraphy may be appropriate.

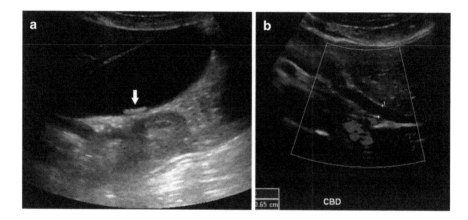

Fig. 5.6 Resolving choledocholithiasis. Abdomen US shows stones within the gallbladder (**a**,
arrow) and a mildly dilated common bile duct (**b**, calipers)

Solution
US evaluates for gallstones and underlying bile duct obstruction.

A 45-year-old woman with right upper quadrant pain. She has no fever or leukocytosis. US shows gallstones but no other evidence for acute cholecystitis.

a. X-ray abdomen and pelvis
b. CT abdomen with contrast
c. MRI abdomen without and with contrast
d. Cholescintigraphy
e. No ideal imaging exam

No fever or elevated white blood cell count. US shows only gallstones.

a. X-ray abdomen and pelvis is usually not appropriate.
b. *CT abdomen with contrast* is the most appropriate.
c. MRI abdomen without and with contrast may be appropriate.
d. Cholescintigraphy may be appropriate.

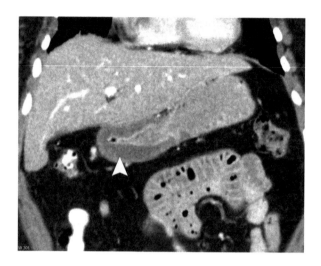

Fig. 5.7 Gastritis secondary to ulcer. Abdomen CT with contrast coronal reconstruction image shows wall thickening and submucosal edema (arrowhead) along the gastric antrum, indicating gastritis

Solution

In patients who have nonspecific abdominal pain, CT with contrast may demonstrate acute cholecystitis as well as diagnose other conditions including chronic cholecystitis, peptic ulcer, pancreatitis, gastroenteritis, and bowel obstruction.

A 38-year-old hospitalized woman with right upper quadrant pain, fever, and leuko-cytosis. Exam reveals a positive Murphy's sign.

a. US abdomen
b. CT abdomen with contrast
c. Cholescintigraphy
d. Percutaneous cholecystostomy
e. No ideal imaging exam

A hospitalized patient with fever, elevated white blood cell count, and positive Murphy sign.

a. *US abdomen* is the most appropriate.
b. CT abdomen with contrast is usually appropriate, but there is a better choice here.
c. Cholescintigraphy may be appropriate. This would follow a US exam indeterminate for acute cholecystitis.
d. Percutaneous cholecystostomy may be appropriate. This procedure can be both diagnostic and therapeutic for acute cholecystitis. It is typically performed on nonoperative patients in whom other causes of sepsis have been excluded.

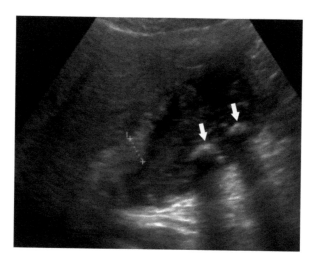

Fig. 5.8 Gangrenous cholecystitis. Abdomen US shows gallstones (arrows) and a thickened gallbladder wall (calipers)

Solution

US is the initial imaging exam for suspected acute cholecystitis. It can be performed at the bedside and detects gallstones and complications of acute cholecystitis. CT is useful in equivocal cases to assess for other diagnoses.

5.3   Right Lower Quadrant Pain: Suspected Appendicitis

A 32-year-old woman with right lower quadrant pain, fever, and leukocytosis. Appendicitis is suspected.

a. X-ray abdomen and pelvis
b. US abdomen right lower quadrant
c. CT abdomen and pelvis with contrast
d. MRI abdomen and pelvis without and with contrast
e. No ideal imaging exam

Fever, leukocytosis, and classic presentation clinically for appendicitis.

a. X-ray abdomen and pelvis may be appropriate. Exam may be useful for the detection of free intraperitoneal air.
b. US abdomen right lower quadrant may be appropriate. Perform exam with graded compression of appendix.
c. *CT abdomen and pelvis with contrast* is the most appropriate. Use of oral or rectal contrast depends on institutional preference.
d. MRI abdomen and pelvis without and with contrast may be appropriate.

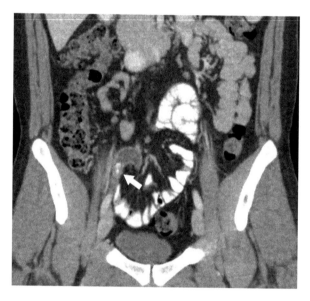

Fig. 5.9 Appendicitis. Abdomen and pelvis CT with contrast coronal reconstruction image shows a dilated appendix containing an appendicolith (arrow)

Solution
CT is the most accurate examination for evaluating patients with suspected appendicitis. While appendicitis can be diagnosed clinically, CT improves the specificity of the diagnosis and the negative appendectomy rate. US is less accurate than CT and has a more variable diagnostic performance.

An 18-year-old woman with right lower quadrant pain, fever, and leukocytosis. She is not pregnant. Appendicitis is a possibility.

a. X-ray abdomen and pelvis
b. US abdomen right lower quadrant
c. CT abdomen and pelvis with contrast
d. MRI abdomen and pelvis without and with contrast
e. No ideal imaging exam

Fever, leukocytosis, possible appendicitis, and atypical presentation.

a. X-ray abdomen and pelvis may be appropriate. Exam may be useful for the detection of free intraperitoneal air.
b. US abdomen right lower quadrant may be appropriate. Perform exam with graded compression of appendix.
c. *CT abdomen and pelvis with contrast* is the most appropriate. Use of oral or rectal contrast depends on institutional preference.
d. MRI abdomen and pelvis without and with contrast may be appropriate.

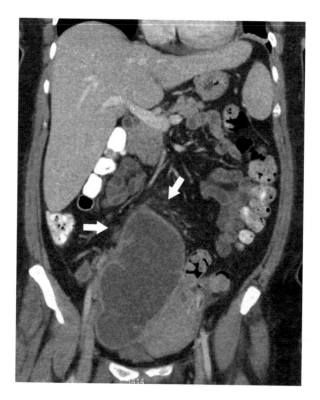

Fig. 5.10 Tubo-ovarian abscess. Abdomen and pelvis CT with contrast coronal reconstruction image shows a right adnexal fluid collection with adjacent fat stranding (arrows) consistent with tubo-ovarian abscess

Solution
CT with contrast can diagnose appendicitis and other causes of right lower quadrant pain such as inflammatory bowel disease, colitis, small bowel obstruction, gynecologic infection, and urinary colic.

A 32-year-old woman with right lower quadrant pain, fever, and leukocytosis. She is pregnant at 26 weeks gestation. Abdominal US is equivocal.

a. X-ray abdomen and pelvis
b. US pelvis
c. CT abdomen and pelvis with contrast
d. MRI abdomen and pelvis without contrast
e. No ideal imaging exam

Fever, leukocytosis, pregnant woman.

a. X-ray abdomen and pelvis is usually not appropriate.
b. US pelvis may be appropriate.
c. CT abdomen and pelvis with contrast may be appropriate. Exam may be useful after negative or equivocal abdominal US and MRI. Use of oral or rectal contrast depends on institutional preference.
d. *MRI abdomen and pelvis without contrast* is the most appropriate. Exam would follow an equivocal US abdomen right lower quadrant.

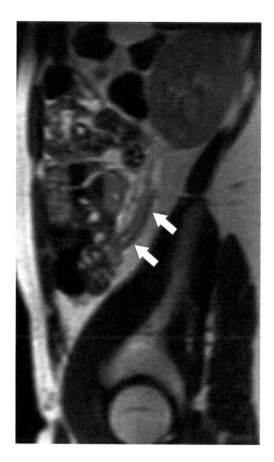

Fig. 5.11 Appendicitis. Abdomen and pelvis MR sagittal image shows a dilated fluid-filled appendix (arrows)

Solution
MRI is used to diagnose appendicitis in pregnant women, often following an inconclusive abdominal US. MRI is much more reliable than US in the detection of the normal appendix to exclude the diagnosis of appendicitis. Abdominopelvic CT exposes the fetus to direct ionizing radiation and should be avoided if possible.

5.4   Left Lower Quadrant Pain: Suspected Diverticulitis

A 51-year-old man with left lower quadrant pain. Diverticulitis is suspected.

a. X-ray abdomen and pelvis
b. X-ray contrast enema
c. CT abdomen and pelvis with contrast
d. MRI abdomen and pelvis
e. No ideal imaging exam

Typical or atypical clinical presentations or suspected complications of diverticulitis.

a. X-ray abdomen and pelvis may be appropriate.
b. X-ray contrast enema may be appropriate.
c. *CT abdomen and pelvis with contrast* is the most appropriate. Oral and/or colonic contrast may be helpful for visualizing the bowel lumen.
d. MRI abdomen and pelvis may be appropriate.

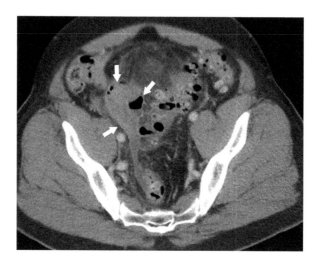

Fig. 5.12 Diverticulitis with perforation. Pelvis CT with contrast shows sigmoid colon diverticulitis, adjacent fat stranding indicating inflammation, and an extraluminal collection of fluid and air (arrows)

Solution

CT is the examination of choice for diverticulitis, as it is highly accurate and can assess for extra-colonic complications. MRI may be an appropriate alternative in younger patients with recurrent episodes if they are undergoing repeat imaging and limiting overall radiation dose is a consideration.

5.5   Acute Abdominal Pain and Fever or Suspected Abdominal Abscess

A 57-year-old man status post recent abdominal surgery with pain and fever. Abscess is suspected.

a. X-ray abdomen and pelvis
b. US abdomen
c. CT abdomen and pelvis with contrast
d. MRI abdomen and pelvis without and with contrast
e. No ideal imaging exam

Postoperative patient with fever.

a. X-ray abdomen and pelvis may be appropriate. Exam evaluates for bowel perforation with free air.
b. US abdomen may be appropriate.
c. *CT abdomen and pelvis with contrast* is the most appropriate.
d. MRI abdomen and pelvis without and with contrast may be appropriate.

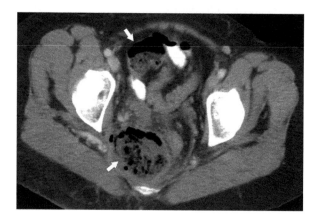

Fig. 5.13 Postoperative abscess. Pelvis CT with contrast shows two extraluminal collections (arrows) containing air and fluid

Solution

CT abdomen is the best examination to assess postoperative patients for suspected abscess. US could be used to detect certain diagnoses (e.g., cholecystitis, liver abscess, or gynecologic infections) but overall demonstrates lower accuracies than CT.

A 46-year-old woman status post recent pelvic surgery with persistent pain and fever. No abscess was seen on a CT exam 7 days ago.

a. X-ray abdomen and pelvis
b. US abdomen
c. CT abdomen and pelvis with contrast
d. MRI abdomen and pelvis without and with contrast
e. No ideal imaging exam

Postoperative patient with persistent fever and no abscess seen on CT scan within the last 7 days.

a. X-ray abdomen and pelvis may be appropriate. Exam evaluates for bowel perforation.
b. US abdomen may be appropriate.
c. *CT abdomen and pelvis with contrast* is the most appropriate.
d. MRI abdomen and pelvis without and with contrast may be appropriate.

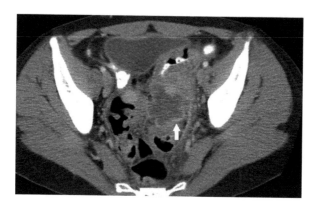

Fig. 5.14 Postoperative abscess. Pelvis CT with contrast shows a rim-enhancing extraluminal fluid collection (arrow)

Solution

CT abdomen and pelvis with contrast is appropriate for repeat imaging following an initial negative CT in a postoperative patient where abscess is suspected. Abscess, bowel ischemia, or leak can be occult and present in a delayed fashion.

A 52-year-old man with non-localizing abdominal pain and fever. He has no history of recent surgery.

a. X-ray abdomen and pelvis
b. US abdomen
c. CT abdomen and pelvis with contrast
d. MRI abdomen and pelvis without and with contrast
e. No ideal imaging exam

Patient presenting with fever and no recent operation.

a. X-ray abdomen and pelvis may be appropriate. Exam evaluates for bowel perforation with free air.
b. US abdomen may be appropriate.
c. *CT abdomen and pelvis with contrast* is the most appropriate.
d. MRI abdomen and pelvis without and with contrast may be appropriate.

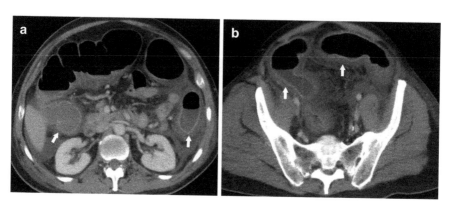

Fig. 5.15 Pseudomembranous colitis. Abdomen and pelvis CT with contrast shows diffuse
colonic wall thickening (arrows) at the level of the kidneys (**a**) and pelvis (**b**)

Solution
CT with contrast is the preferred imaging modality to assess abdominal pain, particularly in patients with fever. Most common diagnoses in the urgent setting are
appendicitis, acute cholecystitis, small bowel obstruction, pancreatitis, renal colic,
perforated peptic ulcer, and diverticulitis.

A 19-year-old pregnant woman with abdominal pain and fever.

a. X-ray abdomen and pelvis
b. US abdomen
c. CT abdomen and pelvis with contrast
d. MRI abdomen and pelvis without contrast
e. No ideal imaging exam

Pregnant patient.

a. X-ray abdomen and pelvis may be appropriate.
b. *US abdomen* is the most appropriate.
c. CT abdomen and pelvis with contrast may be appropriate. Use only after exams without ionizing radiation.
d. MRI abdomen and pelvis without contrast is usually appropriate, but there is a better choice here.

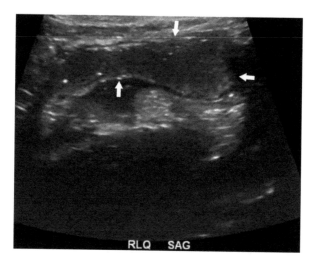

Fig. 5.16 Abscess. Abdomen US shows a loculated fluid collection (arrows) in the right lower quadrant

Solution
In pregnant patients, US and MRI are the preferred initial imaging modalities for evaluating abdominal pain and fever. MRI is frequently used after an inconclusive US examination and demonstrates high accuracies for the detection of appendicitis and abscess.

5.6   Suspected Small Bowel Obstruction

An 84-year-old woman with suspected acute small bowel obstruction.

a. X-ray abdomen and pelvis
b. X-ray small bowel follow-through
c. CT abdomen and pelvis with contrast
d. MRI abdomen and pelvis without and with contrast
e. No ideal imaging exam

Suspected small bowel obstruction with an acute presentation.

a. X-ray abdomen and pelvis may be appropriate.
b. X-ray small bowel follow-through may be appropriate.
c. *CT abdomen and pelvis with contrast* is the most appropriate.
d. MRI abdomen and pelvis without and with contrast may be appropriate.

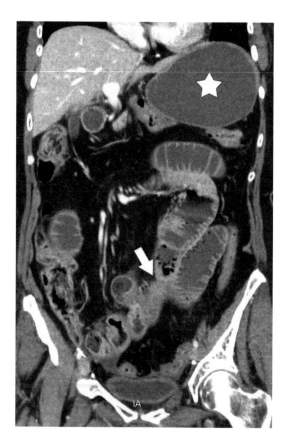

Fig. 5.17 Small bowel obstruction. Abdomen and pelvis CT with contrast coronal reconstruction image shows a distended stomach (star), dilated proximal small bowel, and decompressed colon with a caliber transition (arrow) in the jejunum. Oral contrast was not used

Solution
CT is preferred for diagnosing acute small bowel obstruction. Omit oral contrast as it can cause vomiting and aspiration, and since intrinsic contrast is already provided by the fluid in distended bowel loops. MRI may be used in pregnant and younger patients to avoid ionizing radiation. X-ray abdomen and pelvis and small bowel follow-through are both of limited use in this setting as radiography cannot differentiate mechanical obstruction from ileus.

A 70-year-old woman with suspected intermittent small bowel obstruction.

a. X-ray abdomen and pelvis
b. X-ray small bowel follow-through
c. CT abdomen and pelvis with contrast
d. MRI abdomen and pelvis without and with contrast
e. No ideal imaging exam

Suspected intermittent or low-grade small bowel obstruction with an indolent presentation.

a. X-ray abdomen and pelvis is usually not appropriate.
b. X-ray small bowel follow-through may be appropriate.
c. *CT abdomen and pelvis with contrast* is the most appropriate.
d. MRI abdomen and pelvis without and with contrast may be appropriate.

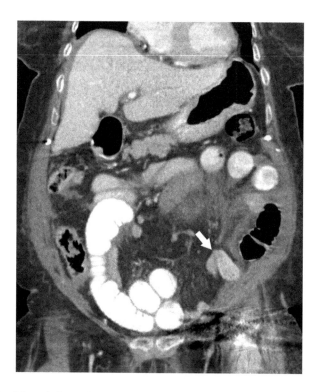

Fig. 5.18 Small bowel obstruction. Abdomen and pelvis CT with intravenous and oral contrast coronal reconstruction image shows dilated proximal small bowel and decompressed colon with a caliber transition (arrow) in the jejunum

Solution
CT is preferred for evaluating small bowel obstruction. With low-grade or intermittent obstruction, oral contrast can help improve visualization of the obstruction.

5.7   Jaundice

A 52-year-old woman with jaundice, fever and acute abdominal pain. She has a known history of gallstones.

a. US abdomen
b. CT abdomen with contrast
c. MRI abdomen without and with contrast and MRCP
d. ERCP
e. No ideal imaging exam

Acute abdominal pain and at least one of the following: fever, history of biliary surgery, known cholelithiasis.

a. *US abdomen* is the most appropriate.
b. CT abdomen with contrast is usually appropriate, but there is a better choice here. Addition of non-contrast images may be useful in detecting choledocholithiasis.
c. MRI abdomen with MRCP is usually appropriate, but there is a better choice here. Contrast is useful in evaluating for cholangitis.
d. ERCP may be appropriate. For high suspicion of common bile duct stones, this procedure should be the initial exam.

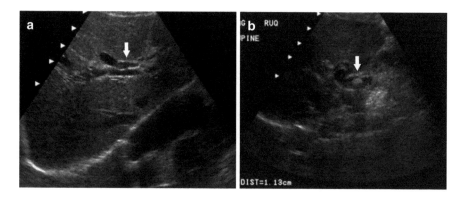

Fig. 5.19 Biliary obstruction from choledocholithiasis. Abdomen US shows dilated intrahepatic bile ducts (**a**, arrow). The common bile duct is also dilated and contains a stone (**b**, arrow)

Solution
US is the first-line modality to confirm mechanical obstruction of the bile ducts and assess for choledocholithiasis. It is used to direct the choice of the second-line test, which could be CT, MRI with MRCP or ERCP.

A 60-year-old man with painless jaundice and a history of unexplained weight loss over the past 4 months.

a. CT abdomen with contrast
b. MRI abdomen without and with contrast and MRCP
c. ERCP
d. US abdomen endoscopic
e. No ideal imaging exam

Painless and one or more of the following: weight loss, fatigue, anorexia, duration of symptoms greater than 3 months.

a. *CT abdomen with contrast* is the most appropriate.
b. MRI abdomen with contrast and with MRCP is usually appropriate. If malignancy is known or likely, exam allows for treatment planning.
c. ERCP may be appropriate.
d. US abdomen endoscopic may be appropriate. Procedure may diagnose and treat bile duct ampullary or pancreatic mass.

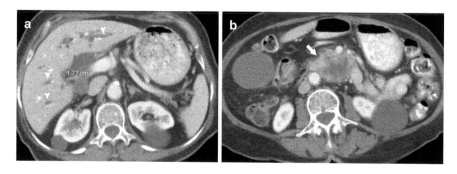

Fig. 5.20 Biliary obstruction from pancreatic cancer. Abdomen CT with contrast shows intrahepatic biliary ductal dilatation (**a**, arrowheads), a dilated common bile duct (**a**, calipers), and a pancreatic mass (**b**, arrow)

Solution

In cases of biliary obstruction with high suspicion of malignancy, CT abdomen with pancreatic and portal venous phase contrast imaging through the liver, biliary tree, and pancreas can detect the mass causing the obstruction, assess for resectability and metastatic disease. MRI demonstrates similar accuracy for depicting malignancy but is slightly superior to CT for detecting stone disease.

A 27-year-old man with jaundice. Clinical evaluation and laboratory values are not consistent with mechanical biliary obstruction.

a. US abdomen
b. CT abdomen with contrast
c. MRI abdomen without and with contrast and MRCP
d. ERCP
e. No ideal imaging exam

Clinical condition and laboratory examination make mechanical obstruction unlikely.

a. *US abdomen* is the most appropriate. Exam evaluates for cirrhosis.
b. CT abdomen with contrast is usually appropriate, but there is a better choice here.
c. MRI abdomen with MRCP is usually appropriate. Use exam when US is equivocal. Exam can evaluate for cirrhosis and for hepatic fat or iron deposition.
d. ERCP is usually not appropriate.

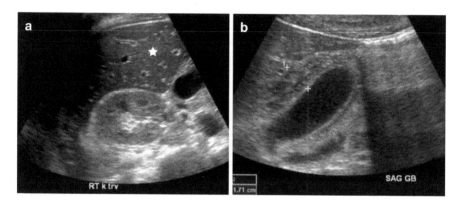

Fig. 5.21 Hepatitis. Abdomen US shows a hypoechoic liver (**a**, star) and a thick gallbladder wall (**b**, calipers), findings seen with hepatitis

Solution

If mechanical biliary obstruction is unlikely, US or MRI with MRCP is an appropriate first-line imaging technique. Both evaluate for diffuse hepatic parenchymal liver disease. MRI with MRCP is more tissue specific and may help direct the subsequent biopsy.

5.8   Acute Pancreatitis

A 41-year-old patient with acute upper abdominal pain and elevated amylase and lipase.

a. X-ray abdomen and pelvis
b. US abdomen
c. CT abdomen with contrast
d. MRI abdomen without and with contrast and MRCP
e. No ideal imaging exam

First-time presentation with high clinical certainty of diagnosis; typical abdominal pain, increased amylase and lipase and <48–72 hours after onset of symptoms.

a. X-ray abdomen and pelvis is usually not appropriate.
b. *US abdomen* is the most appropriate.
c. CT abdomen with contrast may be appropriate. Exam may be used if US is equivocal.
d. MRI abdomen without and with contrast and MRCP may be appropriate. Exam may be used if US is equivocal or if choledocholithiasis is suspected.

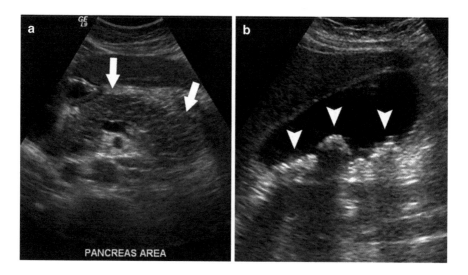

Fig. 5.22 Pancreatitis from gallstones. Abdomen US shows a hypoechoic diffusely enlarged pancreas (**a**, arrows) consistent with pancreatitis and stones (**b**, arrowheads) within the gallbladder

Solution

US assesses for gallstones and should be performed in patients who present for the first time with pancreatitis where the cause for pancreatitis is uncertain.

A 36-year-old man critically ill with multiple organ failure from acute pancreatitis >48 hours after onset of symptoms.

a. X-ray abdomen and pelvis
b. US abdomen
c. CT abdomen with contrast
d. MRI abdomen without and with contrast and MRCP
e. No ideal imaging exam

Critically ill with systemic inflammatory response syndrome, severe clinical scores and >48–72 h after onset of symptoms.

a. X-ray abdomen and pelvis is usually not appropriate.
b. US abdomen may be appropriate.
c. *CT abdomen with contrast* is the most appropriate.
d. MRI abdomen without and with contrast and MRCP is usually appropriate, but there is a better choice here. Exam is a reasonable alternative to CT, but it is less feasible in critically ill patients.

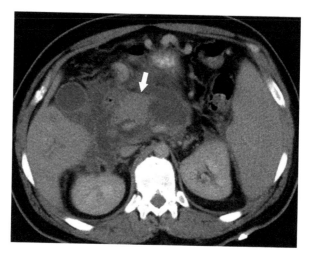

Fig. 5.23 Pancreatitis with pancreatic necrosis. Abdomen CT with contrast shows a mixed fluid- and soft tissue collection replacing much of the pancreas. Residual enhancing normal pancreatic head (arrow) is seen

Solution

CT with contrast after 48–72 h from the onset of symptoms will detect pancreatic necrosis as well as peri-pancreatic fluid collections. Exam assesses the size, extent, and character of the necrotic fluid collections and enables planning for aspiration and culture.

An 84-year-old man with upper abdominal pain, renal insufficiency, and amylase and lipase values equivocal for pancreatitis.

a. X-ray abdomen and pelvis
b. US abdomen
c. CT abdomen without contrast
d. MRI abdomen without and with contrast and MRCP
e. No ideal imaging exam

Initial presentation with atypical signs and symptom, equivocal amylase and lipase values, and when alternative diagnoses (e.g., bowel ischemia etc.) are possible.

a. X-ray abdomen and pelvis is usually not appropriate.
b. US abdomen may be appropriate.
c. *CT abdomen without contrast* is the most appropriate. If renal function allows, contrast-enhanced imaging is preferable.
d. MRI abdomen without and with contrast and MRCP may be appropriate. Exam has limited role if contrast is contraindicated.

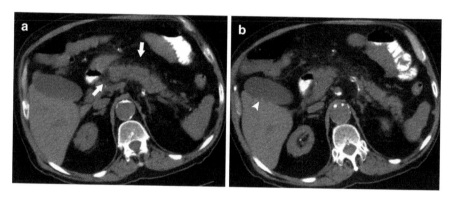

Fig. 5.24 Pancreatitis. Abdomen CT without contrast shows peri-pancreatic fat stranding (**a**, arrows) consistent with pancreatitis and gallstones (**b**, arrowhead)

Solution

CT provides the best abdominal survey for equivocal or uncertain presentations when diagnoses other than acute pancreatitis are being considered (e.g., acute kidney injury, bowel ischemia). Although use of contrast is preferred when possible, non-contrast CT is a good alternative when contrast is contraindicated.

A 54-year-old man with known necrotizing pancreatitis now with abrupt decrease in serum hematocrit and hypotension.

a. X-ray abdomen
b. US abdomen
c. CT abdomen with contrast
d. MRI abdomen without and with contrast and MRCP
e. No ideal imaging exam

Known necrotizing pancreatitis with significant deterioration in clinical status (e.g., decrease in hemoglobin/hematocrit, hypotension, or increase in white blood cell count).

a. X-ray abdomen and pelvis is usually not appropriate.
b. US abdomen may be appropriate.
c. *CT abdomen with contrast* is the most appropriate.
d. MRI abdomen without and with contrast and MRCP may be appropriate. Exam is often not feasible in critically ill patients.

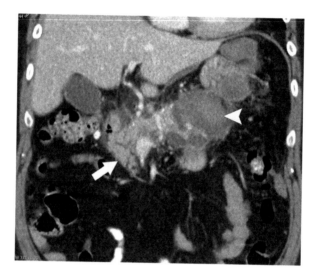

Fig. 5.25 Hemorrhagic necrotizing pancreatitis. Abdomen CT coronal reconstruction image shows replacement of the pancreatic tail with hyperdense fluid (arrowhead) consistent with hemorrhage. The pancreatic head and uncinate process are preserved (arrow)

Solution

CT with contrast should be performed when there is a significant deterioration of the patient's condition. Exam can identify complications such an abscess or new hemorrhage and occasionally the underlying ruptured pseudoaneurysm that is the cause.

5.9   Dysphagia

A 69-year-old man recovering from recent stroke now with oropharyngeal dysphagia.

a. X-ray pharynx dynamic and static imaging
b. X-ray esophagram with double and single contrast
c. X-ray barium swallow modified
d. Tc-99m transit scintigraphy esophagus
e. No ideal imaging exam

Oropharyngeal dysphagia with an attributable cause.

a. X-ray pharynx dynamic and static imaging may be appropriate.
b. X-ray esophagram with double and single contrast may be appropriate.
c. *X-ray barium swallow modified* is the most appropriate.
d. Tc-99m transit scintigraphy esophagus is usually not appropriate.

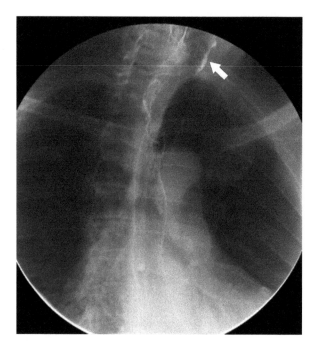

Fig. 5.26 Aspiration. X-ray modified barium swallow spot image shows contrast in the upper trachea (arrow)

Solution

X-ray modified barium swallow is the best examination when oropharyngeal dysphagia has an attributable cause. The exam tests a variety of barium consistencies to assess therapeutic options. X-ray pharynx with dynamic and static imaging and biphasic or single-contrast esophagram examinations evaluate for a cause of abnormal swallowing function.

A 49-year-old woman with unexplained oropharyngeal dysphagia.

a. X-ray pharynx dynamic and static imaging
b. X-ray esophagram with double and single contrast
c. X-ray barium swallow modified
d. Tc-99m transit scintigraphy esophagus
e. No ideal imaging exam

Unexplained oropharyngeal dysphagia.

a. *X-ray pharynx dynamic and static imaging* and choice (b) are equally the most appropriate and should be performed together.
b. *X-ray esophagram with double and single contrast* and choice (a) are equally the most appropriate and should be performed together.
c. X-ray barium swallow modified may be appropriate.
d. Tc-99m transit scintigraphy esophagus may be appropriate.

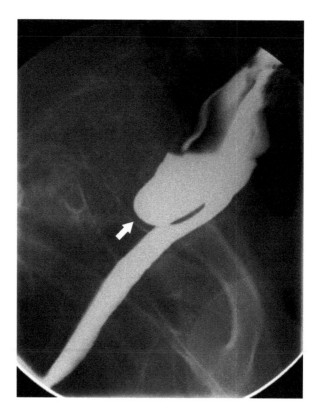

Fig. 5.27 Zenker's diverticulum. X-ray esophagram spot image shows a large outpouching (arrow) of the posterior hypopharynx

Solution

X-ray pharynx with dynamic and static imaging and an X-ray esophagram with double and single contrast should be performed on patients with unexplained oropharyngeal dysphagia. The former evaluates for functional and structural abnormalities of the pharynx while the latter detects lesions in the esophagus or at the gastric cardia that can cause referred symptoms.

A 74-year-old man with retrosternal dysphagia.

a. X-ray pharynx dynamic and static imaging
b. X-ray esophagram with double and single contrast
c. X-ray barium swallow modified
d. Tc-99m transit scintigraphy esophagus
e. No ideal imaging exam

Retrosternal dysphagia in immunocompetent patients.

a. X-ray pharynx dynamic and static imaging may be appropriate.
b. *X-ray esophagram with double and single contrast* is the most appropriate.
c. X-ray barium swallow modified may be appropriate.
d. Tc-99m transit scintigraphy esophagus may be appropriate.

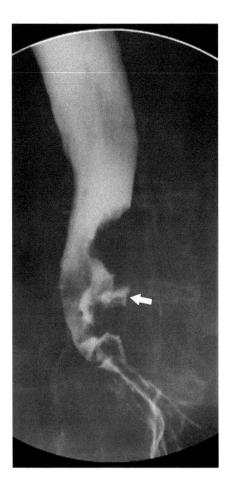

Fig. 5.28 Esophageal cancer. X-ray esophagram spot image shows irregular narrowing in the distal esophagus with ulceration (arrow)

Solution

The biphasic esophagram is the preferred examination to assess retrosternal dysphagia in immunocompetent patients. Double-contrast views best detect mucosal lesions, whereas single-contrast views best detect lower esophageal rings or strictures and assess motility. This exam evaluates the entire esophagus and the gastric cardia more fully than the other exam options.

55-year-old woman with retrosternal dysphagia. She is immunocompromised.

a. X-ray pharynx dynamic and static imaging
b. X-ray esophagram with double and single contrast
c. X-ray barium swallow modified
d. Tc-99m transit scintigraphy esophagus
e. No ideal imaging exam

Substernal dysphagia in immunocompromised patients.

a. X-ray pharynx dynamic and static imaging is usually not appropriate.
b. *X-ray esophagram with double and single contrast* is the most appropriate.
c. X-ray barium swallow modified may be appropriate.
d. Tc-99m transit scintigraphy esophagus is usually not appropriate.

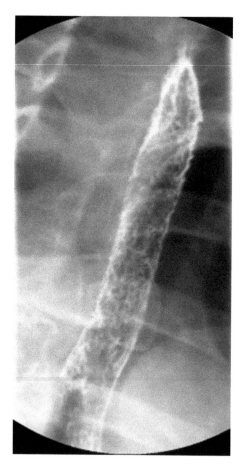

Fig. 5.29 Candida esophagitis. X-ray esophagram spot image shows a "shaggy" esophagus caused by confluent mucosal plaques and ulcers

Solution

X-ray esophagram with double and single contrast is the preferred initial exam to assess for the mucosal changes associated with infectious esophagitis. If abnormal, endoscopy is performed to obtain tissue for microbiology and pathology and to direct further management.

5.10   Crohn's Disease

A 21-year-old man with fever, severe abdominal pain, vomiting, and leukocytosis.
Crohn's disease is suspected.

a. X-ray small bowel follow through
b. CT abdomen and pelvis with contrast
c. CT enterography
d. MR enterography
e. No ideal imaging exam

Acute initial presentation. Fever, severe abdominal pain, vomiting, leukocytosis. Suspected Crohn's disease.

a. X-ray small bowel follow through is usually not appropriate.
b. *CT abdomen and pelvis with contrast* and choice (c) are equally the most appropriate. It may be better tolerated than choice (c) in the acute setting.
c. *CT enterography* and choice (b) are equally the most appropriate. However, in the acute setting, patients may be unable to tolerate the large volume of oral contrast required for this exam.
d. MR enterography may be appropriate. This exam may not be well tolerated in the acute setting.

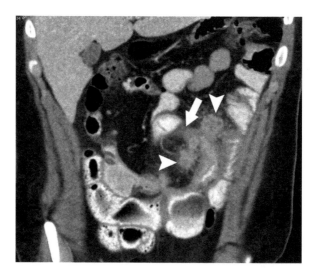

Fig. 5.30 Crohn's disease. Abdomen CT coronal reconstruction image shows loops of small bowel with wall thickening surrounded by fat stranding, phlegmon (arrowheads), and fistula formation (arrow)

Solution

CT enterography is optimized to detect pathology in the small bowel but requires ingestion of large amounts of oral contrast. Standard CT abdomen and pelvis with contrast is an alternative for initial diagnosis.

A 21-year-old woman with known Crohn's disease now presenting with acute symptoms suggesting acute exacerbation.

a. X-ray small bowel follow through
b. CT abdomen and pelvis with contrast
c. CT enterography
d. MR enterography
e. No ideal imaging exam

Known Crohn's disease; acute exacerbation such as fever or increasing abdominal pain or leukocytosis.

a. X-ray small bowel follow through may be appropriate.
b. CT abdomen and pelvis with contrast is usually appropriate, but there is a better choice here.
c. *CT enterography* is the most appropriate.
d. MR enterography is usually appropriate, but there is a better choice here. Image quality may be degraded in the severely ill patient.

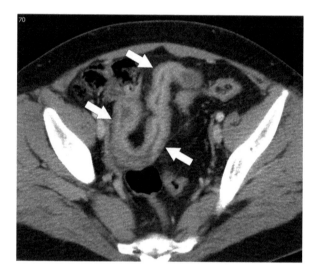

Fig. 5.31 Crohn's disease flare. CT enterography with contrast shows mucosal hyper-enhancement and wall thickening (arrows) along the distal ileum

Solution
CT enterography and standard CT with contrast are both appropriate for detection of Crohn's disease complications. CT enterography may not be feasible in severely ill patients or those with obstructive symptoms as these patients may not be able to tolerate the large volume of oral contrast needed for the exam. MR enterography is a suitable alternative to CT, if the necessary technology and expertise are available.

A 24-year-old woman being treated for Crohn's disease now stable and presenting for follow-up.

a. X-ray small bowel follow through
b. CT abdomen and pelvis with contrast
c. CT enterography
d. MR enterography
e. No ideal imaging exam

Known Crohn's disease; stable, mild symptoms, or surveillance.

a. X-ray small bowel follow through may be appropriate.
b. CT abdomen and pelvis with contrast may be appropriate.
c. CT enterography is usually appropriate, but there is a better choice here.
d. *MR enterography* is the most appropriate.

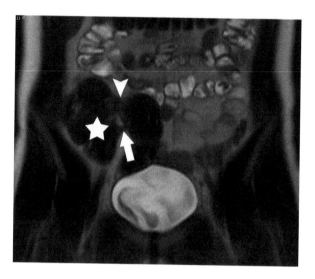

Fig. 5.32 Chronic Crohn's disease. MR enterography coronal T2-weighted image shows a short segment stricture of the distal ileum (arrowhead) with pre-stenotic dilatation and a fistula (long arrow) between the cecum (star) and the distal ileum

Solution

MR enterography, which avoids ionizing radiation, is preferable to CT for surveillance imaging in young patients. CT enterography and standard CT (if the patient cannot tolerate large amounts of oral contrast) would also be appropriate if MR enterography is not available.

5.11   Liver Lesion Characterization

A 75-year-old woman with 2.5 cm indeterminate liver lesion seen on US. She has no evidence of underlying liver disease or extrahepatic malignancy.

a. CT abdomen with contrast
b. MRI abdomen without and with contrast
c. FDG-PET/CT skull base to mid-thigh
d. Percutaneous biopsy
e. No ideal imaging exam

Indeterminate >1 cm lesion on US. No suspicion or evidence of extrahepatic malignancy or underlying liver disease.

a. CT abdomen with contrast is usually appropriate, but there is a better option here. Consider this if the lesion is not cystic on US and MRI is not available or contraindicated.
b. *MRI abdomen without and with contrast* is the most appropriate.
c. FDG-PET/CT skull base to mid-thigh is usually not appropriate. Exam is not indicated unless there is a known malignancy.
d. Percutaneous biopsy may be appropriate. Consider this procedure if imaging is inconclusive or suspicious for malignancy.

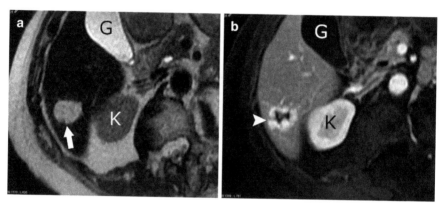

Fig. 5.33 Hemangioma. Abdomen MR axial T2-weighted (**a**) and post-contrast (**b**) images show a T2-hyperintense lesion (arrow) with peripheral nodular enhancement (arrowhead) in the liver. *G* gallbladder, *K* kidney

Solution
MRI without and with contrast is the best exam for the characterization of liver lesions. CT with contrast is a suitable alternative if MRI is contraindicated. For most scenarios, a CT with contrast is preferred to an MRI without contrast.

A 37-year-old woman with 4.5 cm indeterminate liver lesion seen on CT. She has no evidence of underlying liver disease or extrahepatic malignancy.

a. US abdomen
b. MRI abdomen without and with contrast
c. FDG-PET/CT skull base to mid-thigh
d. Percutaneous biopsy
e. No ideal imaging exam

Indeterminate >1 cm lesion on CT. No suspicion or evidence of extrahepatic malignancy or underlying liver disease.

a. US abdomen may be appropriate. Exam can distinguish between a cyst vs. solid lesion and guide percutaneous biopsy.
b. *MRI abdomen without and with contrast* is the most appropriate.
c. FDG-PET/CT skull base to mid-thigh is usually not appropriate. Exam is not indicated unless there is a known malignancy.
d. Percutaneous biopsy may be appropriate. Consider this procedure if imaging is inconclusive or suspicious for malignancy.

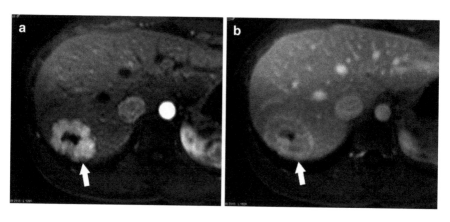

Fig. 5.34 Focal nodular hyperplasia. Abdomen MR axial post-contrast images of the liver in the arterial (**a**) and portal venous phase (**b**) of enhancement show a lesion (arrow) with intense early enhancement, rapid washout, and a central relatively hypo-vascular scar

Solution
MRI without and with contrast is the best exam for characterizing liver lesions.

A 70-year-old woman with a history of lung cancer now with 2.0 cm indeterminate liver lesion seen on US.

a. CT abdomen with contrast
b. MRI abdomen without and with contrast
c. FDG-PET/CT skull base to mid-thigh
d. Percutaneous biopsy
e. No ideal imaging exam

Indeterminate >1 cm lesion on US. Known history of an extrahepatic malignancy.

a. CT abdomen with contrast is usually appropriate, but there is a better option here. Consider this if MRI is contraindicated.
b. *MRI abdomen without and with contrast* is the most appropriate. Use this exam if US shows that the lesion is not a cyst.
c. FDG-PET/CT skull base to mid-thigh may be appropriate. Exam is indicated in the context of staging the primary malignancy.
d. Percutaneous biopsy may be appropriate. Consider this procedure if imaging is inconclusive or to histologically confirm metastasis.

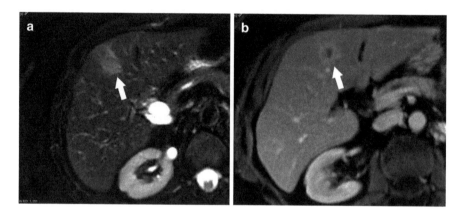

Fig. 5.35 Lung cancer metastasis. Abdomen MR axial T2-weighted (**a**) and post-contrast (**b**) images of the liver in a patient with lung cancer show a mildly T2-hyperintense enhancing lesion (arrow)

Solution
MRI abdomen without and with contrast can be used to characterize a liver lesion and identify additional lesions in the setting of metastatic disease. CT with contrast is a suitable alternative if MRI is contraindicated. Percutaneous image-guided liver biopsy may be used for histologic confirmation of disease.

A 58-year-old woman with a history of colon cancer now with 1.5 cm indeterminate liver lesion seen on CT.

a. US abdomen
b. MRI abdomen without and with contrast
c. FDG-PET/CT skull base to mid-thigh
d. Percutaneous biopsy
e. No ideal imaging exam

Indeterminate >1 cm lesion on CT. Known history of an extrahepatic malignancy.

a. US may be appropriate. Use if CT was performed without contrast and MRI is contraindicated.
b. *MRI abdomen without and with contrast* is the most appropriate.
c. FDG-PET/CT skull base to mid-thigh may be appropriate. Exam is indicated in the context of staging the primary malignancy.
d. Percutaneous biopsy may be appropriate. Consider this procedure if imaging is inconclusive or to histologically confirm metastasis.

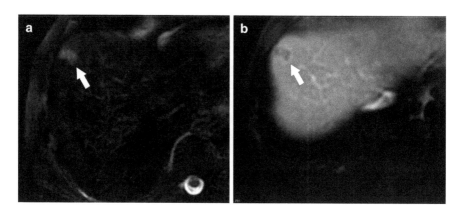

Fig. 5.36 Colon cancer metastasis. Abdomen MR axial T2-weighted (**a**) and post-contrast (**b**) images of the liver in a patient with colon cancer show a mildly T2-hyperintense enhancing lesion (arrow)

Solution
MRI abdomen without and with contrast can be used to characterize a liver lesion and identify additional lesions in the setting of metastatic disease. Percutaneous image-guided liver biopsy may be used for histologic confirmation of disease. FDG-PET/CT is used for whole-body staging.

A 51-year-old man with a history of chronic hepatitis now with 4.0 cm indeterminate liver lesion seen on US.

a. CT abdomen with contrast
b. MRI abdomen without and with contrast
c. FDG-PET/CT skull base to mid-thigh
d. Percutaneous biopsy
e. No ideal imaging exam

Indeterminate >1 cm lesion on US. Known or suspected liver disease associated with a high risk of hepatocellular carcinoma (chronic hepatitis, cirrhosis, hemochromatosis, etc.).

a. CT abdomen with contrast may be appropriate.
b. *MRI abdomen without and with contrast* is the most appropriate.
c. FDG-PET/CT skull base to mid-thigh is usually not appropriate. Exam is not useful for staging hepatocellular carcinoma.
d. Percutaneous biopsy may be appropriate. Consider this procedure if imaging is suspicious for malignancy.

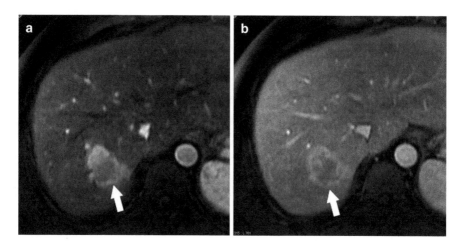

Fig. 5.37 Hepatocellular carcinoma. Abdomen MR axial post-contrast images of the liver in the arterial (**a**) and equilibrium phase (**b**) of enhancement in a patient with hepatitis C viral infection shows a lesion (arrow) with early enhancement (**a**), rapid washout (**b**), and a persistently enhancing pseudocapsule

Solution
MRI without and with contrast is the exam of choice for the characterization of liver lesions in patients with chronic liver disease. CT with contrast is a suitable alternative if MRI is contraindicated.

A 50-year-old man with a history of cirrhosis and prior therapy for hepatocellular carcinoma now with 4.5 cm indeterminate liver lesion seen on CT.

a. US abdomen
b. MRI abdomen without and with contrast
c. FDG-PET/CT skull base to mid-thigh
d. Percutaneous biopsy
e. No ideal imaging exam

Indeterminate >1 cm lesion on CT. Known or suspected liver disease associated with a high risk of hepatocellular carcinoma (chronic hepatitis, cirrhosis, hemochromatosis, etc.).

a. US may be appropriate. Exam can distinguish between a cyst vs. solid lesion and guide percutaneous biopsy.
b. *MRI abdomen without and with contrast* is the most appropriate. Use if CT is inconclusive and for follow-up of image-guided hepatocellular therapy (e.g., chemoembolization, ablation).
c. FDG-PET/CT skull base to mid-thigh is usually not appropriate.
d. Percutaneous biopsy may be appropriate.

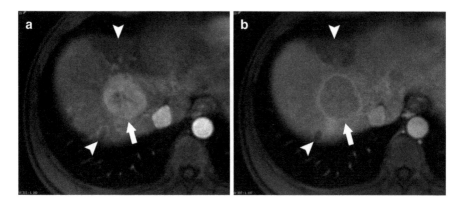

Fig. 5.38 Hepatocellular carcinoma recurrence. Abdomen MR axial post-contrast images of the liver in arterial (**a**) and equilibrium phase (**b**) of enhancement show a lesion (arrow) with early enhancement (**a**), rapid washout (**b**), and a persistently enhancing pseudocapsule. Lesions treated with transarterial chemoembolization (arrowheads) do not enhance

Solution
MRI abdomen without and with contrast may better characterize lesions seen with CT and is especially useful when there has been prior intervention (i.e., thermal ablation, chemoembolization).

5.12 Colorectal Cancer Screening

A 51-year-old woman presents for colorectal cancer screening. She is at average risk.

a. X-ray barium enema single contrast every 5 years after negative screen
b. X-ray barium enema double contrast every 5 years after negative screen
c. CT colonography every 5 years after negative screen
d. MR colonography every 5 years after negative screen
e. No ideal imaging exam

Average risk, age >50 years.

a. X-ray barium enema single contrast every 5 years after negative screen may be appropriate.
b. X-ray barium enema double contrast every 5 years after negative screen may be appropriate.
c. *CT colonography every 5 years after negative screen* is the most appropriate.
d. MR colonography every 5 years after negative screen may be appropriate.

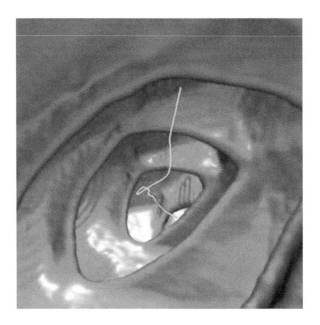

Fig. 5.39 Normal colon. CT colonography 3D "fly through" reconstruction image shows no polyps or masses. The line indicates the course of the lumen

Solution
CT colonography is the preferred imaging exam for colorectal cancer screening. If this is unavailable, then double-contrast barium enema is a suitable alternative. Single-contrast barium enema is inferior to double contrast for screening. MR colonography has lower spatial resolution than CT and has limited sensitivity from polyps <6 mm.

A 54-year-old man presents for colorectal cancer screening. He is at average risk, but fetal occult blood test is positive.

a. X-ray barium enema single contrast
b. X-ray barium enema double contrast
c. CT colonography
d. MR colonography
e. No ideal imaging exam

An average-risk individual after positive fecal occult blood test indicating a relative elevation in risk.

a. X-ray barium enema single contrast may be appropriate.
b. X-ray barium enema double contrast may be appropriate.
c. *CT colonography* is the most appropriate.
d. MR colonography may be appropriate.

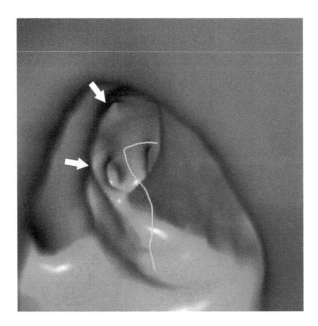

Fig. 5.40 Colonic diverticulitis. CT colonography 3D "fly through" reconstruction image shows diverticulitis (arrows) but no polyps or masses. The line indicates the course of the lumen

Solution
CT colonography is the preferred imaging exam for colorectal cancer screening. If this is unavailable, then double-contrast barium enema is a suitable alternative. Single-contrast barium enema is inferior to double contrast for screening. MR colonography has lower spatial resolution than CT and has limited sensitivity from polyps <6 mm.

A 60-year-old woman with incomplete screening colonoscopy.

a. X-ray barium enema single contrast
b. X-ray barium enema double contrast
c. CT colonography
d. MR colonography
e. No ideal imaging exam

Average, moderate, or high-risk individual after incomplete colonoscopy.

a. X-ray barium enema single contrast may be appropriate.
b. X-ray barium enema double contrast may be appropriate.
c. *CT colonography* is the most appropriate.
d. MR colonography is usually not appropriate.

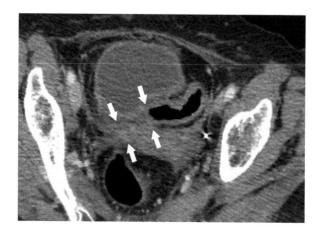

Fig. 5.41 Colonic stricture. CT colonography axial image shows luminal narrowing (arrows) in the sigmoid colon through which the colonoscope could not pass. Remainder of the colon was otherwise unremarkable

Solution

CT colonography is the preferred exam to follow an incomplete colonoscopy. Double-contrast barium enema is an appropriate alternative if CT colonography is unavailable.

A 54-year-old man presents for colon cancer screening. He is at moderate risk with a history of an adenomatous polyp.

a. X-ray barium enema single contrast every 5 years after negative screen
b. X-ray barium enema double contrast every 5 years after negative screen
c. CT colonography every 5 years after negative screen
d. MR colonography every 5 years after negative screen
e. No ideal imaging exam

A moderate-risk individual: personal history of adenoma or carcinoma or first-degree family history of cancer or adenoma.

a. X-ray barium enema single contrast every 5 years after negative screen may be appropriate.
b. X-ray barium enema double contrast every 5 years after negative screen may be appropriate.
c. *CT colonography every 5 years after negative screen* is the most appropriate.
d. MR colonography every 5 years after negative screen may be appropriate.

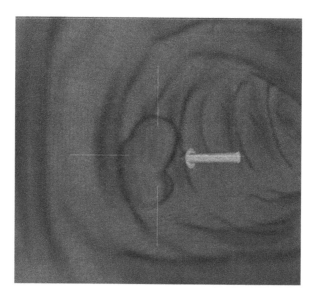

Fig. 5.42 Colonic adenoma. CT colonography 3D "fly through" reconstruction image shows a 2.1 cm polyp (arrow)

Solution
CT colonography is the preferred imaging technique for colorectal cancer screening in moderate-risk individuals. Recommended screening interval after a negative screening exam is 5 years.

A 30-year-old man presents for colon cancer screening. He is at high risk with hereditary nonpolyposis colorectal cancer syndrome.

a. X-ray barium enema single contrast
b. X-ray barium enema double contrast
c. CT colonography
d. MR colonography
e. No ideal imaging exam

A high-risk individual: hereditary nonpolyposis colorectal cancer.

a. X-ray barium enema single contrast is usually not appropriate.
b. X-ray barium enema double contrast is usually not appropriate.
c. CT colonography is usually not appropriate.
d. MR colonography is usually not appropriate.
e. *No ideal imaging exam* is the correct answer. Colonoscopy is recommended.

Solution

Imaging, including CT colonography and barium enema, is usually not appropriate for colorectal cancer screening in high-risk patients with hereditary nonpolyposis colorectal cancer and inflammatory bowel disease. Colonoscopy is the preferred exam in these cases.

A 43-year-old woman presents for colon cancer screening. She is at high risk with a diagnosis of ulcerative colitis.

a. X-ray barium enema single contrast
b. X-ray barium enema double contrast
c. CT colonography
d. MR colonography
e. No ideal imaging exam

A high-risk individual: ulcerative colitis or Crohn's colitis.

a. X-ray barium enema single contrast is usually not appropriate.
b. X-ray barium enema double contrast is usually not appropriate.
c. CT colonography is usually not appropriate.
d. MR colonography is usually not appropriate.
e. *No ideal imaging exam* is the correct answer. Colonoscopy is recommended.

Solution

Imaging, including CT colonoscopy and barium enema, is usually not appropriate for colorectal cancer screening in high-risk patients with colitis. Optical colonoscopy is the preferred test as it enables biopsies to look for dysplasia.

5.13   Colorectal Cancer Staging

A 55-year-old man with the diagnosis of rectal cancer presents for loco-regional staging. Clinical exam suggests advanced stage.

a. US pelvis transrectal
b. CT abdomen and pelvis with contrast
c. MRI pelvis without and with contrast
d. CT colonography
e. No ideal imaging exam

Rectal cancer. Locoregional staging.

a. US pelvis transrectal is usually appropriate, but there is a better choice here. Use for suspected early stage disease.
b. CT abdomen and pelvis with contrast may be appropriate. Use if MRI is contraindicated.
c. *MRI pelvis without and with contrast* is the most appropriate.
d. CT colonography is usually not appropriate.

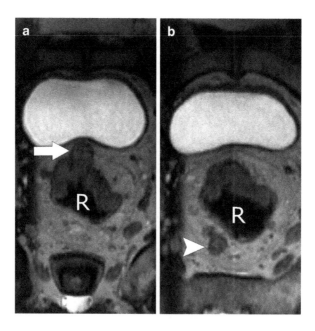

Fig. 5.43 Rectal cancer. Pelvic MR axial T2-weighted images show a mass involving the anterior and lateral walls of the rectum (R) extending into the mesorectal fascia (**a**, arrow) and lymphadenopathy (**b**, arrowhead)

Solution
Pelvic MRI and US are accurate and complementary modalities for local staging of colorectal cancer. Transrectal US may perform better for early stage tumors and MRI for more advanced. CT abdomen and pelvis with contrast may be performed when MRI is contraindicated.

A 71-year-old woman with the diagnosis of colon cancer presents for staging for distant metastases.

a. US abdomen
b. CT chest, abdomen, and pelvis with contrast
c. MRI abdomen and pelvis without and with contrast
d. FDG-PET/CT skull base to mid-thigh
e. No ideal imaging exam

Colorectal cancer. Staging for distant metastases.

a. US abdomen is usually not appropriate
b. *CT chest, abdomen, and pelvis with contrast* is the most appropriate.
c. MRI abdomen and pelvis without and with contrast is usually appropriate, but there is a better answer here. Usually performed with a chest CT.
d. FDG-PET/CT skull base to mid-thigh may be appropriate.

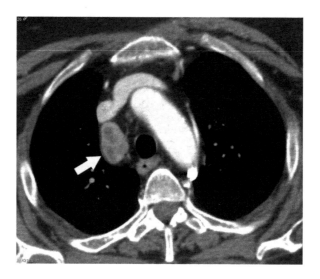

Fig. 5.44 Colon cancer metastasis. Chest CT with contrast in a patient with colon cancer shows mediastinal lymphadenopathy (arrow)

Solution

MRI without and with contrast (usually in combination with a CT chest) or CT chest, abdomen, and pelvis with contrast are options to assess for suspected colorectal cancer metastases. FDG-PET/CT is usually not indicated, though it may be useful for planning before treating suspected loco-regional disease.

Urologic Imaging

6

6.1   Renal Trauma

A 30-year-old man with blunt abdominal trauma and microscopic hematuria. Isolated renal trauma is suspected.

a. X-ray abdomen and pelvis
b. US kidneys and bladder
c. US abdomen for free fluid
d. CT abdomen and pelvis with contrast
e. No ideal imaging exam

G. X. Wang et al., *Choosing the Correct Radiologic Test*,
https://doi.org/10.1007/978-3-030-65185-5_6

Blunt abdominal trauma with microscopic hematuria; no suspicion of associated abdominal injury.

a. X-ray abdomen and pelvis may be appropriate.
b. US kidneys and bladder is usually not appropriate.
c. US abdomen for free fluid may be appropriate.
d. CT abdomen and pelvis with contrast may be appropriate.
e. *No ideal imaging exam* is the correct answer.

Solution

Microscopic hematuria alone is not sufficient to indicate significant renal injury in patients with blunt abdominal trauma. Imaging is more appropriate in patients experiencing gross hematuria, shock, signs associated with renal injury (e.g., flank ecchymoses, or fractures of the lower ribs or thoracolumbar spine), or penetrating trauma to the upper abdomen or lower thorax.

A 30-year-old man with blunt abdominal trauma and hematuria. Renal trauma associated with multisystem injury is suspected.

a. X-ray abdomen and pelvis
b. US kidneys and bladder
c. US abdomen for free fluid
d. CT abdomen and pelvis with contrast
e. No ideal imaging exam

Blunt abdominal trauma; suspicion of multisystem trauma with hematuria.

a. X-ray abdomen and pelvis is usually appropriate, but there is a better choice here. Exam detects fractures but not renal injury.
b. US kidneys and bladder is usually not appropriate.
c. US abdomen for free fluid may be appropriate.
d. *CT abdomen and pelvis* with contrast is the most appropriate. Exam detects renal trauma and associated injuries.

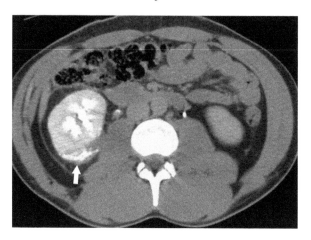

Fig. 6.1 Renal fracture with urine leak from blunt trauma. Abdomen CT with contrast in the delayed phase reveals leakage of excreted contrast into the perirenal space (arrow)

Solution
CT with multidetector technology is the gold standard for imaging hemodynamically stable patients with suspected blunt intra-abdominal injuries. CT is a rapid and accurate method for detecting and grading the extent of abdominal injuries.

A 30-year-old man with penetrating abdominal injury. Renal trauma is suspected.

a. X-ray abdomen and pelvis
b. US kidneys and bladder
c. US abdomen for free fluid
d. CT abdomen and pelvis with contrast
e. No ideal imaging exam

Penetrating abdominal injury; suspicion of multisystem trauma, with or without hematuria.

a. X-ray abdomen and pelvis may be appropriate. Use for question of retained foreign body.
b. US kidneys and bladder is usually not appropriate.
c. US abdomen for free fluid may be appropriate.
d. *CT abdomen and pelvis* with contrast is the most appropriate.

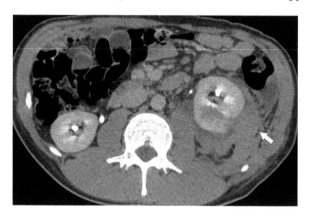

Fig. 6.2 Renal injury from penetrating trauma. Abdomen CT with contrast shows perinephric hematoma (arrow) and renal injury from a stab wound

Solution
CT with multidetector technology is the gold standard for imaging hemodynamically stable patients with suspected penetrating intra-abdominal injuries. CT is a rapid and accurate method for detecting and grading the extent of abdominal injuries.

6.2   Lower Urinary Tract Trauma

A 24-year-old man with penetrating trauma to the lower abdomen and pelvis. Bladder injury is suspected.

a. X-ray pelvis
b. X-ray retrograde urethrography
c. US pelvis transabdominal (bladder and urethra)
d. CT pelvis with bladder contrast (CT cystography)
e. No ideal imaging exam

Penetrating trauma, lower abdomen or pelvis.

a. X-ray pelvis may be appropriate. Use for question of retained foreign body.
b. X-ray retrograde urethrography may be appropriate. Use if urethral injury is suspected.
c. US pelvis transabdominal (bladder and urethra) is usually not appropriate.
d. *CT pelvis with bladder contrast (CT cystography)* is the most appropriate.

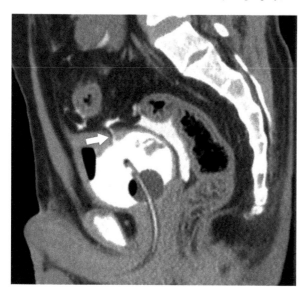

Fig. 6.3 Intraperitoneal bladder rupture. Pelvis CT cystogram sagittal reconstruction image shows a contrast-filled bladder containing a Foley balloon and extravasation of contrast through a defect in the bladder dome (arrow) into the intraperitoneal space

Solution
CT cystography is the preferred exam to assess for bladder rupture after penetrating trauma to the lower abdomen or pelvis. Rupture is identified by extravasation of contrast. X-ray retrograde urethrography should be performed when pelvic fracture is present and in cases of gross hematuria to exclude urethral injury before bladder catheterization.

A 34-year-old man with blunt trauma to the lower abdomen and pelvis. Bladder injury is suspected.

a. X-ray retrograde urethrography
b. US pelvis transabdominal (bladder and urethra)
c. CT pelvis with bladder contrast (CT cystography)
d. Angiography of pelvis
e. No ideal imaging exam

Blunt trauma, lower abdomen, or pelvis.

a. X-ray retrograde urethrography may be appropriate. Perform if pelvic fracture is present.
b. US pelvis transabdominal (bladder and urethra) is usually not appropriate.
c. *CT pelvis with bladder contrast (CT cystography)* is the most appropriate.
d. Angiography of pelvis is usually not appropriate. It can be used for persistent bleeding prior to embolotherapy.

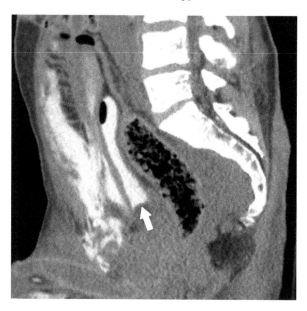

Fig. 6.4 Extraperitoneal bladder rupture. Pelvis CT cystogram sagittal reconstruction image shows a contrast-filled bladder (arrow) and extravasation of contrast into the pre-vesicular space

Solution
CT cystography is the preferred exam to assess for bladder rupture following a blunt trauma to the lower abdomen or pelvis. Rupture is identified by extravasation of contrast. X-ray retrograde urethrography should be performed when pelvic fracture is present and in cases of gross hematuria to exclude urethral injury before bladder catheterization.

A 19-year-old man with blunt trauma to the perineum. Urethral injury is suspected.

a. X-ray retrograde urethrography
b. US pelvis transabdominal (bladder and urethra)
c. CT pelvis with contrast
d. Angiography pelvis
e. No ideal imaging exam

Blunt perineal trauma in the male (straddle injury).

a. *X-ray retrograde urethrography* is the most appropriate.
b. US pelvis transabdominal (bladder and urethra) is usually not appropriate.
c. CT pelvis with contrast is usually appropriate, but there is a better choice here.
d. Angiography pelvis is usually not appropriate.

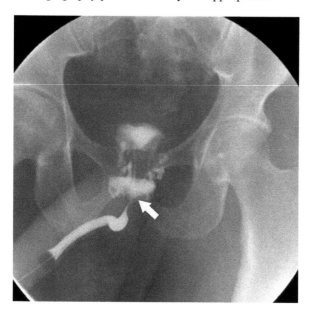

Fig. 6.5 Urethral tear. X-ray retrograde urethrography oblique anteroposterior view shows contrast extravasation (arrow) from a tear at the membranous urethra

Solution
X-ray retrograde urethrography is the best exam for suspected blunt perineal trauma in men presenting with a straddle injury and for suspected urethral injury from a penetrating trauma. CT pelvis with contrast may be appropriate to further assess for injury to the lower abdomen and pelvis.

6.3   Acute Onset Flank Pain or Suspected Urolithiasis

A 32-year-old man presents with acute onset of left flank pain suspicious for urolithiasis. He reports no such prior episodes.

a. X-ray abdomen and pelvis
b. X-ray intravenous urography
c. US kidneys and bladder with Doppler
d. CT abdomen and pelvis without contrast
e. No ideal imaging exam

Suspicion of stone disease.

a. X-ray abdomen and pelvis is usually not appropriate.
b. X-ray intravenous urography may be appropriate.
c. US kidneys and bladder with Doppler may be appropriate.
d. *CT abdomen and pelvis without contrast* is the most appropriate. This can be performed with reduced radiation dose techniques.

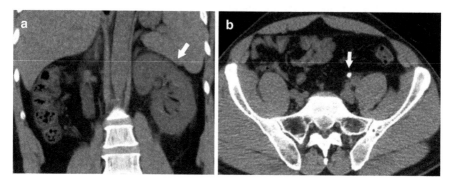

Fig. 6.6 Obstructive urolithiasis. Abdomen and pelvis CT without contrast coronal reconstruction image (**a**) shows moderate left hydronephrosis (arrow). An axial image through the mid pelvis (**b**) reveals a left ureteral stone (arrow)

Solution

CT abdomen and pelvis without contrast is the preferred imaging modality to assess for urolithiasis. Virtually all stones are radiopaque on CT, which can be used to measure stone size, plan treatment, and predict outcome.

A 32-year-old man presents with acute onset of left flank pain suspicious for uroli-thiasis. He reports previous episodes of symptomatic kidney stones.

a. X-ray abdomen and pelvis
b. X-ray intravenous urography
c. US kidneys and bladder with Doppler
d. MRI abdomen and pelvis
e. No ideal imaging exam

Symptoms of recurrent stone disease.

a. X-ray abdomen and pelvis may be appropriate. Perform with US if CT is not available.
b. X-ray intravenous urography is usually not appropriate.
c. *US kidneys and bladder with Doppler* is the most appropriate.
d. MRI abdomen and pelvis may be appropriate.

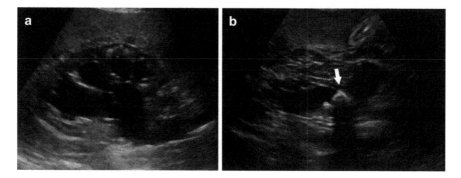

Fig. 6.7 Obstructive urolithiasis. Kidney US sagittal view of the right kidney (**a**) and ureter (**b**) shows hydronephrosis and obstructing stone (arrow) in the mid ureter

Solution

In patients presenting with symptoms of recurrent stone disease, US evaluates for hydronephrosis, which would indicate ureteral obstruction. If positive, CT is complementary to accurately measure the size of the stone and for treatment planning.

A 35-year-old pregnant woman presents with acute onset of left flank pain suspicious for urolithiasis.

a. X-ray abdomen and pelvis
b. X-ray intravenous urography
c. US kidneys and bladder with Doppler
d. CT abdomen and pelvis without contrast
e. No ideal imaging exam

Suspicion of stone disease.

a. X-ray abdomen and pelvis is usually not appropriate.
b. X-ray intravenous urography is usually not appropriate.
c. *US kidneys and bladder with Doppler* is the most appropriate.
d. CT abdomen and pelvis without contrast may be appropriate.

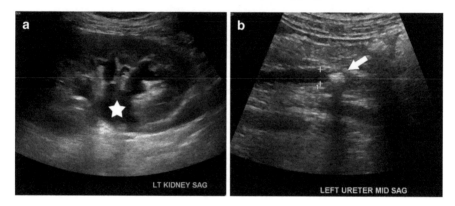

Fig. 6.8 Obstructive urolithiasis in pregnancy. Kidney US sagittal view of the left kidney (**a**) and ureter (**b**) in a woman at 34 weeks of pregnancy shows hydronephrosis (star) and an obstructive stone (arrow) in a dilated ureter (calipers)

Solution
US is the preferred imaging modality for diagnosing hydronephrosis in pregnant patients. It does not expose the patient or fetus to ionizing radiation and may also be able to visualize a stone.

6.4   Acute Pyelonephritis

A 22-year-old previously healthy woman with acute pyelonephritis.

a. X-ray intravenous urography
b. US kidneys and bladder
c. CT abdomen and pelvis with contrast
d. MRI abdomen and pelvis without and with contrast
e. No ideal imaging exam

Uncomplicated patient.

a. X-ray intravenous urography is usually not appropriate.
b. US kidneys and bladder is usually not appropriate.
c. CT abdomen and pelvis with contrast is usually not appropriate.
d. MRI abdomen and pelvis without and with contrast is usually not appropriate.
e. *No ideal imaging exam* is the correct answer.

Solution
Imaging is unnecessary in otherwise healthy patients with uncomplicated pyelone-phritis if they respond to antibiotic therapy within 72 h.

A 24-year-old diabetic woman with acute pyelonephritis. She re-presents with worsening symptoms while being treated.

a. X-ray intravenous urography
b. US kidneys and bladder
c. CT abdomen and pelvis with contrast
d. MRI abdomen and pelvis without and with contrast
e. No ideal imaging exam

Complicated patient (e.g., diabetes, immunocompromised, history of stones, prior renal surgery, or not responding to therapy).

a. X-ray intravenous urography is usually not appropriate.
b. US kidneys and bladder may be appropriate. X-ray abdomen and pelvis should be performed concurrently.
c. *CT abdomen and pelvis with contrast* is the most appropriate.
d. MRI abdomen and pelvis without and with contrast may be appropriate.

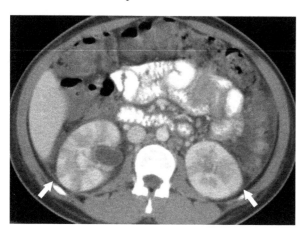

Fig. 6.9 Pyelonephritis. Abdomen and pelvis CT with contrast shows enlarged kidneys with striated nephrogram (arrows) consistent with pyelonephritis

Solution

CT abdomen and pelvis with contrast is the preferred exam for complicated patients (e.g., diabetes, immunocompromised, history of stones, prior renal surgery or not responding to therapy) presenting with pyelonephritis. MR of the abdomen and pelvis without and with contrast is an alternative in cases where CT with contrast is contraindicated.

6.5   Acute Onset Scrotal Pain

A 28-year-old male patient with acute onset left scrotal pain. He reports no history of scrotal trauma or mass.

a. US scrotum with Doppler
b. MRI pelvis scrotum without and with contrast
c. Tc-99m scintigraphy scrotum
d. Ga-67 or In-111 white blood cell scintigraphy scrotum
e. No ideal imaging exam

Patients without history of trauma or antecedent mass.

a. *US scrotum with Doppler* is the most appropriate. Exam shows high sensitivity and specificity.
b. MRI pelvis scrotum without and with contrast may be appropriate. Consider this if US indicates torsion is unlikely.
c. Tc-99m scintigraphy scrotum is usually not appropriate.
d. Ga-67 or In-111 white blood cell scan scrotum is usually not appropriate.

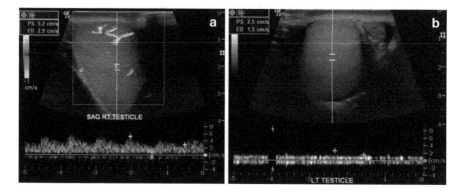

Fig. 6.10 Left testicular torsion. Scrotal US with Doppler demonstrates pulsatile arterial waveforms in the right (**a**) but not in the left (**b**) testicle

Solution

In patients presenting with scrotal pain, US scrotum with Doppler can diagnose testicular torsion with a high degree of sensitivity and can detect other causes of scrotal pain and swelling such as orchitis.

6.6   Hematuria

A 32-year-old woman presents with hematuria after completing a marathon earlier in the day.

a. X-ray abdomen and pelvis
b. US kidneys and bladder
c. CT abdomen and pelvis without and with contrast (CT urography)
d. MRI abdomen and pelvis without and with contrast (MR urography)
e. No ideal imaging exam

Patients following vigorous exercise, presence of infection, or recent menstruation.

a. X-ray abdomen and pelvis is usually not appropriate.
b. US kidneys and bladder is usually not appropriate.
c. CT abdomen and pelvis without and with contrast (CT urography) is usually not appropriate.
d. MRI abdomen and pelvis without and with contrast (MR urography) is usually not appropriate.
e. *No ideal imaging exam* is the correct answer.

Solution

In cases where a patient presents with hematuria following vigorous exercise, infection, or menstruation, an imaging assessment is unlikely to be beneficial. However, chronic hematuria requires further workup, which should include imaging.

A 22-year-old man with a history of glomerulonephropathy, now with hematuria.

a. X-ray abdomen and pelvis
b. US kidneys and bladder
c. CT abdomen and pelvis without and with contrast (CT urography)
d. MRI abdomen and pelvis without and with contrast (MR urography)
e. No ideal imaging exam

Patients with parenchymal renal disease.

a. X-ray abdomen and pelvis is usually not appropriate.
b. *US kidneys and bladder* is the most appropriate.
c. CT abdomen and pelvis without and with contrast (CT urography) is usually not appropriate.
d. MRI abdomen and pelvis without and with contrast (MR urography) is usually not appropriate.

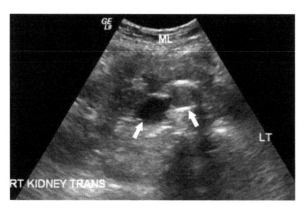

Fig. 6.11 Horseshoe kidney. Kidney US transverse image of the midline abdomen shows a fused right and left kidney (ML) anterior to the aorta and inferior vena cava (arrows)

Solution
US is the preferred exam for patients with hematuria suspected to be caused by renal parenchymal disease. In this setting, US can help assess for abnormalities in renal morphology.

A 50-year-old presents with new onset hematuria. He is otherwise healthy, with no history of renal disease or recent vigorous exercise.

a. X-ray abdomen and pelvis
b. US kidneys and bladder
c. CT abdomen and pelvis without and with contrast (CT urography)
d. MRI abdomen and pelvis without and with contrast (MR urography)
e. No ideal imaging exam

All patients except those with recent vigorous exercise, ongoing infection, menstruation, or generalized renal parenchymal disease.

a. X-ray abdomen is usually not appropriate.
b. US kidneys and bladder may be appropriate.
c. *CT abdomen and pelvis without and with contrast (CT urography)* is the most appropriate.
d. MRI abdomen and pelvis without and with contrast (MR urography) may be appropriate.

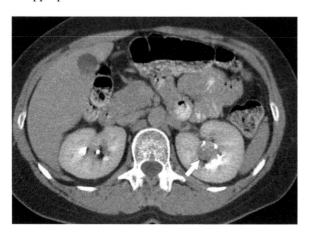

Fig. 6.12 Transitional cell carcinoma. Abdomen CT with contrast shows a soft tissue mass (arrow) in the left renal pelvis

Solution

For cases where hematuria cannot be attributed to recent infection, menstruation, vigorous exercise, or known disease of the renal parenchyma, CT abdomen and pelvis without and with contrast, performed as a CT urogram, is the preferred imaging modality. CT is more sensitive in detecting renal and urothelial masses compared to US or MRI.

6.7   Hematospermia

A 24-year-old man with transient, episodic hematospermia. He is otherwise healthy.

a. US prostate transrectal
b. CT pelvis with contrast
c. MRI pelvis without contrast
d. Angiography pelvis
e. No ideal imaging exam

A man <40 years of age, transient or episodic hematospermia, and no other symptoms or signs of disease.

a. US prostate transrectal is usually not appropriate.
b. CT pelvis with contrast is usually not appropriate.
c. MRI pelvis without contrast is usually not appropriate.
d. Angiography pelvis is usually not appropriate.
e. *No ideal imaging exam* is the correct answer.

Solution

In patients with hematospermia who are <40 years of age, imaging assessment is not generally indicated, as the symptom is usually not associated with a significant underlying disease. Imaging may be useful following a period of watchful waiting or in the presence of new symptoms.

A 42-year-old man with persistent hematospermia. He is symptomatic for urinary retention.

a. US prostate transrectal
b. CT pelvis with contrast
c. MRI pelvis without contrast
d. Angiography pelvis
e. No ideal imaging exam

Man 40 years of age or older, or man of any age with persistent hematospermia or hematospermia accompanied by symptoms or signs of disease.

a. *US prostate transrectal* is the most appropriate.
b. CT pelvis with contrast is usually not appropriate.
c. MRI pelvis without contrast is usually appropriate, but there is a better choice here. It evaluates for suspected prostate cancer or ejaculatory duct obstruction if transrectal US is inconclusive.
d. Angiography pelvis is usually not appropriate.

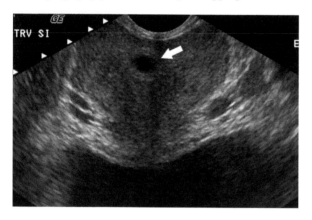

Fig. 6.13 Utricle cyst. Prostate US transverse view demonstrates a midline cyst (arrow) in the prostate

Solution

In patients ≥40 years of age and in patients with persistent or refractory hematospermia, transrectal US of the prostate assesses for abnormalities (e.g., cysts or calculi in the prostate, ejaculatory ducts, or seminal vesicles; benign prostatic hypertrophy; prostatitis; and Cowper gland masses). MRI pelvis without contrast may be appropriate if US is negative or inconclusive.

6.8   **Recurrent Lower Urinary Tract Infections in Women**

A 25-year-old woman presents with recurrent bladder infections. She is otherwise healthy.

a. X-ray intravenous urography
b. US kidneys and bladder
c. CT abdomen and pelvis without and with contrast
d. MRI pelvic without and with contrast
e. No ideal imaging exam

Uncomplicated with no underlying risk factors.

a. X-ray intravenous urography is usually not appropriate.
b. US kidneys and bladder is usually not appropriate.
c. CT abdomen and pelvis without and with contrast is usually not appropriate.
d. MRI pelvis without and with contrast is usually not appropriate. May be indicated if urinary diverticulum is suspected.
e. *No ideal imaging exam* is the correct answer.

Solution

Recurrent uncomplicated urinary tract infections do not routinely require cystoscopy or imaging, as most women with this complaint have normal urinary tracts.

A 50-year-old woman presents with recurrent bladder infections that has been increasing in frequency and is unresponsive to conventional therapy.

a. X-ray intravenous urography
b. US kidneys and bladder
c. CT abdomen and pelvis without and with contrast
d. MRI pelvic without and with contrast
e. No ideal imaging exam

Patients who do not respond to conventional therapy, get frequent re-infections, or have known underlying risk factors.

a. X-ray intravenous urography is usually not appropriate.
b. US kidneys and bladder is usually not appropriate.
c. *CT abdomen and pelvis without and with contrast* is the most appropriate. CT urography protocol is preferred.
d. MRI pelvic without and with contrast may be appropriate. Consider this for suspected urethral diverticulum or pelvic organ prolapse.

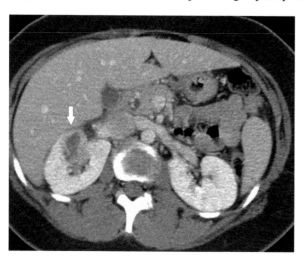

Fig. 6.14 Renal abscess. Abdomen CT with contrast shows an abscess (arrow) in the right kidney

Solution

CT without and with contrast is recommended for recurrent lower urinary tract infections, persistent infection despite adequate therapy, or known underlying risk factors for complications. CT urography is preferred and can assess disease extent and identify complications (e.g., renal abscess) or congenital anomalies of the urinary tract.

6.9 Benign Prostatic Hyperplasia

A 60-year-old man with prostatic hypertrophy with symptoms of bladder outlet obstruction.

a. X-ray intravenous urography
b. US kidneys
c. US pelvis (bladder and prostate)
d. MRI pelvis without contrast
e. No ideal imaging exam

Lower urinary tract symptoms.

a. X-ray intravenous urography is usually not appropriate. Exam has largely been replaced by CT urography.
b. US kidneys may be appropriate. Exam can evaluate for hydronephrosis.
c. US pelvis (bladder and prostate) may be appropriate. Exam measures bladder residual and estimates prostate size and bladder wall thickness.
d. MRI pelvis without contrast is usually not appropriate. Exam assesses prostate size, bladder wall thickness, and hydronephrosis.
e. *No ideal imaging exam* is the correct answer.

Solution
Imaging is not necessary for patients with lower symptoms of bladder outlet obstruction but who have normal renal function.

6.10   Renal Failure

A 43-year-old woman with acute kidney injury.

a. US kidneys and bladder
b. CT abdomen without contrast
c. MRA abdomen without contrast
d. Tc-99m MAG3 scan kidneys
e. No ideal imaging exam

Acute renal failure, unspecified.

a. *US kidneys and bladder* is the most appropriate. Excludes bilateral obstruction in high-risk groups.
b. CT abdomen without contrast is usually not appropriate. Exam may be helpful in detecting calculi or to search for retroperitoneal mass as the cause of the obstruction.
c. MRA abdomen without contrast is usually not appropriate. Exam evaluates for vascular stenosis or thrombosis.
d. Tc-99m MAG3 scan kidneys may be appropriate. Useful if creatinine level is high.

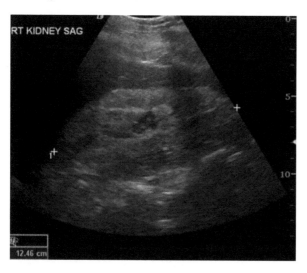

Fig. 6.15 Acute tubular necrosis. Kidney US shows a normal-sized right kidney (calipers) with an echogenic cortex consistent with acute medical renal disease. The left kidney looked similar

Solution
In cases of acute renal failure, US kidneys and bladder can assess renal size and parenchyma as well as evaluate for bilateral obstruction.

A 75-year-old man with chronic renal failure.

a. US kidneys and bladder
b. CT abdomen without contrast
c. MRA abdomen without contrast
d. Tc-99m MAG3 scan kidneys
e. No ideal imaging exam

Chronic renal failure.

a. *US kidneys and bladder* is the most appropriate. Doppler may be useful in assessing for renal artery stenosis.
b. CT abdomen without contrast may be appropriate. Exam may be helpful in detecting calculi or to search for retroperitoneal mass as the cause of the obstruction.
c. MRA abdomen may be appropriate. Exam can be used to evaluate for renal artery stenosis.
d. Tc-99m MAG3 scan kidneys is usually not appropriate. It assesses global and differential renal function and prognosis for recovery.

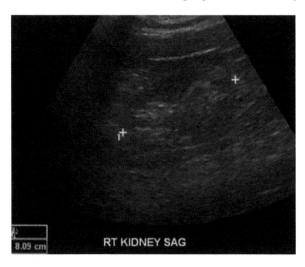

Fig. 6.16 Renal atrophy. Kidney US demonstrates small right kidney (calipers) with an echogenic cortex consistent with chronic medical renal disease. The left kidney looked similar

Solution
US kidneys and bladder is the preferred exam to assess the extent of chronic renal disease. Doppler may be useful for renal artery stenosis evaluation.

6.11   Renal Transplant Dysfunction

A 59-year-old man with a renal transplant and rising serum creatinine.

a. US kidney with Doppler
b. CTA abdomen and pelvis
c. MRA abdomen and pelvis without and with contrast
d. Tc-99m MAG3 scan kidney
e. No ideal imaging exam

Renal transplant dysfunction.

a. *US kidney with Doppler* is the most appropriate.
b. CTA abdomen and pelvis may be appropriate.
c. MRA abdomen without and with contrast may be appropriate.
d. Tc-99m MAG3 scan kidney is usually appropriate, but there is a better choice here. It is complementary to US kidney with Doppler.

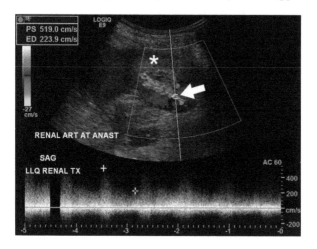

Fig. 6.17 Renal artery stenosis in a transplanted kidney. Kidney US with Doppler demonstrates the transplanted kidney (star) and elevated peak systolic velocity at the renal artery anastomosis (arrow)

Solution

US kidney with Doppler is the most appropriate first-line imaging exam to look for causes of renal transplant dysfunction (e.g., renal artery stenosis, hydronephrosis). Tc-99m MAG3 scan kidney is complementary to US kidney to assess the three sequential phases of renal function.

6.12   Renovascular Hypertension

A 52-year-old man with hypertension suspected of renovascular origin. His renal function is normal.

a. US kidneys with Doppler
b. CTA abdomen
c. Angiotensin-converting enzyme inhibitor renal scan
d. Angiography kidneys
e. No ideal imaging exam

High index of suspicion for renovascular hypertension and normal renal function.

a. US kidneys with Doppler may be appropriate. It is useful if there is a dedicated team skilled in the exam.
b. *CTA abdomen* is the most appropriate.
c. Angiotensin-converting enzyme inhibitor renal scan may be appropriate. This exam has relatively high sensitivity and specificity in patients with normal renal function.
d. Angiography kidneys may be appropriate. It is the gold standard for diagnosing renal artery stenosis but is invasive. It is used to guide angioplasty or stent placement.

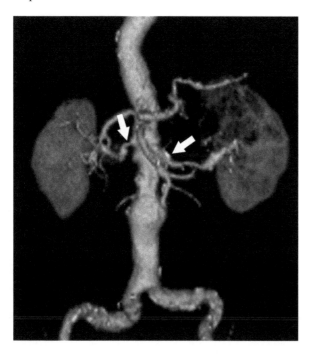

Fig. 6.18 Bilateral renal artery stenoses. Abdomen CTA 3D reconstruction image shows stenoses (arrows) at both renal artery origins

Solution
CTA abdomen should be performed for suspected renovascular disease. This exam is highly sensitive for renal artery stenosis, and normal results usually exclude this pathology.

A 51-year-old man with hypertension suspected of renovascular origin. He has decreased renal function, with eGFR <30 mL/min/1.73 m^2.

a. CTA abdomen
b. MRA abdomen without contrast
c. Angiotensin-converting enzyme inhibitor renal scan
d. Angiography kidneys
e. No ideal imaging exam

High index of suspicion of renovascular hypertension and diminished renal function.

a. CTA abdomen may be appropriate.
b. *MRA abdomen without contrast* is the most appropriate. Useful in older patients with atherosclerotic vascular disease with diminished renal function as they are the most likely to have proximal renal artery stenosis.
c. Angiotensin-converting enzyme inhibitor renal scan is usually not appropriate.
d. Angiography kidneys is usually not appropriate.

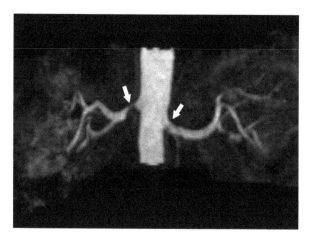

Fig. 6.19 Bilateral renal artery stenoses. Abdomen MRA without contrast MIP image shows narrowing (arrows) at the origins of the renal arteries bilaterally

Solution
MRA abdomen without contrast enables assessment of the renal arteries.

A 50-year-old man with hypertension. Renovascular etiology is considered unlikely.

a. US kidneys with Doppler
b. CTA abdomen
c. MRA abdomen without and with contrast
d. Angiotensin-converting enzyme inhibitor renal scan
e. No ideal imaging exam

Low index of suspicion of renovascular hypertension (i.e., likely "essential" hypertension).

a. US kidneys with Doppler is usually not appropriate.
b. CTA abdomen is usually not appropriate.
c. MRA abdomen without and with contrast is usually not appropriate.
d. Angiotensin-converting enzyme inhibitor renal scan is usually not appropriate.
e. *No ideal imaging exam* is the correct answer.

Solution

Imaging is not indicated in patients with low index of suspicion for renovascular hypertension.

6.13   **Incidentally Discovered Adrenal Mass**

A 62-year-old man with a 2 cm left adrenal mass incidentally detected on spine MRI. He has no history of malignancy.

a. CT abdomen without and with contrast
b. MIBG scan
c. FDG-PET whole body
d. Biopsy adrenal gland
e. No ideal imaging exam

No history of malignancy; mass 1–4 cm in diameter, initial evaluation.

a. *CT abdomen without and with contrast* is the most appropriate. Delayed imaging post contrast is obtained to calculate washout.
b. MIBG scan is usually not appropriate. Use only when pheochromocytoma is suspected.
c. FDG-PET whole body is usually not appropriate.
d. Biopsy adrenal gland is usually not appropriate.

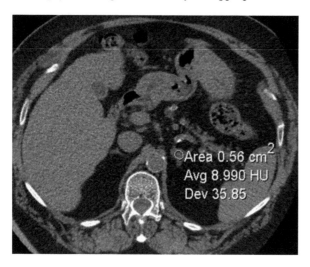

Fig. 6.20 Adrenal adenoma. Abdomen CT without contrast shows a 2 cm mass in the left adrenal gland with density (circle) of <10 Hounsfield units

Solution
CT abdomen without and with contrast is the most appropriate imaging to characterize an incidentally detected adrenal mass. In particular, delayed enhanced CT and use of washout percentages are better able to distinguish adenomas from metastases than unenhanced CT alone.

A 29-year-old man with 3.5 cm left incidentally detected adrenal mass thought to be benign on evaluation a year ago. He has no history of malignancy and now presents for follow-up.

a. CT abdomen without contrast
b. CT abdomen without and with contrast
c. MRI abdomen without and with contrast
d. FDG-PET whole body
e. No ideal imaging exam

No history of malignancy; mass 1–4 cm in diameter, follow-up evaluation after 12 months.

a. *CT abdomen without contrast* is the most appropriate.
b. CT abdomen without and with contrast is usually not appropriate. Contrast is unnecessary to assess for interval changes in size.
c. MRI abdomen without and with contrast is usually not appropriate.
d. FDG-PET whole body is usually not appropriate.

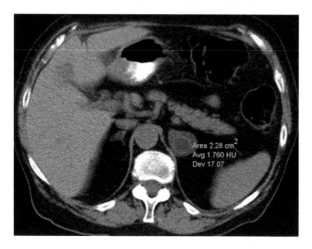

Fig. 6.21 Adrenal adenoma. Abdomen CT without contrast shows a 3.5 cm mass in the left adrenal gland which demonstrates 1-year stability and a density of <10 Hounsfield units (circle)

Solution

CT abdomen without contrast is the most appropriate exam to follow-up an incidentally detected adrenal mass. Contrast is unnecessary as the exam is used to assess for changes in lesion size.

A 60-year-old man with 5 cm left adrenal mass incidentally detected on spine MRI. He has no history of malignancy.

a. CT abdomen with contrast
b. CT abdomen without and with contrast
c. FDG-PET/CT skull base to mid-thigh
d. Biopsy adrenal gland
e. No ideal imaging exam

No history of malignancy; mass >4 cm in diameter.

a. *CT abdomen with contrast* is the most appropriate.
b. CT abdomen without and with contrast is usually not appropriate. Exam is used to characterize 1–4 cm adrenal nodules.
c. FDG-PET/CT skull base to mid-thigh may be appropriate.
d. Biopsy adrenal gland is usually not appropriate.

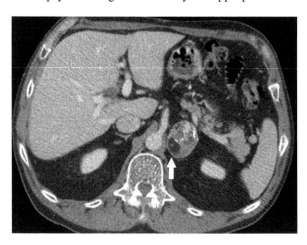

Fig. 6.22 Adrenal myelolipoma. Abdomen CT with contrast shows a 5 cm left adrenal mass containing fat (arrow)

Solution

Adrenal masses >4 cm are more likely to be malignant (e.g., primary adrenal cortical carcinoma or metastasis) than smaller ones. CT abdomen with contrast helps characterize the mass and serves as a part of preoperative staging. If mass is not typical for adenoma, myelolipoma, hemorrhage, or simple cyst, then resection should be considered.

A 50-year-old man with a 2.5 cm left adrenal mass detected on an abdomen CT. He has been diagnosed with lung cancer.

a. MRI abdomen without contrast
b. MRI abdomen without and with contrast
c. MIBG scan
d. Biopsy adrenal gland
e. No ideal imaging exam

History of malignancy; mass <4 cm in diameter, initial evaluation.

a. *MRI abdomen without contrast* is the most appropriate. CT without and with contrast is an alternative.
b. MRI abdomen without and with contrast is usually not appropriate.
c. MIBG scan is usually not appropriate. Use only when pheochromocytoma is suspected.
d. Biopsy adrenal gland may be appropriate. It should only be performed on a mass with characteristics suspicious for metastasis that cannot be characterized as benign on imaging.

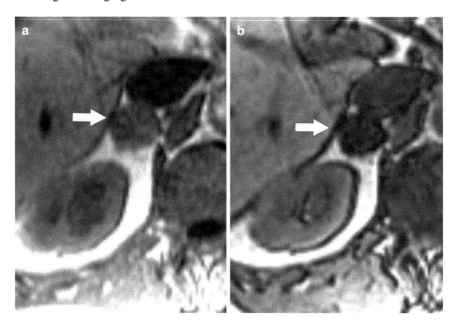

Fig. 6.23 Adrenal adenoma. Abdomen MR T1-weighted axial images show a 2.5 cm adrenal mass (arrows) that drops in signal from in-phase (**a**) to out-of-phase (**b**), indicating high lipid content within the nodule

Solution
Adrenal masses <4 cm are likely benign even in patients with a primary malignancy. MRI abdomen without contrast can help determine whether the incidentally detected adrenal mass is benign. This exam uses chemical-shift (in- and out-of-phase) imaging to characterize the mass's lipid content, with high lipid content being a benign feature.

A 54-year-old man with a 5 cm left adrenal mass detected on a chest CT. He has been treated for lung cancer.

a. CT abdomen without contrast
b. MRI abdomen without contrast
c. MIBG scan
d. Biopsy adrenal gland
e. No ideal imaging exam

History of malignancy; mass >4 cm in diameter.

a. CT abdomen without contrast is usually not appropriate.
b. MRI abdomen without contrast is usually not appropriate.
c. MIBG scan is usually not appropriate. Use only when pheochromocytoma is suspected.
d. *Biopsy adrenal gland* is the most appropriate.

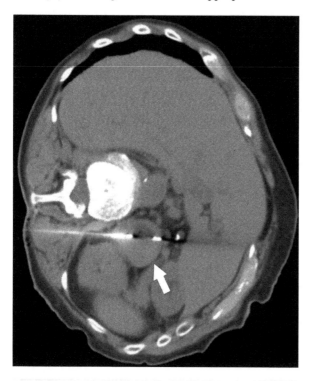

Fig. 6.24 Adrenal nodule biopsy. Adrenal gland biopsy under CT guidance shows a core biopsy needle in the left adrenal mass (arrow)

Solution

Adrenal masses measuring >4 cm are more likely to be malignant compared to smaller ones. In a patient with a history of a primary malignancy, a biopsy is most appropriate to evaluate for metastasis.

6.14   Indeterminate Renal Mass

A 46-year-old man with an indeterminate renal mass incidentally detected on abdominal CT.

a. US kidneys with Doppler
b. CT abdomen without and with contrast
c. MRI abdomen without and with contrast
d. Biopsy kidney
e. No ideal imaging exam

Patient with indeterminate renal mass and normal renal function.

a. US kidneys with Doppler is usually appropriate, but there is a better choice here.
b. *CT abdomen without and with contrast* is the most appropriate.
c. MRI abdomen without and with contrast is usually appropriate, but there is a better choice here.
d. Biopsy kidney may be appropriate.

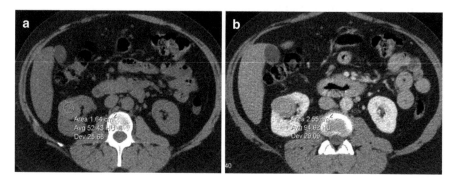

Fig. 6.25 Renal cell carcinoma. Abdomen CT without (**a**) and with (**b**) contrast shows a 3.5 cm right renal mass that increases by ≥20 Hounsfield units in attenuation (circle) with contrast, which indicates enhancement

Solution
CT abdomen without and with contrast can characterize both solid and cystic lesions presenting as an indeterminate renal mass. MRI without and with contrast can substitute for CT. US may also be useful in the characterization of simple cysts, though complex masses will require further evaluation with CT or MRI.

A 38-year-old woman with severe renal insufficiency presents for characterization of an indeterminate renal mass incidentally found on US.

a. CT abdomen without contrast
b. MRI abdomen without contrast
c. Biopsy kidney
d. Angiography kidney
e. No ideal imaging exam

A patient with severe renal insufficiency with contraindication to intravenous contrast.

a. CT abdomen without contrast may be appropriate. It may be useful to detect fat in an angiomyolipoma or to evaluate attenuation value of a cyst.
b. *MRI abdomen without contrast* is the most appropriate.
c. Biopsy kidney may be appropriate.
d. Angiography kidney is usually not appropriate.

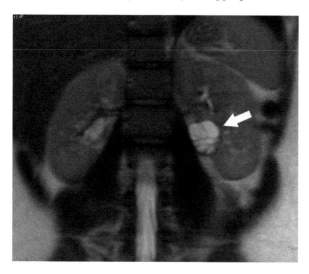

Fig. 6.26 Clear cell renal cell carcinoma. Abdomen MR T2-weighted coronal image shows a complex multi-septated cystic lesion (arrow) in the left kidney

Solution

MRI abdomen without contrast is the most appropriate imaging modality for characterizing renal masses in patients who have contraindications to both iodinated and gadolinium-based contrast. The exam differentiates solid from cystic tissue and fat from other types of soft tissue.

6.15 Prostate Cancer Detection, Staging, and Surveillance

6.15.1 American Joint Committee on Cancer (AJCC) Prostate Cancer Staging

Stage	Sub-stage	Definition
Primary tumor (T)		
TX		Primary tumor cannot be assessed
T0		No evidence of primary tumor
T1		Clinically inapparent tumor, neither palpable nor visible by imaging
	T1a	Incidental histologic finding; ≤5% of tissue resected during TURP
	T1b	Incidental histologic finding; >5% of tissue resected during TURP
	T1c	Tumor identified by needle biopsy (e.g., because of elevated PSA)
T2		Tumor confined within the prostate[a]
	T2a	Tumor involves half of one lobe or less
	T2b	Tumor involves more than half of one lobe but not both lobes
	T2c	Tumor involves both lobes
T3		Tumor extends through the prostate capsule[b]
	T3a	Extracapsular extension (unilateral or bilateral)
	T3b	Tumor invades seminal vesicle(s)
T4		Tumor is fixed or invades adjacent structures other than seminal vesicles: bladder, external sphincter, rectum, levator muscles, and/or pelvic wall
Regional lymph nodes (N)		
N0		No lymph node metastasis
N1		Metastasis in regional lymph node(s)
Distant metastasis (M)		
M0		No distant metastasis
M1		Distant metastasis
	M1a	Nonregional lymph node metastasis
	M1b	Bone metastasis
	M1c	Metastasis at other sites with or without bone disease

[a]Tumor found in one or both lobes by needle biopsy, but not palpable or reliably visible by imaging, is classified as T1c

[b]Invasion into the prostatic apex or into (but not beyond) the prostatic capsule is classified not as T3 but as T2

Edge et al. 2010

6.15.2 Prostate Cancer Risk Stratification

Low risk: 10-year PSA failure-free survival rate of ~80%

- AJCC clinical stage T1c or T2a *and*
- PSA ≤10 ng/ml *and*
- Biopsy Gleason score ≤6

Intermediate risk: 10-year PSA failure-free survival rate of ~50%

- AJCC clinical stage T2b *or*
- PSA >10 and ≤20 ng/ml *or*
- Biopsy Gleason score 7

High risk: 10-year PSA failure-free survival rate of ~33%

- AJCC clinical stage T2c disease *or*
- PSA >20 ng/ml *or*
- Gleason score ≥8

D'Amico et al. 2002

A 66-year-old man diagnosed with prostate cancer is categorized as low risk for locally advanced disease and metastases.

a. CT abdomen and pelvis with contrast
b. MRI pelvis without and with contrast
c. Tc-99m bone scan whole body
d. FDG-PET/CT whole body
e. No ideal imaging exam

Prostate cancer diagnosed on biopsy, patient at low risk for locally advanced disease and metastases.

a. CT abdomen and pelvis with contrast is usually not appropriate.
b. MRI pelvis without and with contrast may be appropriate. It could be used for active surveillance of the prostate.
c. Tc-99m bone scan whole body is usually not appropriate.
d. FDG-PET/CT whole body is usually not appropriate.
e. *No ideal imaging exam* is the best choice here.

Solution
For prostate cancer patients with low risk for locally advanced disease or metastases, imaging is unlikely to provide additional information to guide treatment. There may be a role for MRI if the management choice is active surveillance.

A 69-year-old man diagnosed with prostate cancer is categorized as intermediate risk for locally advanced disease and metastases.

a. CT abdomen and pelvis with contrast
b. MRI pelvis without and with contrast
c. Tc-99m bone scan whole body
d. FDG-PET/CT whole body
e. No ideal imaging exam

Prostate cancer diagnosed on biopsy, patient at intermediate risk for locally advanced disease and metastases.

a. CT abdomen and pelvis with contrast may be appropriate.
b. *MRI pelvis without and with contrast* is the most appropriate.
c. Tc-99m bone scan whole body may be appropriate.
d. FDG-PET/CT whole body is usually not appropriate.

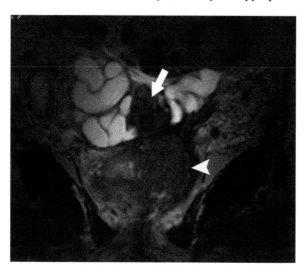

Fig. 6.27 Locally invasive prostate cancer. Pelvis MR T2-weighted coronal oblique image shows a soft tissue mass within the left prostate (arrowhead) that invades the seminal vesicles (arrow)

Solution
MRI pelvis without and with contrast is the most appropriate imaging modality for assessing the extent of disease in prostate cancer patients with intermediate risk of locally advanced disease and metastases. It detects extra-glandular tumor growth and evaluates for pelvic lymphadenopathy.

A 62-year-old man diagnosed with prostate cancer is categorized as high risk for locally advanced disease and metastases.

a. CT abdomen and pelvis with contrast
b. MRI pelvis without and with contrast
c. Tc-99m bone scan whole body
d. FDG-PET/CT whole body
e. No ideal imaging exam

Prostate cancer, high risk for locally advanced disease and metastases.

a. CT abdomen and pelvis with contrast is usually appropriate, but there is a better choice here.
b. *MRI pelvis without and with contrast* and choice (c) are equally the most appropriate.
c. *Tc-99m bone scan whole body* and choice (b) are equally the most appropriate.
d. FDG-PET/CT whole body may be appropriate.

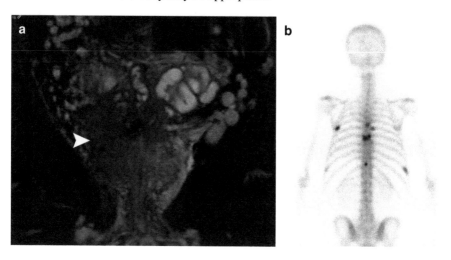

Fig. 6.28 Metastatic prostate cancer. (**a**) Prostate MR T2-weighted coronal oblique image shows a soft tissue mass in the right prostate (arrowhead) that invades the seminal vesicles. (**b**) Whole-body Tc-99m bone scan posterior view shows multiple foci of tracer uptake in the thoracic spine, left scapula, and bilateral ribs

Solution
In prostate cancer patients at high risk for locally advanced disease and metastases, MRI pelvis without and with contrast evaluates for extra-glandular tumor growth and pelvic lymphadenopathy, and Tc-99m bone scan whole body evaluates for skeletal metastases.

A 74-year-old man with rising serum PSA concerning for prostate cancer, but with multiple negative prostate biopsies.

a. CT abdomen and pelvis with contrast
b. MRI pelvis without and with contrast
c. Tc-99m bone scan whole body
d. FDG-PET/CT whole body
e. No ideal imaging exam

Multiple negative prostate biopsies, but there is concern for prostate cancer based upon rising or persistently elevated serum markers.

a. CT abdomen and pelvis with contrast is usually not appropriate.
b. *MRI pelvis without and with contrast* is the most appropriate.
c. Tc-99m bone scan whole body is usually not appropriate.
d. FDG-PET/CT whole body is usually not appropriate.

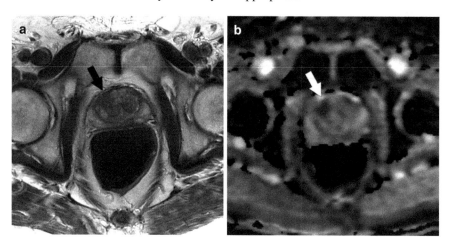

Fig. 6.29 Prostate cancer. Pelvis MR axial T2-weighted (**a**) and apparent diffusion coefficient (**b**) images show a T2-hypointense soft tissue mass in the right transition zone (arrows) demonstrating restricted diffusion restriction

Solution

MRI pelvis without and with contrast is the most sensitive imaging exam for detecting prostate cancer.

6.16   Renal Cell Carcinoma Staging

A 65-year-old man diagnosed with renal cell carcinoma for pretreatment staging evaluation.

a. X-ray chest
b. CT chest with contrast
c. CT abdomen without and with contrast
d. MRI abdomen without and with contrast

Renal cell carcinoma staging.

a. X-ray chest is usually appropriate, but there is a better choice here. It is complementary to abdominal CT.
b. CT chest with contrast may be appropriate.
c. *CT abdomen without and with contrast* is the most appropriate. It is complementary to chest X-ray.
d. MRI abdomen without and with contrast is usually appropriate, but there is a better choice here. It is an alternative to abdominal CT.

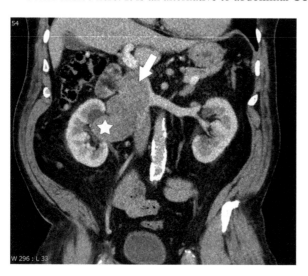

Fig. 6.30 Renal cell carcinoma with vascular invasion. Abdomen CT with contrast coronal reconstruction image shows an enhancing right renal mass (star) that extends into the inferior vena cava (arrow)

Solution

CT abdomen without and with contrast is the most appropriate imaging modality for staging renal cell carcinoma. MRI may be substituted for CT if iodinated contrast is contraindicated. Chest X-ray is complementary to evaluate for pulmonary metastases.

6.17   Invasive Bladder Cancer Staging

A 71-year-old man diagnosed with muscle-invasive bladder for pretreatment staging evaluation.

a. X-ray chest
b. CT chest with contrast
c. CT abdomen without and with contrast
d. MRI abdomen without and with contrast

Pretreatment staging of invasive bladder cancer.

a. *X-ray chest* is the most appropriate.
b. CT chest with contrast may be appropriate.
c. CT abdomen without and with contrast is usually appropriate, but there is a better choice here. Perform as a CT urogram to include an excretory phase for locoregional staging and upper-tract screening.
d. MRI abdomen without and with contrast is usually appropriate, but there is a better choice here.

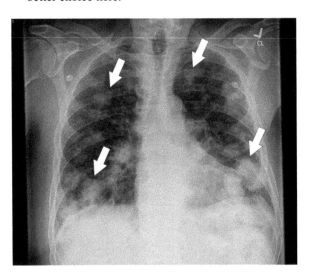

Fig. 6.31 Metastatic bladder cancer. Chest radiograph posteroanterior view shows multiple bilateral masses (arrows)

Solution
Staging for invasive bladder cancer should include a chest X-ray to assess for pulmonary metastases. Additional imaging modalities that may be appropriate for assessing locoregional disease include CT abdomen without and with contrast, performed as a CT urogram or MRI abdomen without and with contrast.

6.18   Testicular Cancer Staging

A 54-year-old man status post-orchiectomy with the diagnosis of testicular cancer.

a. X-ray chest
b. CT chest with contrast
c. CT abdomen and pelvis with contrast
d. MRI abdomen and pelvis without and with contrast

Staging testicular tumor diagnosed by orchiectomy.

a. X-ray chest is usually appropriate, but there is a better choice here.
b. CT chest with contrast is usually appropriate, but there is a better choice here. It is complementary to abdomen and pelvic CT.
c. *CT abdomen and pelvis with contrast* is the most appropriate.
d. MRI abdomen without and with contrast is usually appropriate, but there is a better choice here. It is an alternative to CT.

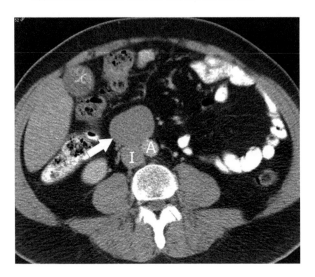

Fig. 6.32 Metastatic testicular cancer. Abdomen CT image shows an enlarged retroperitoneal lymph node (arrow) anterior to the aorta (A) and inferior vena cava (I)

Solution
CT abdomen and pelvis with contrast is the most appropriate imaging modality for assessing the extent of testicular cancer. Chest X-ray or a CT chest with contrast is complementary to evaluate for pulmonary metastases.

Bibliography

D'Amico AV, Cote K, Loffredo M, Renshaw AA, Schultz D. Determinants of prostate cancer-specific survival after radiation therapy for patients with clinically localized prostate cancer. J Clin Oncol. 2002;20(23):4567–73.

Edge SB, Byrd DR, Compton CC, Fritz AG, Greene FL, Trotti A, editors. AJCC cancer staging manual. 7th ed. New York, NY: Springer; 2010.

Women's Imaging

7

7.1   Abnormal Vaginal Bleeding

A 54-year-old postmenopausal woman with vaginal bleeding.

a. US pelvis transabdominal
b. US pelvis transvaginal
c. US sonohysterography
d. MRI pelvis without and with contrast
e. No ideal imaging exam

© The Author(s), under exclusive license to Springer Nature
Switzerland AG 2021
G. X. Wang et al., *Choosing the Correct Radiologic Test*,
https://doi.org/10.1007/978-3-030-65185-5_7

Postmenopausal vaginal bleeding. First study.

a. US pelvis transabdominal is usually appropriate, but there is a better choice here.
b. *US pelvis transvaginal* is the most appropriate.
c. US sonohysterography may be appropriate.
d. MRI pelvis without and with contrast is usually not appropriate.

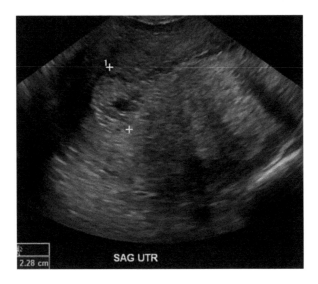

Fig. 7.1 Endometrial cancer. Transvaginal pelvis US sagittal view of the uterus reveals an abnormally thick endometrium (calipers)

Solution
Endometrial thickness of >5 mm on transvaginal US is highly sensitive for endometrial cancer. Transabdominal US can be used but yields less accurate measurements. If cancer has been excluded, sonohysterography is used to evaluate for a focal endometrial lesion, e.g., polyp or submucosal fibroid, or to visualize the endometrium not seen on conventional US.

A 58-year-old postmenopausal woman with vaginal bleeding. Transvaginal US shows endometrial thickness of ≤5 mm.

a. US pelvis transabdominal
b. US sonohysterography
c. CT pelvis with contrast
d. MRI pelvis without and with contrast
e. No ideal imaging exam

Postmenopausal vaginal bleeding, endometrium ≤5 mm by transvaginal US.

a. US pelvis transabdominal may be appropriate.
b. US sonohysterography is usually not appropriate.
c. CT pelvis with contrast is usually not appropriate.
d. MRI pelvis without and with contrast is usually not appropriate.
e. *No ideal imaging exam* is the correct answer.

Solution

Endometrial thickness ≤5 mm with transvaginal US indicates <1:100 chance of underlying for cancer in postmenopausal patients with bleeding. Imaging with transabdominal US may be helpful when there is poor visualization of the endometrium. Further workup, should bleeding persist, would involve nonfocal biopsy, not imaging.

A 52-year-old postmenopausal woman with vaginal bleeding. Transvaginal US shows endometrial thickness of >5 mm.

a. US pelvis transabdominal
b. US pelvis with Doppler
c. US sonohysterography
d. MRI pelvis without and with contrast
e. No ideal imaging exam

Postmenopausal vaginal bleeding, endometrium >5 mm by transvaginal US.

a. US pelvis transabdominal may be appropriate.
b. US pelvis with Doppler may be appropriate.
c. *US sonohysterography* is the most appropriate.
d. MRI pelvis without and with contrast may be appropriate. Appropriate when sonohysterography is not available.

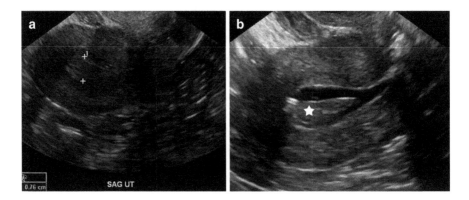

Fig. 7.2 Endometrial polyp. Transvaginal US (**a**) shows an abnormally thick endometrium (calipers). The concurrent sonohysterography (**b**) reveals an underlying endometrial polyp (star) originating from the fundal endometrium

Solution
Sonohysterography allows for better delineation of the endometrial lining compared to transvaginal US alone and enables improved differentiation of focal lesions such as polyps from diffuse abnormalities such as endometrial hyperplasia. This exam should be performed after cancer has been excluded with a nonfocal endometrial biopsy.

A 36-year-old premenopausal woman with abnormal vaginal bleeding.

a. US pelvis transabdominal
b. US pelvis transvaginal
c. US sonohysterography
d. MRI pelvis without and with contrast
e. No ideal imaging exam

Premenopausal vaginal bleeding. First study.

a. US pelvis transabdominal is usually appropriate, but there is a better choice here.
b. *US pelvis transvaginal* is the most appropriate. 3D imaging may be a useful adjunct.
c. US sonohysterography may be appropriate.
d. MRI pelvis without and with contrast is usually not appropriate.

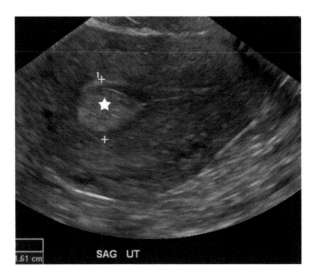

Fig. 7.3 Endometrial polyp. Transvaginal US sagittal view of the uterus shows endometrium which is of normal thickness (calipers) but contains a focal lesion (star) corresponding to a polyp

Solution
Transvaginal US should be used to evaluate abnormal vaginal bleeding. Endometrial thickness is not a reliable indicator of endometrial pathology in premenopausal women, but it is helpful in the detection of endometrial polyps or submucosal fibroids that could be a cause for bleeding.

A 34-year-old premenopausal woman with abnormal vaginal bleeding. Transvaginal US shows endometrial thickness <16 mm.

a. US pelvis transabdominal
b. US pelvis with Doppler
c. US sonohysterography
d. MRI pelvis without and with contrast
e. No ideal imaging exam

Premenopausal vaginal bleeding, endometrium <16 mm by transvaginal US.

a. US pelvis transabdominal may be appropriate.
b. US pelvis with Doppler may be appropriate.
c. US sonohysterography may be appropriate.
d. MRI pelvis without and with contrast is usually not appropriate.
e. *No ideal imaging exam* is the correct answer.

Solution
Endometrial thickness of <16 mm is within normal limits, and, hence, the cause for bleeding is unlikely to be malignancy. US sonohysterography may be appropriate following transvaginal US to assess focal abnormalities within the endometrial cavity to guide biopsy or resection. US pelvis Doppler may help in detection of a focal or diffuse endometrial abnormality.

A 47-year-old premenopausal woman with abnormal vaginal bleeding. Transvaginal US shows endometrial thickness ≥16 mm.

a. US pelvis with Doppler
b. US sonohysterography
c. CT pelvis with contrast
d. MRI pelvis without and with contrast
e. No ideal imaging exam

Premenopausal vaginal bleeding, endometrium ≥16 mm by transvaginal US.

a. US pelvis with Doppler may be appropriate. Time exam for the proliferative phase of the menstrual cycle.
b. *US sonohysterography* is the most appropriate.
c. CT pelvis with contrast is usually not appropriate.
d. MRI pelvis without and with contrast may be appropriate.

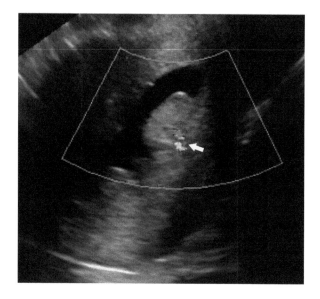

Fig. 7.4 Endometrial polyp. Sagittal view of the uterus on a sonohysterography with color Doppler reveals a polyp originating from the posterior endometrium with a characteristic feeding vessel (arrow)

Solution
Sonohysterography detects focal lesions of the uterine cavity (e.g., endometrial polyp, submucosal fibroid) with greater sensitivity than pelvic US or MRI and enables precise localization for resection planning.

7.2 First-Trimester Bleeding

A 28-year-old woman with vaginal bleeding, a positive serum pregnancy test and in the first trimester of pregnancy.

a. US pelvis transabdominal
b. US pelvis transvaginal
c. US pelvis Doppler
d. MRI pelvis without contrast
e. No ideal imaging exam

Positive urine or serum pregnancy test.

a. US pelvis transabdominal is usually appropriate, but there is a better choice here.
b. *US pelvis transvaginal* is the most appropriate. Include M-mode for fetal heart rate.
c. US pelvis Doppler may be appropriate. Avoid Doppler imaging of the embryo.
d. MRI pelvis is usually not appropriate. Useful when US is nondiagnostic or for the treatment planning of a known ectopic pregnancy.

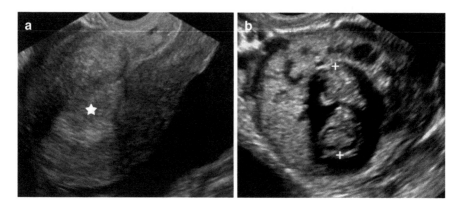

Fig. 7.5 Ectopic pregnancy. Transvaginal pelvis US sagittal view of the uterus (**a**) shows no gestational sac in the endometrial cavity (star). Coronal view of the left adnexa (**b**) reveals the gestational sac with a fetus (calipers)

Solution
Transvaginal US can differentiate an intrauterine from an ectopic pregnancy and confirm status of the fetus. M-mode imaging is used to document embryonic viability and measure heart rate. Transabdominal imaging can be used to assess for free intraperitoneal fluid or hematoma if rupture of an ectopic pregnancy is suspected.

7.3   Acute Pelvic Pain in the Reproductive Age Group

A 32-year-old woman with acute pelvic pain suspected of gynecologic origin. Serum β-hCG is positive.

a. X-ray abdomen
b. US pelvis transvaginal
c. CT pelvis with or without abdomen
d. MRI pelvis with or without abdomen
e. No ideal imaging exam

Gynecological etiology suspected, serum β-hCG positive.

a. X-ray abdomen is not rated for appropriateness.
b. *US pelvis transvaginal* is the most appropriate. Both transvaginal and transabdominal US should be performed if possible.
c. CT pelvis with or without abdomen is usually not appropriate.
d. MRI pelvis with or without abdomen may be appropriate. Perform without contrast. Use if US is inconclusive or nondiagnostic.

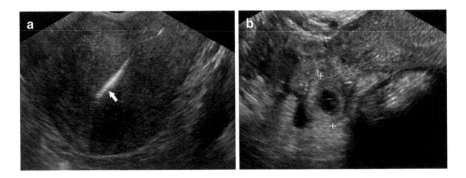

Fig. 7.6 Ectopic pregnancy. Transvaginal pelvis US at midline (**a**) shows no pregnancy and an intrauterine device (arrow) in the endometrial cavity. Image of the right adnexa (**b**) shows a gestational sac with a yolk sac (calipers)

Solution
Transvaginal US is the preferred imaging examination to differentiate an intrauterine from an ectopic pregnancy and confirm the status of the fetus. Transabdominal US is also recommended to provide a larger field of view.

A 32-year-old woman with acute pelvic pain suspected of gynecologic origin. Serum β-hCG is negative.

a. X-ray abdomen
b. US pelvis transvaginal
c. CT pelvis with or without abdomen
d. MRI pelvis with or without abdomen
e. No ideal imaging exam

Gynecological etiology suspected, serum β-hCG negative.

a. X-ray abdomen is not rated for appropriateness.
b. *US pelvis transvaginal* is the most appropriate. Both transvaginal and transabdominal US should be performed if possible.
c. CT pelvis with or without abdomen may be appropriate. Perform with contrast. Use if US is inconclusive or nondiagnostic and MRI is not available. In young women undergoing repeat imaging, cumulative radiation dose should be considered.
d. MRI pelvis with or without abdomen may be appropriate. Perform without and with contrast. Use if US is inconclusive or nondiagnostic.

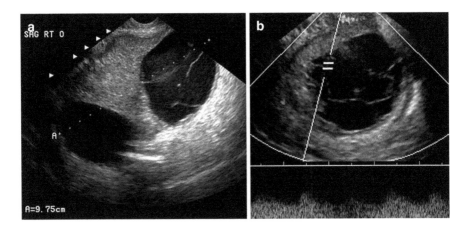

Fig. 7.7 Ovarian torsion. Transvaginal pelvis US on gray scale imaging (**a**) shows an enlarged right ovary (calipers). Doppler imaging (**b**) in torsed ovaries often demonstrates arterial blood flow (spectral scale below) and is therefore not helpful in making this diagnosis

Solution
Transvaginal US can be used to diagnose gynecologic causes of acute pelvic pain such as hemorrhagic cyst, pelvic inflammatory disease, or ovarian torsion. Transabdominal US is also recommended to provide a larger field of view.

A 32-year-old woman with acute pelvic pain suspected of non-gynecologic origin. Serum β-hCG is positive.

a. X-ray abdomen
b. US abdomen and pelvis transabdominal
c. CT abdomen and pelvis with contrast
d. MRI abdomen and pelvis without contrast
e. No ideal imaging exam

Nongynecological etiology suspected, serum β-hCG positive.

a. X-ray abdomen is not rated for appropriateness.
b. *US abdomen and pelvis transabdominal* is the most appropriate. Add transvaginal US as indicated.
c. CT abdomen and pelvis with contrast may be appropriate. Use if US is nondiagnostic and MRI is unavailable or equivocal.
d. MRI abdomen and pelvis without contrast is usually appropriate, but there is a better choice here.

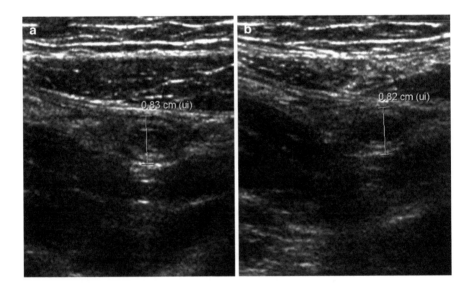

Fig. 7.8 Appendicitis. Transabdominal pelvis US of the right lower quadrant without (**a**) and with (**b**) compression reveals a blind-ending non-compressible loop of bowel (calipers) that measures >6 mm in thickness

Solution
Transabdominal US, with transvaginal US as needed, assesses for gastrointestinal (e.g., appendicitis) or urinary tract (e.g., hydronephrosis) pathology in pregnant patients. MRI is useful when US is inconclusive.

A 30-year-old woman with acute right lower quadrant pelvic pain suspected of non-gynecologic origin. Appendicitis is suspected. Serum β-hCG is negative.

a. X-ray abdomen
b. US pelvis transvaginal
c. CT abdomen and pelvis with contrast
d. MRI abdomen and pelvis without and with contrast
e. No ideal imaging exam

Nongynecological etiology suspected, serum β-hCG negative.

a. X-ray abdomen is not rated for appropriateness.
b. US pelvis transvaginal may be appropriate.
c. *CT abdomen and pelvis* with contrast is the most appropriate.
d. MRI abdomen and pelvis without and with contrast may be appropriate to avoid radiation exposure of CT in a young patient.

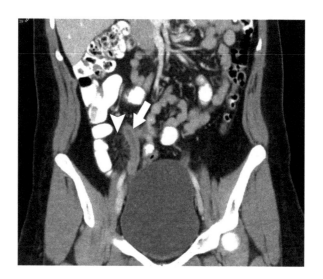

Fig. 7.9 Appendicitis. Abdomen and pelvis CT with contrast coronal reconstruction image shows a dilated appendix (arrow) with thickened walls and which does not fill with enteric contrast. There are inflammatory changes in the adjacent mesentery (arrowhead)

Solution
CT provides the best diagnostic performance in identifying the gastrointestinal (e.g., appendicitis) or urinary tract (e.g., obstructive nephrolithiasis) pathology of acute pelvic pain. CT almost always permits visualization of a normal appendix to exclude the diagnosis of appendicitis.

7.4 Clinically Suspected Adnexal Mass

A 32-year-old premenopausal woman with a clinically suspected adnexal mass. She is not pregnant.

a. US pelvis transvaginal
b. CT pelvis with contrast
c. MRI pelvis without and with contrast
d. FDG-PET/CT whole body
e. No ideal imaging exam

A reproductive age female (not pregnant). Initial evaluation.

a. *US pelvis transvaginal* is the most appropriate. Transabdominal and Doppler US may be added.
b. CT pelvis with contrast is usually not appropriate.
c. MRI pelvis without and with contrast may be appropriate.
d. FDG-PET/CT whole body is usually not appropriate.

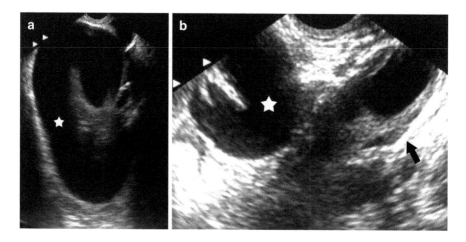

Fig. 7.10 Hydrosalpinx. Transvaginal pelvis US (**a, b**) shows a tubular cystic structure (star) in the left adnexa and a normal separate left ovary (arrow)

Solution

Transvaginal US provides high resolution and transabdominal US a larger field of view, making these in combination the best initial exam. When US is inconclusive, contrast-enhanced MRI allows for soft tissue characterization and assessment of the relationship of the mass to other pelvic structures.

A 32-year-old premenopausal woman with a mixed solid and cystic or completely solid adnexal mass that is persistent on follow-up. She is not pregnant.

a. US pelvis transvaginal
b. CT pelvis with contrast
c. MRI pelvis without and with contrast
d. FDG-PET/CT whole body
e. No ideal imaging exam

A reproductive age female (not pregnant) with complex or solid mass which is persistent or enlarging on pelvic US at short term follow-up.

a. US pelvis transvaginal may be appropriate.
b. CT pelvis with contrast may be appropriate. Use if patient has contraindications to MRI.
c. *MRI pelvis without and with contrast* is the most appropriate. Use if non-surgical management is elected and malignancy cannot be excluded.
d. FDG-PET/CT whole body is usually not appropriate, as it is not appropriate for tissue characterization of adnexal lesions.

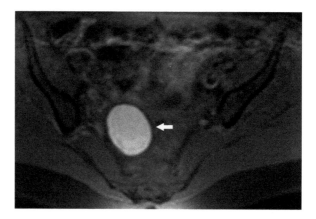

Fig. 7.11 Endometrioma. Pelvis MR axial T1-weighted image shows a homogeneous, intensely bright cyst (arrow) in the right ovary

Solution

Vast majority of incidental adnexal masses in premenopausal women are benign (e.g., fibroid, endometrioma, dermoid, and fibroma). MRI, with its superior ability to characterize soft tissue, is the best modality to establish the diagnosis. If lesion is suspected to be malignant, CT is used to evaluate for the extent of tumor spread.

A 62-year-old postmenopausal woman with clinically suspected adnexal mass.

a. US pelvis transvaginal
b. CT pelvis with contrast
c. MRI pelvis without and with contrast
d. FDG-PET/CT whole body
e. No ideal imaging exam

A postmenopausal female (>12 months amenorrhea). Initial evaluation.

a. *US pelvis transvaginal* is the most appropriate. Transabdominal and Doppler US may be added.
b. CT pelvis with contrast is usually not appropriate.
c. MRI pelvis without and with contrast may be appropriate.
d. FDG-PET/CT whole body is usually not appropriate.

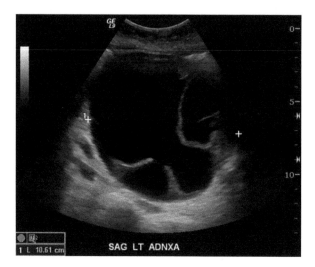

Fig. 7.12 Ovarian cystadenoma. Transvaginal pelvis US shows a mixed solid and cystic mass in the left adnexa. A normal left ovary was not seen

Solution
Transvaginal and transabdominal US with Doppler are sensitive in detecting malignant adnexal masses. MRI may be used when US is inconclusive for soft tissue characterization of masses suspected to be benign.

7.5 Infertility

A 33-year-old woman with infertility and suspected endometriosis.

a. Hysterosalpingography
b. US pelvis transabdominal
c. CT pelvis with contrast
d. MRI pelvis without and with contrast
e. No ideal imaging exam

History or clinical suspicion of endometriosis.

a. Hysterosalpingography is usually appropriate, but there is a better choice here.
b. US pelvis transabdominal is usually appropriate, but there is a better choice here.
c. CT abdomen and pelvis is usually not appropriate.
d. *MRI pelvis without and with contrast* is the most appropriate.

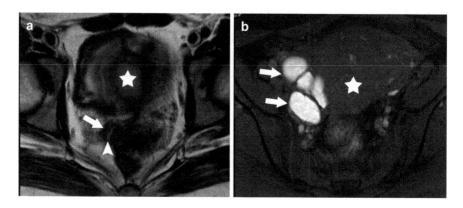

Fig. 7.13 Endometriosis. Pelvic MR axial T2-weighted image (**a**) shows a thickened, scarred right uterosacral ligament (arrow) adjacent to the right lateral vaginal fornix (arrowhead). Axial T1-weighted image (**b**) shows right hematosalpinx (arrows). Uterus (star) appears normal

Solution
MRI offers high sensitivity and specificity in the diagnosis of endometriosis. Pelvic US is less sensitive in the detection of endometriomas and usually does not detect extra-ovarian implants. Hysterosalpingography may be useful for an infertility workup to evaluate tubal patency and the uterine cavity contour.

A 34-year-old woman with infertility and suspected tubal occlusion.

a. Hysterosalpingography
b. US pelvis transvaginal
c. CT abdomen and pelvis with contrast
d. MRI pelvis without and with contrast
e. No ideal imaging exam

Suspicion of tubal occlusion, pelvic inflammatory disease, or history of pelvic surgery.

a. *Hysterosalpingography* is the most appropriate.
b. US pelvis transvaginal is usually appropriate, but there is a better choice here.
c. CT abdomen and pelvis is usually not appropriate.
d. MRI pelvis without and with contrast is usually appropriate, but there is a better choice here.

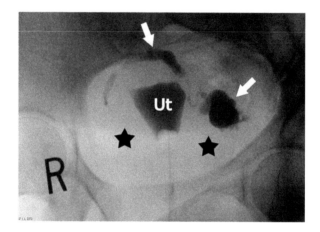

Fig. 7.14 Hydrosalpinx. Hysterosalpingography antero-posterior view shows bilateral dilated fallopian tubes (arrows). Lack of free contrast spill into the peritoneal cavity (stars) indicates tubal occlusion. The uterus (Ut) is normal

Solution
Hysterosalpingography allows for the direct evaluation of fallopian tube caliber and patency. While pelvic US and MRI enable visualization of an abnormally dilated tube, neither exam directly evaluates for tubal occlusion.

A 22-year-old woman with infertility and recurrent pregnancy loss.

a. Hysterosalpingography
b. US pelvis transvaginal
c. CT abdomen and pelvis with contrast
d. MRI pelvis
e. No ideal imaging exam

Recurrent pregnancy loss.

a. Hysterosalpingography may be appropriate.
b. US pelvis transvaginal is usually appropriate, but there is a better choice here.
c. CT abdomen and pelvis is usually not appropriate.
d. *MRI pelvis* is the most appropriate.

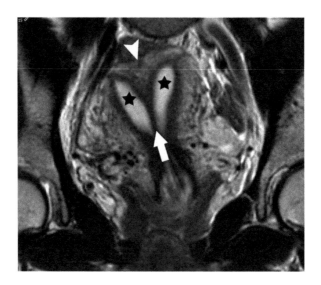

Fig. 7.15 Septate uterus. Pelvic MR FSE T2-weighted image through the uterine long axis shows two endometrial cavities (stars) separated by a thick septum (arrow) and a normal uterine fundal contour (arrowhead)

Solution
MRI allows for the assessment of common anatomic causes of recurrent pregnancy loss, including Müllerian anomalies, synechiae, and leiomyomas. MRI is more accurate than transvaginal US and hysterosalpingography in the evaluation of Müllerian anomalies. Pelvic US may be used to monitor follicle development in treating infertility.

7.6   Pelvic Floor Dysfunction

A 69-year-old woman with incomplete urinary voiding and incontinence.

a. X-ray fluoroscopic cystocolpoproctography
b. US pelvis transabdominal
c. CT pelvis
d. MRI pelvis dynamic
e. No ideal imaging exam

Urinary dysfunction. Urinary leakage, frequency, or urgency. Straining or incomplete voiding.

a. X-ray fluoroscopic cystocolpoproctography is usually appropriate, but there is a better choice here. It evaluates the overall pelvic floor function.
b. US pelvis transabdominal may be appropriate. It evaluates bladder post-void residual.
c. CT pelvis is usually not appropriate.
d. *MRI pelvis dynamic* is the most appropriate. Patient is imaged at rest and with Valsalva maneuvers.

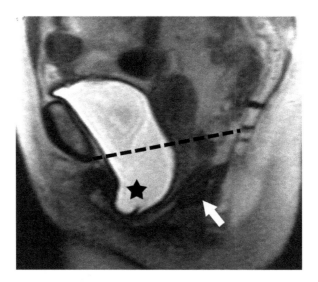

Fig. 7.16 Cystocele. Pelvis MR sagittal T2-weighted image with Valsalva maneuver demonstrates abnormal descent of the bladder (star) and puborectalis muscle (arrow) below the expected position of the pelvic floor (dashed line)

Solution
MRI offers superior tissue contrast and 3D volumetric data compared to fluoroscopic cystocolpoproctography, which provides functional and 2D anatomic information. Dynamic MRI during patient straining shows mobility of the pelvic organs and changes in the pelvic floor hiatus.

A 64-year-old woman with constipation and incomplete defecation.

a. X-ray fluoroscopic defecography
b. US pelvis transperineal
c. CT pelvis
d. MRI pelvis dynamic with rectal contrast
e. No ideal imaging exam

Defecatory dysfunction. Straining during defecation, incomplete evacuation or splinting, or digital maneuvers to defecate.

a. *X-ray fluoroscopic defecography* is the most appropriate.
b. US pelvis transperineal may be appropriate.
c. CT pelvis is usually not appropriate.
d. MRI pelvis dynamic with rectal contrast may be appropriate. The patient is imaged at rest and with Valsalva maneuvers.

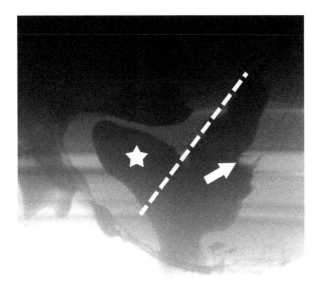

Fig. 7.17 Rectocele and rectal intussusception. Defecography lateral view demonstrates a rectocele bulge (star) beyond the expected location of the anterior rectal wall (dashed line) and an infolding of the rectal wall (arrow) indicating an intussusception

Solution
X-ray fluoroscopic defecography images the process of rectal evacuation and identifies associated structural abnormalities in the pelvic floor. Defecography may be particularly valuable to assess for abnormalities in patients with discordant results on manometry and balloon expulsion test.

7.7   Ovarian Cancer Screening

A 51-year-old woman with an average risk for ovarian cancer presents for screening.

a. US pelvis transabdominal
b. US pelvis transvaginal
c. CT abdomen and pelvis
d. MRI pelvis
e. No ideal imaging exam

A premenopausal or postmenopausal female with an average risk of ovarian cancer.

a. US pelvis transabdominal is usually not appropriate.
b. US pelvis transvaginal is usually not appropriate.
c. CT abdomen and pelvis is usually not appropriate.
d. MRI pelvis is usually not appropriate.
e. *No ideal imaging exam* is the correct answer.

Solution
Ovarian cancer screening is not recommended in average-risk populations. There is no change in the distribution of ovarian cancer stage at diagnosis or in cancer-specific mortality with the use of screening US.

A 38-year-old premenopausal woman with a family history of ovarian cancer presents for screening.

a. US pelvis transabdominal
b. US pelvis transvaginal
c. CT abdomen and pelvis
d. MRI pelvis
e. No ideal imaging exam

A premenopausal female with high risk of ovarian cancer (personal history or family history).

a. US pelvis transabdominal may be appropriate.
b. US pelvis transvaginal may be appropriate.
c. CT abdomen and pelvis is usually not appropriate.
d. MRI pelvis is usually not appropriate.
e. *No ideal imaging exam* is the correct answer.

Solution
Women with a known or probable genetic predisposition for ovarian cancer should be counseled that, even in high-risk settings, no evidence supports the effectiveness of ovarian cancer screening. However, transvaginal US with or without Doppler may be appropriate for BRCA1 and BRCA2 mutation carriers for the assessment of ovarian pathology and treatment planning for prophylactic salpingo-oophorectomy.

7.8 Ovarian Cancer Pretreatment Imaging and Follow-Up

A 65-year-old woman with ovarian cancer presents for pretreatment evaluation.

a. US abdomen and pelvis
b. CT chest with contrast
c. CT abdomen and pelvis with contrast
d. MRI abdomen and pelvis without and with contrast
e. No ideal imaging exam

Pretreatment staging of ovarian cancer.

a. US abdomen and pelvis is usually not appropriate.
b. CT chest with contrast is usually appropriate, but there is a better choice here. Use if chest X-ray is abnormal.
c. *CT abdomen and pelvis with contrast* is the most appropriate.
d. MRI abdomen and pelvis without and with contrast is usually appropriate, but there is a better choice here. Use if CT with contrast is contraindicated.

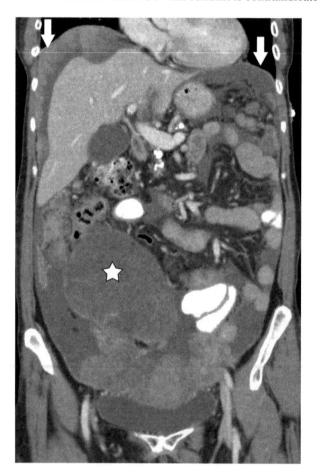

Fig. 7.18 Ovarian cancer. Abdomen and pelvis CT with contrast coronal reconstruction image shows a multilobulated pelvic mass (star), tumor that extends to both hemidiaphragms (arrows), and ascites

Solution
CT is preferred for ovarian cancer staging and treatment planning as it detects both local and distant tumor involvement. Chest CT should be performed when chest radiography is abnormal. MRI is recommended for patients with a contraindication to iodinated contrast agents.

A 80-year-old woman with a history of ovarian cancer with concern for recurrence.

a. US abdomen and pelvis
b. CT abdomen and pelvis with contrast
c. MRI abdomen and pelvis without and with contrast
d. FDG-PET/CT whole body
e. No ideal imaging exam

Rule out recurrent ovarian cancer.

a. US abdomen and pelvis is usually not appropriate.
b. *CT abdomen and pelvis* with contrast is the most appropriate.
c. MRI abdomen and pelvis without and with contrast is usually appropriate, but there is a better choice here. Use if CT with contrast is contraindicated.
d. FDG-PET/CT whole body is usually appropriate, but there is a better choice here. Use if CT is negative, but recurrence is still clinically suspected or for treatment planning.

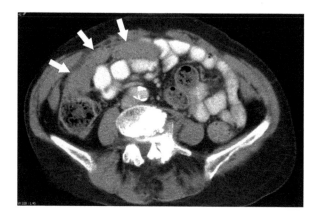

Fig. 7.19 Recurrent ovarian cancer. Abdomen and pelvis CT with contrast shows multiple peritoneal soft tissue nodules (arrows)

Solution

CT is preferred for detecting ovarian cancer recurrence as it is widely available and sufficiently accurate. In cases where CT is negative and the serum tumor marker CA-125 is rising, FDG-PET/CT has been shown to be more sensitive and specific than CT alone.

7.9 Endometrial Cancer of the Uterus

A 54-year-old woman with newly diagnosed endometrial cancer. Pretreatment evaluation to assess the depth of myometrial invasion by tumor.

a. US pelvis transvaginal
b. US sonohysterography
c. CT pelvis with contrast
d. MRI pelvis without and with contrast
e. No ideal imaging exam

Assessing the depth of myometrial invasion.

a. US pelvis transvaginal is usually not appropriate.
b. US sonohysterography may be appropriate. It carries a very low risk of malignant cell dissemination into peritoneal cavity.
c. CT pelvis with contrast is usually not appropriate.
d. *MRI pelvis without and with contrast* is the most appropriate.

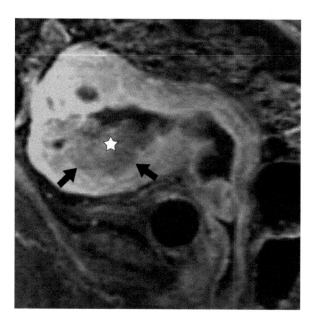

Fig. 7.20 Endometrial cancer. Pelvic MR sagittal post-contrast image shows a tumor (star) in the endometrial cavity with myometrial invasion (arrows)

Solution

Contrast-enhanced MRI performs significantly better than pelvic US or CT for evaluating the depth of myometrial invasion.

A 78-year-old woman with newly diagnosed endometrial cancer. Pretreatment evaluation to assess for lymph node metastases.

a. US pelvis transabdominal
b. CT abdomen and pelvis with contrast
c. MRI abdomen and pelvis without and with contrast
d. FDG-PET/CT whole body
e. No ideal imaging exam

Lymph node evaluation in newly diagnosed endometrial cancer.

a. US pelvis transabdominal is usually not appropriate.
b. CT abdomen and pelvis with contrast is usually appropriate, but there is a better choice here.
c. MRI abdomen and pelvis without and with contrast is usually appropriate, but there is a better choice here.
d. *FDG-PET/CT whole body* is the most appropriate.

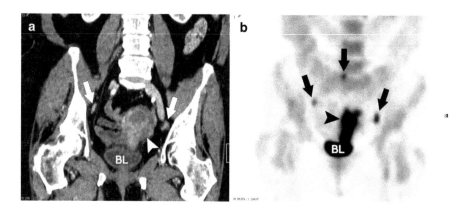

Fig. 7.21 Endometrial cancer lymphadenopathy. Abdomen and pelvis CT with contrast coronal reconstruction image (**a**) and whole-body FDG-PET/CT coronal MIP image (**b**) show normal-sized lymph nodes (arrows) with tracer avidity, indicating tumor involvement. The primary uterine tumor (arrowhead) is also hypermetabolic. The bladder (BL) contains excreted tracer

Solution
FDG-PET/CT is more sensitive than CT alone for detecting lymph node involvement by tumor. CT and MRI both use morphologic criteria alone and perform comparably in detecting lymphadenopathy.

A 82-year-old woman with newly diagnosed endometrial cancer. Pretreatment evaluation to assess for endocervical tumor extension.

a. US pelvis transvaginal
b. US sonohysterography
c. CT pelvis with contrast
d. MRI pelvis without and with contrast
e. No ideal imaging exam

Assessing endocervical tumor extent in newly diagnosed endometrial cancer.

a. US pelvis transvaginal may be appropriate. Use if MRI is contraindicated.
b. US sonohysterography is usually not appropriate.
c. CT pelvis with contrast is usually not appropriate.
d. *MRI pelvis without and with contrast* is the most appropriate.

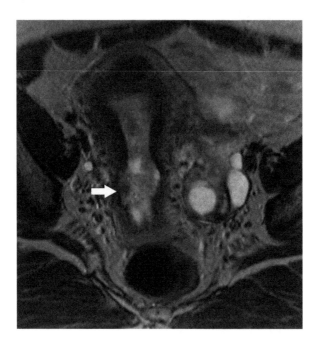

Fig. 7.22 Endometrial cancer with cervical extension. Pelvic MR axial T2-weighted image shows tumor extending from the endometrial cavity into the cervix (arrow)

Solution
MRI allows for the most accurate evaluation of the extent of pelvic tumor compared to CT or US. MRI is superior to US in evaluating for tumor extension into the cervix.

A 54-year-old woman with a history of endometrial cancer, now with suspected recurrence.

a. CT abdomen and pelvis with contrast
b. CT chest with contrast
c. MRI abdomen and pelvis without and with contrast
d. FDG-PET/CT whole body
e. No ideal imaging exam

Posttherapy evaluation of a patient with clinically suspected recurrence of endometrial cancer.

a. CT abdomen and pelvis with contrast is usually appropriate, but there is a better choice here.
b. CT chest with contrast may be appropriate.
c. MRI abdomen and pelvis without and with contrast may be appropriate.
d. *FDG-PET/CT whole body* is the most appropriate.

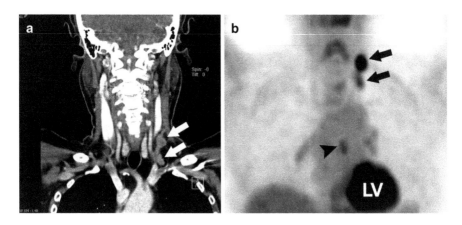

Fig. 7.23 Endometrial cancer recurrence. Neck CT with contrast coronal reconstruction image (**a**) and whole-body FDG-PET/CT coronal MIP image (**b**) show normal sized supraclavicular lymph nodes (arrows) with avid tracer uptake, indicating tumor involvement. Also seen is mediastinal lymphadenopathy (arrowhead) and a normally FDG-avid left ventricle (LV)

Solution
FDG-PET fused with CT or MRI performs better than CT, MRI, or tumor markers alone in the diagnosis of recurrent endometrial cancer.

7.10   Staging of Invasive Cancer of the Cervix

A 30-year-old woman with cervical cancer FIGO stage IB1 with tumor size ≤4 cm.

a. X-ray chest
b. CT abdomen and pelvis with contrast
c. MRI pelvis without and with contrast
d. FDG-PET/CT whole body
e. No ideal imaging exam

FIGO stage IB1, tumor size ≤4 cm.

a. X-ray chest may be appropriate.
b. CT abdomen and pelvis with contrast may be appropriate.
c. *MRI pelvis without and with contrast* and choice (d) are equally the most appropriate. These exams are complementary.
d. *FDG-PET/CT whole body* and choice (c) are equally the most appropriate. These exams are complementary.

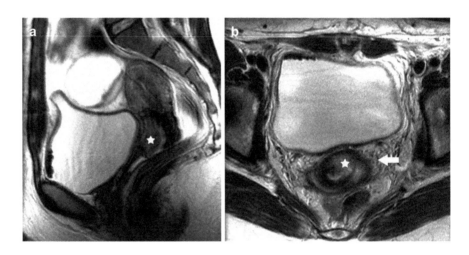

Fig. 7.24 Cervical cancer with parametrial extension. Pelvic MR sagittal (**a**) and axial (**b**) T2-weighted images show cervical tumor (star) extending to the left parametrium (arrow)

Solution
MRI and FDG-PET/CT are complementary exams for cervical cancer staging. MRI is accurate in determining tumor size and extent of pelvic spread. PET imaging assesses lymph node and extra-pelvic metastases.

A 34-year-old woman with cervical cancer FIGO stage IB2 with tumor size >4 cm.

a. X-ray chest
b. CT abdomen and pelvis with contrast
c. MRI pelvis without and with contrast
d. FDG-PET/CT whole body
e. No ideal imaging exam

FIGO stage IB2, tumor size >4 cm.

a. X-ray chest may be appropriate.
b. CT abdomen and pelvis with contrast is usually appropriate, but there is a better choice here.
c. *MRI pelvis without and with contrast* and choice (d) are equally the most appropriate. These exams are complementary.
d. *FDG-PET/CT whole body* and choice (c) are equally the most appropriate. These exams are complementary.

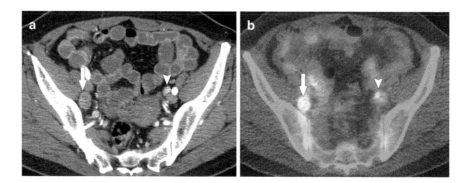

Fig. 7.25 Cervical cancer lymphadenopathy. Pelvis CT (**a**) shows an enlarged right (arrow) and a normal-sized left (arrowhead) pelvic node. Concurrent whole-body FDG-PET/CT fusion image (**b**) reveals that both nodes are hypermetabolic, indicating tumor involvement

Solution
MRI and FDG-PET/CT are complementary exams for cervical cancer staging. MRI is accurate in determining the tumor size and the extent of pelvic spread. PET imaging assesses lymph node and extra-pelvic metastases.

A 54-year-old woman with cervical cancer, FIGO stage II or greater.

a. CT abdomen and pelvis with contrast
b. CT chest with contrast
c. MRI pelvis without and with contrast
d. FDG-PET/CT whole body
e. No ideal imaging exam

FIGO stage greater than Ib.

a. CT abdomen and pelvis with contrast is usually appropriate, but there is a better choice here.
b. CT chest with contrast may be appropriate.
c. *MRI pelvis without and with contrast* and choice (d) are equally the most appropriate. These exams are complementary.
d. *FDG-PET/CT whole body* and choice (c) are equally the most appropriate. These exams are complementary.

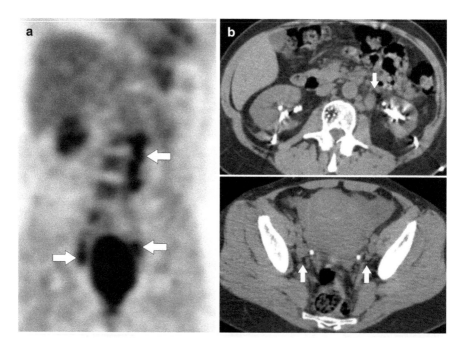

Fig. 7.26 Cervical cancer with metastases. Whole-body FDG-PET/CT coronal MIP image (**a**) shows hypermetabolic foci (arrows) in the upper abdomen and pelvis. Concurrent abdomen and pelvis CT images (**b**) show these foci to correspond to pelvic and para-aortic nodes (arrows)

Solution
MRI and FDG-PET/CT are complementary exams for staging tumors which may have spread beyond the confines of the cervix (greater than stage Ib). MRI evaluates tumor for size and local invasion and PET detects lymphadenopathy.

Pediatric Imaging

8

8.1 Head Trauma in a Child

8.1.1 Glasgow Coma Scale (GCS)

Eye opening response

- Spontaneous (open with blinking at baseline): 4 points
- To verbal stimuli, command, speech: 3 points
- To pain only (not applied to face): 2 points
- No response: 1 point

Verbal response

- Oriented: 5 points
- Confused conversation, but able to answer questions: 4 points
- Inappropriate words: 3 points
- Incomprehensible speech: 2 points
- No response: 1 point

Motor response

- Obeys commands for movement: 6 points
- Purposeful movement to painful stimulus: 5 points
- Withdraws in response to pain: 4 points
- Flexion in response to pain (decorticate posturing): 3 points
- Extension response in response to pain (decerebrate posturing): 2 points
- No response: 1 point

Teasdale et al. 1974

© The Author(s), under exclusive license to Springer Nature
Switzerland AG 2021
G. X. Wang et al., *Choosing the Correct Radiologic Test*,
https://doi.org/10.1007/978-3-030-65185-5_8

8.1.2 Pediatric Emergency Care Network (PECARN) Clinical Criteria for Minor Head Trauma

Risk stratification for clinically important brain injury after head trauma for children with GCS scores of 14–15.

PECARN criteria for children *younger than 2 years of age*

Very low risk	GCS = 15 with *none* of the following: Palpable skull fracture, occipital or parietal or temporal scalp hematoma, loss of consciousness $\geq$5 s, severe mechanism of injury[a], not acting normally per parents, or other signs of altered mental status[b]
Intermediate risk	GCS = 15 with *any* of the following: Occipital or parietal or temporal scalp hematoma, loss of consciousness $\geq$5 s, severe mechanism of injury[a], not acting normally per parents. No other signs of altered mental status[b] or palpable skull fracture
High risk	GCS = 14 or with other signs of altered mental status[b] or palpable skull fracture

[a]Severe mechanism of injury: motor vehicle crash with patient ejection, death of another passenger, or rollover; pedestrian or bicyclist without helmet struck by a motorized vehicle; falls of more than 0.9 m (3 ft) (or more than 1.5 m [5 ft] for age $\geq$2 years); or head struck by a high-impact object
[b]Other signs of altered mental status: agitation, somnolence, repetitive questioning, or slow response to verbal communication

PECARN criteria for children *2 years of age or older*

Very low risk	GCS = 15 with *none* of the following: Signs of basilar skull fracture, any loss of consciousness, vomiting, severe injury mechanism[a], severe headache, or other signs of altered mental status[b]
Intermediate risk	GCS = 15 with *any* of the following: History of any loss of consciousness, vomiting, severe mechanism of injury[a], or severe headache. No altered mental status[b] or signs of basilar skull fracture
High risk	GCS = 14 or with other signs of altered mental status,[b] or signs of basilar skull fracture

[a]Severe mechanism of injury: motor vehicle crash with patient ejection, death of another passenger, or rollover; pedestrian or bicyclist without helmet struck by a motorized vehicle; falls of more than 0.9 m (3 ft) (or more than 1.5 m [5 ft] for age $\geq$2 years); or head struck by a high-impact object
[b]Other signs of altered mental status: agitation, somnolence, repetitive questioning, or slow response to verbal communication

Kuppermann et al. 2009

A 5-year-old child with minor acute head trauma and at very low risk for clinically important brain injury per PECARN criteria. Abusive trauma is not suspected.

a. X-ray skull
b. CT head without contrast
c. CT head with contrast
d. MRI head without contrast
e. No ideal imaging exam

Minor acute head trauma. Very low risk for clinically important brain injury per PECARN criteria. Abusive trauma is not suspected.

a. X-ray skull is usually not appropriate.
b. CT head without contrast is usually not appropriate.
c. CT head with contrast is usually not appropriate.
d. MRI head without contrast is usually not appropriate.
e. *No ideal imaging exam* is the correct answer.

Solution

The PECARN clinical decision rules have been robustly validated. Those meeting the very low-risk criteria have virtually no risk for clinically important brain injury following acute head trauma. Therefore, imaging can be safely avoided in this scenario.

A 6-year-old child with minor acute head trauma and at intermediate risk for clinically important brain injury per PECARN criteria. Abusive trauma is not suspected.

a. X-ray skull
b. CT head without contrast
c. CT head with contrast
d. MRI head without contrast
e. No ideal imaging exam

Minor acute head trauma. Intermediate risk for clinically important brain injury per PECARN criteria. Abusive trauma is not suspected.

a. X-ray skull is usually not appropriate.
b. CT head without contrast may be appropriate.
c. CT head with contrast is usually not appropriate.
d. MRI head without contrast is usually not appropriate.
e. *No ideal imaging exam* is the correct answer.

Solution
Children with minor acute head trauma with intermediate risk for clinically important brain injury per PECARN criteria are best managed with close clinical observation rather than imaging. However, CT head without contrast may be appropriate in patients with worsening clinical symptoms or signs during observation, for those with parental preference for imaging or in young infants where observational assessment is more challenging.

A 1-year-old child with minor acute head trauma and at high risk for clinically important brain injury per PECARN criteria. Abusive trauma is not suspected.

a. X-ray skull
b. CT head without contrast
c. CT head with contrast
d. MRI head without contrast
e. No ideal imaging exam

Minor acute head trauma. High risk for clinically important brain injury per
PECARN criteria. Abusive trauma is not suspected.

a. X-ray skull is usually not appropriate.
b. *CT head without contrast* is the most appropriate.
c. CT head with contrast is usually not appropriate.
d. MRI head without contrast is usually not appropriate.

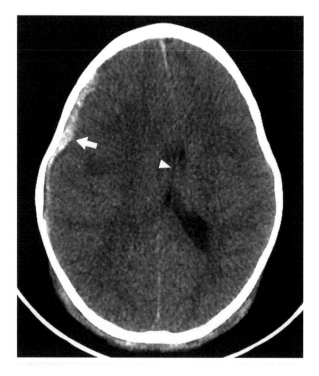

Fig. 8.1 Head trauma. Head CT shows subdural hematoma (arrow) with mass effect manifested
as right-to-left midline shift (arrowhead) and complete effacement of the right lateral ventricle

Solution
In children with minor acute head trauma at high risk for clinically important brain
injury per PECARN criteria, head CT without contrast is recommended. Image
acquisition is rapid, and the exam demonstrates excellent sensitivity for acute intracranial hemorrhage and fractures.

A 4-year-old child with acute head trauma and GCS of 12. Abusive head trauma is not suspected.

a. X-ray skull
b. CT head without contrast
c. CT head with contrast
d. MRI head without contrast
e. No ideal imaging exam

Moderate or severe acute blunt head trauma (GCS ≤13). Abusive head trauma is not suspected.

a. X-ray skull is usually not appropriate.
b. *CT head without contrast* is the most appropriate.
c. CT head with contrast is usually not appropriate.
d. MRI head without contrast is usually not appropriate.

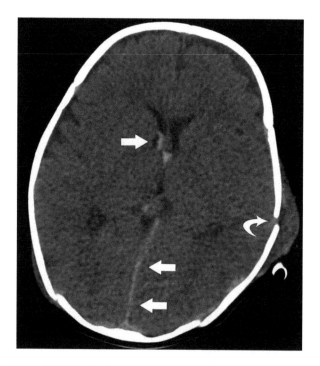

Fig. 8.2   Head trauma. Head CT shows intracranial blood (arrows) and a skull fracture with associated scalp hematoma (curved arrow)

Solution

Head CT without contrast is recommended for patients with moderate or severe acute blunt head trauma (GCS ≤13). CT has rapid acquisition time and excellent sensitivity for traumatic injuries, including herniation or hemorrhage, that require prompt intervention.

8.2   Seizures

A 3-day-old premature infant, born at 30 weeks gestational age, presents with seizures.

a. US head
b. CT head without contrast
c. MRI head without contrast
d. FDG-PET head
e. No ideal imaging exam

Neonatal seizures.

a. *US head* is the most appropriate.
b. CT head without contrast is usually not appropriate.
c. MRI head without contrast may be appropriate.
d. FDG-PET head is usually not appropriate.

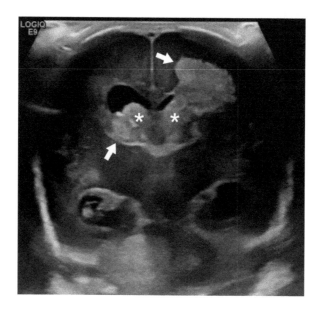

Fig. 8.3 Germinal matrix hemorrhage. Head US shows hemorrhage within enlarged left and right lateral ventricles (stars) with extension into the brain parenchyma bilaterally (arrows) consistent with grade 4 germinal matrix hemorrhage

Solution

The most common cause of seizure in this setting is hypoxic ischemic encephalopathy followed by intracranial hemorrhage. US is the preferred initial imaging exam as it can be performed at the bedside and is sensitive for hematoma. MRI can help define the extent of injury and assess for developmental abnormalities associated with seizures.

A 9-month-old girl presents with a single episode of febrile seizure lasting 5 min.

a. US head
b. CT head without contrast
c. MRI head without contrast
d. FDG-PET head
e. No ideal imaging exam

Simple febrile seizures.

a. US head is usually not appropriate.
b. CT head without contrast is usually not appropriate.
c. MRI head without contrast is usually not appropriate.
d. FDG-PET head is usually not appropriate.
e. *No ideal imaging exam* is the correct answer.

Solution
Febrile seizures occur between 3 months and 5 years of age and are not associated with intracranial infection or other defined cause. Imaging is not indicated for simple febrile seizures, defined as lasting <15 min and not recurring within 24 h. In patients with complex febrile seizures (i.e., prolonged, occurring more than once in 24 h, or focal) or with seizures associated with meningitis/encephalitis or underlying trauma, imaging should be considered.

An 8-year-old girl with posttraumatic seizures.

a. US head
b. CT head without contrast
c. MRI head without contrast
d. FDG-PET head
e. No ideal imaging exam

Posttraumatic seizures.

a. US head is usually not appropriate.
b. *CT head without contrast* is the most appropriate.
c. MRI head without contrast may be appropriate.
d. FDG-PET head is usually not appropriate.

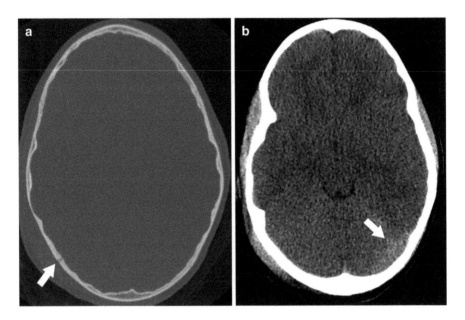

Fig. 8.4 Intracranial hemorrhage with skull fracture. Head CT bone window (**a**) shows a right parietal skull fracture (arrow). Soft tissue window (**b**) shows left subdural blood (arrow)

Solution

CT is the preferred imaging exam to assess for intracranial injury as the cause of a seizure. MRI can also effectively assess for intracranial trauma but may be less readily available or feasible in the acute posttraumatic setting.

A 6-year-old boy with partial seizures.

a. US head
b. CT head without contrast
c. MRI head without contrast
d. FDG-PET head
e. No ideal imaging exam

Partial seizures.

a. US head is usually not appropriate.
b. CT head without contrast may sometimes be appropriate. Use if MRI unavailable or contraindicated.
c. *MRI head without contrast* is the most appropriate.
d. FDG-PET head may be appropriate. Use in children with recurrent seizures.

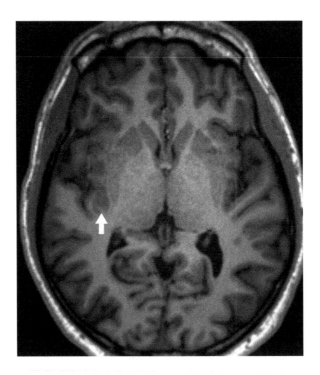

Fig. 8.5 Gray matter heterotopia. Head MR axial T1-weighted image shows thickening of the right insula with abnormal extension of gray matter medially (arrow)

Solution
Brain imaging is often positive with partial seizures and can reveal causative lesions including developmental abnormalities, hemorrhage, neoplasm, and gliosis. MRI is the preferred modality due to its high sensitivity.

A 4-year-old girl with the first episode of generalized seizure. She is otherwise normal neurologically.

a. US head
b. CT head without contrast
c. MRI head without contrast
d. FDG-PET head
e. No ideal imaging exam

First episode of generalized seizure in a child who is otherwise neurologically normal.

a. US head is usually not appropriate.
b. CT head without contrast may be appropriate.
c. MRI head without contrast may be appropriate.
d. FDG-PET head is usually not appropriate.
e. *No ideal imaging exam* is the correct answer.

Solution

In this setting, imaging is not recommended as it rarely reveals any intracranial abnormalities.

A 5-year-old boy with the first episode of generalized seizure and a history of developmental delay.

a. US head
b. CT head without contrast
c. MRI head without contrast
d. FDG-PET head
e. No ideal imaging exam

Generalized seizure in a child with a history of neurologic abnormality.

a. US head is usually not appropriate.
b. CT head without contrast may be appropriate.
c. *MRI head without contrast* is the most appropriate.
d. FDG-PET head is usually not appropriate.

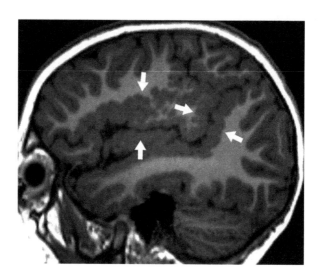

Fig. 8.6 Polymicrogyria. Head MR sagittal T1-weighted image shows abnormally small fine undulating cortical gyri (arrows) diffusely along the Sylvian fissure

Solution
A generalized seizure in a pediatric patient with a history of neurologic abnormality should be evaluated with head MRI to assess for an underlying lesion.

A 12-year-old boy with intractable seizures.

a. US head
b. CT head without contrast
c. MRI head without contrast
d. FDG-PET head
e. No ideal imaging exam

Intractable or refractory seizures.

a. US head is usually not appropriate.
b. CT head without contrast may be appropriate.
c. *MRI head without contrast* is the most appropriate.
d. FDG-PET head may be appropriate.

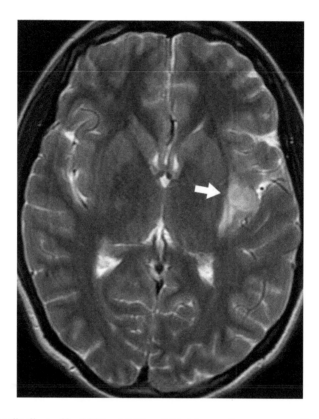

Fig. 8.7 Ganglioglioma. Head MR axial T2-weighted image shows an expansile mass (arrow) along the left insula

Solution
Brain imaging with MRI is the preferred initial exam in a child with intractable seizures to identify lesions that are potentially treatable with surgery. FDG-PET can complement anatomic imaging to prognosticate the outcome of epilepsy surgery.

8.3   Headache

A 12-year-old boy with isolated episode of headache, consistent with tension head-ache on clinical evaluation.

a. CT head without contrast
b. CT head with contrast
c. MRI head without contrast
d. MRI head without and with contrast
e. No ideal imaging exam

Child with primary headache.

a. CT head without contrast is usually not appropriate.
b. CT head with contrast is usually not appropriate.
c. MRI head without contrast is usually not appropriate.
d. MRI head without and with contrast is usually not appropriate.
e. *No ideal imaging exam* is the correct answer.

Solution

Imaging rarely reveals findings that contribute to the diagnosis and treatment of primary headaches such as chronic or recurrent migraine or tension headaches.

A 9-year-old boy with headaches. Intracranial neoplasm is suspected.

a. CT head without contrast
b. CT head with contrast
c. MRI head without contrast
d. MRI head without and with contrast
e. No ideal imaging exam

A child with secondary headache.

a. CT head without contrast may be appropriate.
b. CT head with contrast is usually not appropriate.
c. *MRI head without contrast* and choice (d) are equally the most appropriate.
d. *MRI head without and with contrast* and choice (c) are equally the most appropriate.

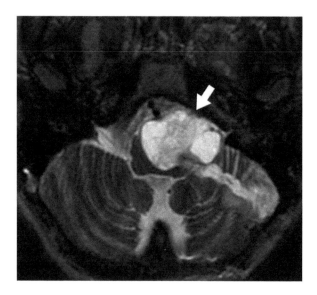

Fig. 8.8 Pilocytic astrocytoma. Head MR axial T2-weighted image shows a mixed cystic and solid expansile mass (arrow) in the medulla

Solution

MRI is the preferred modality for comprehensive evaluation of the brain parenchyma and other intracranial soft tissues and can be performed initially without contrast. However, if an abnormality is seen on non-contrast imaging, addition of contrast is recommended to improve the detection and characterization of neoplasm and inflammation. If MRI is unavailable or contraindicated, CT without contrast may be used to screen for and assess the extent of intracranial injury or pathology.

A 11-year-old girl with sudden severe ("thunderclap") headache.

a. CT head without contrast
b. CTA head
c. MRI head without contrast
d. MRA head without contrast
e. No ideal imaging exam

A child with sudden severe ("thunderclap") headache.

a. *CT head without contrast* and choices (c) and (d) are equally the most appropriate.
b. CTA head may be appropriate.
c. *MRI head without contrast* and choices (a) and (d) are equally the most appropriate.
d. *MRA head without contrast* and choice (a) and (c) are equally the most appropriate.

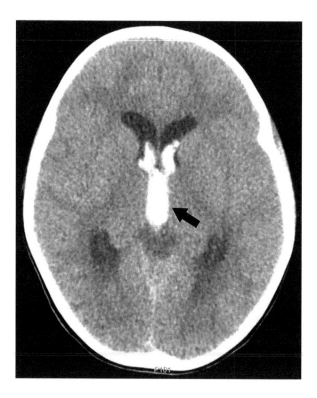

Fig. 8.9 Intracranial hemorrhage. Head CT without contrast demonstrates blood in the ventricles (arrow)

Solution
Severe sudden headaches can be associated with intracranial hemorrhage from vascular malformations or arterial dissection. CT is generally preferred since it is widely available, does not require patient sedation, and is highly sensitive for acute hemorrhage. MRI is also useful particularly when arterial dissection is suspected as it is more sensitive than CT for acute infraction and can be performed with an MRA to assess the vessels.

An 11-year-old boy with headache. An intracranial infection is suspected.

a. CT head without contrast
b. CT head with contrast
c. MRI head without contrast
d. MRI head without and with contrast
e. No ideal imaging exam

A child with headache attributed to infection.

a. CT head without contrast may be appropriate.
b. CT head with contrast may be appropriate.
c. MRI head without contrast may be appropriate.
d. *MRI head without and with contrast* is the most appropriate.

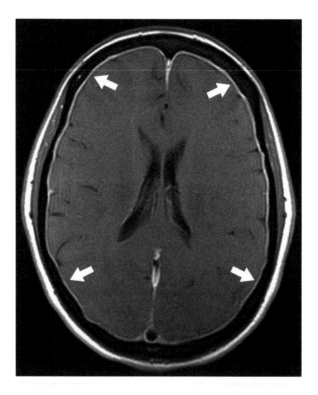

Fig. 8.10 Meningitis. Head MR axial post-contrast image shows diffuse thickening and enhancement of the pachymeninges

Solution
MRI is the preferred modality to evaluate for intracranial infections such as meningitis, encephalitis, and abscess. CT is less sensitive than MRI for intracranial infections but may be useful in the acute setting or to assess for suspected extracranial infections such as sinusitis and mastoiditis.

8.4   Sinusitis

A 4-year-old girl with uncomplicated acute sinusitis.

a. X-ray paranasal sinuses
b. CT paranasal sinuses without contrast
c. CT paranasal sinuses with contrast
d. MRI paranasal sinuses without contrast
e. No ideal imaging exam

A child with uncomplicated acute sinusitis.

a. X-ray paranasal sinuses is usually not appropriate.
b. CT paranasal sinuses without contrast is usually not appropriate.
c. CT paranasal sinuses with contrast is usually not appropriate.
d. MRI paranasal sinuses without contrast is usually not appropriate.
e. *No ideal imaging exam* is the correct answer.

Solution

For acute sinusitis without suspected complications, such as orbital or intracranial involvement, imaging is not recommended. The diagnosis of acute sinusitis is based on clinical evaluation. Furthermore, since paranasal sinus opacification is a common incidental finding in asymptomatic children, imaging abnormalities are not useful in making the diagnosis.

A 13-year-old boy with chronic sinusitis being considered for endoscopic surgery.

a. X-ray paranasal sinuses
b. CT paranasal sinuses without contrast
c. CT paranasal sinuses with contrast
d. MRI paranasal sinuses without contrast
e. No ideal imaging exam

A child with persistent (worsening course or not responding to treatment), recurrent, or chronic sinusitis. Define paranasal sinus anatomy before functional endoscopic sinus surgery.

a. X-ray paranasal sinuses is usually not appropriate.
b. *CT paranasal sinuses without contrast* is the most appropriate.
c. CT paranasal sinuses with contrast is usually not appropriate.
d. MRI paranasal sinuses without contrast is usually not appropriate.

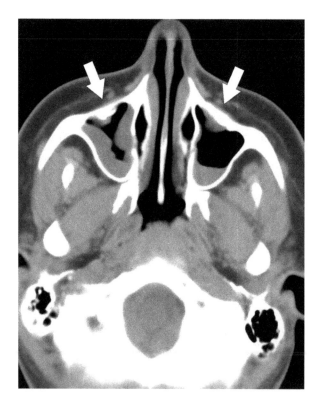

Fig. 8.11 Sinusitis. Sinus CT shows bilateral mucosal thickening of the maxillary sinuses (arrows) consistent with chronic sinusitis. Air-fluid level in the left maxillary sinus indicates acute sinusitis

Solution
CT accurately depicts sinus anatomy, soft tissue changes, and associated complications. MRI is less useful in this setting as it may require sedation or general anesthesia for young children and is inferior to CT for depicting bony anatomy and abnormalities.

8.5   Pneumonia in the Immunocompetent Child

A 1-year-old child with suspected uncomplicated community acquired pneumonia not requiring hospitalization.

a. X-ray chest
b. US chest
c. CT chest
d. MRI chest
e. No ideal imaging exam

A child 3 months of age and older. Suspected uncomplicated community-acquired pneumonia in a well-appearing child who does not require hospitalization.

a. X-ray chest is usually not appropriate.
b. US chest is usually not appropriate.
c. CT chest is usually not appropriate.
d. MRI chest is usually not appropriate.
e. *No ideal imaging exam* is the correct answer.

Solution
Routine use of imaging in this setting is not recommended. Radiography does not reliably distinguish between viral and bacterial community-acquired pneumonia or differentiate between bacterial pathogens. In addition, use of radiography may lead to unnecessary antibiotic use.

A 6-year-old child with community acquired pneumonia that does not respond to initial outpatient treatment.

a. X-ray chest
b. US chest
c. CT chest
d. MRI chest
e. No ideal imaging exam

Child 3 months of age and older. Community-acquired pneumonia that does not respond to initial outpatient treatment or requires hospitalization.

a. *X-ray chest* is the most appropriate.
b. US chest may be appropriate.
c. CT chest is usually not appropriate.
d. MRI chest is usually not appropriate.

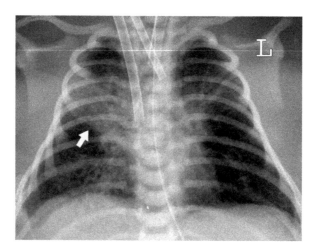

Fig. 8.12 Pneumonia. Chest X-ray anteroposterior view shows focal opacification in the right upper lobe

Solution
Radiography is recommended in this setting to determine the presence, size, and character of the air space disease and to identify complications that may require a change in clinical management.

A 7-year-old child with pneumonia and a moderate parapneumonic effusion seen on chest X-ray. Next imaging exam.

a. X-ray chest decubitus view
b. US chest
c. CT chest with contrast
d. MRI chest
e. No ideal imaging exam

Pneumonia complicated by moderate or large parapneumonic effusion on chest radiograph. Next imaging exam.

a. X-ray chest decubitus view may be appropriate.
b. *US chest* is the most appropriate.
c. CT chest with contrast may be appropriate.
d. MRI chest is usually not appropriate.

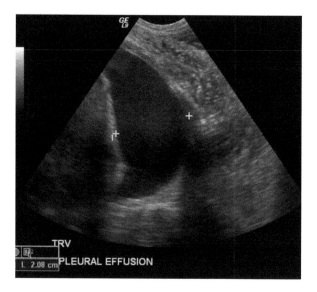

Fig. 8.13 Pleural effusion. Chest US shows a moderate size simple-appearing pleural effusion (calipers)

Solution

US can assess the size of a pleural effusion and evaluate for complexity. US can also guide thoracentesis, if needed.

A 12-year-old child presenting with pneumonia and a history of recurrent localized pneumonia on chest X-ray. Next imaging exam.

a. US chest
b. CT chest without contrast
c. CT chest with contrast
d. MRI chest
e. No ideal imaging exam

A 12-year-old child with pneumonia with a history of recurrent localized pneumonia on chest X-ray. Next imaging exam.

a. US chest is usually not appropriate.
b. CT chest without contrast may be appropriate.
c. *CT chest with contrast* is the most appropriate.
d. MRI chest is usually not appropriate.

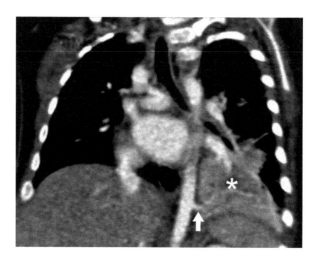

Fig. 8.14 Pulmonary sequestration. Chest CT with contrast coronal oblique reconstruction image shows a consolidated left lower lobe (star) with abnormal arterial supply from the aorta (arrow)

Solution
CT helps identify factors that predispose to recurrent localized pneumonia, such as foreign bodies, congenital lobular over-inflation, and bronchopulmonary dysplasia. Use of contrast is recommended to improve the assessment of additional causes such as bronchial tumors, pulmonary sequestration, and bronchopulmonary foregut malformation.

8.6   Vomiting in Infants

A 3-day-old boy with bilious vomiting.

a. X-ray abdomen
b. X-ray contrast enema
c. X-ray fluoroscopy upper GI series
d. US abdomen
e. No ideal imaging exam

Bilious vomiting in neonate up to 1-week old.

a. *X-ray abdomen* is the most appropriate.
b. X-ray contrast enema is usually appropriate, but there is a better choice here.
c. X-ray fluoroscopy upper GI series is usually appropriate, but there is a better choice here.
d. US abdomen may be appropriate.

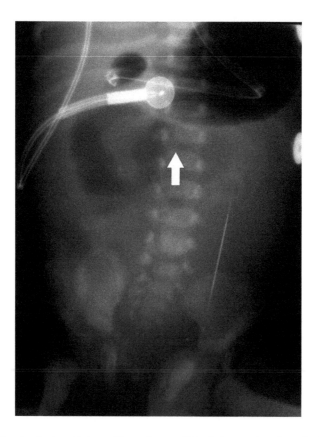

Fig. 8.15 Midgut volvulus. Abdomen X-ray shows a distended stomach and proximal duodenum with an abrupt transition (arrow) to collapsed bowel in the distal duodenum

Solution
In this setting, a congenital gastrointestinal tract abnormality is the primary consideration. The pattern of bowel distention on abdominal radiography can help distinguish between proximal and distal obstruction, and thus direct further evaluation with either an upper GI series or contrast enema, respectively. Note that negative radiography does not exclude the diagnosis of malrotation.

A 4-week-old boy with bilious vomiting.

a. X-ray abdomen
b. X-ray fluoroscopy upper GI series
c. US abdomen
d. Radionuclide gastric motility scan
e. No ideal imaging exam

Bilious vomiting in an infant 1 week to 3 months old.

a. X-ray abdomen may sometimes be appropriate.
b. *X-ray fluoroscopy upper GI series* is the most appropriate.
c. US abdomen is usually not appropriate.
d. Radionuclide gastric motility scan is usually not appropriate.

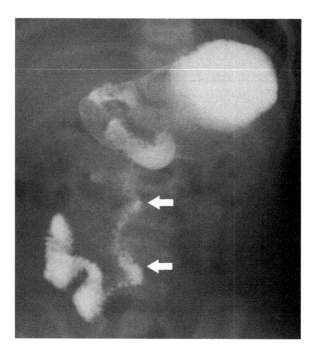

Fig. 8.16 Midgut volvulus. Upper GI series X-ray anteroposterior view shows small bowel that does not cross the midline and spirals caudally (arrows)

Solution

An upper GI series is recommended to evaluate for malrotation and midgut volvulus. This exam assesses the esophagus, stomach, pylorus, and the duodenum to the duodenojejunal junction.

A 6-week-old girl with intermittent nonbilious vomiting since birth.

a. X-ray abdomen
b. X-ray fluoroscopy upper GI series
c. US abdomen
d. Radionuclide gastric motility scan
e. No ideal imaging exam

Intermittent nonbilious vomiting since birth, in infants up to 3 months of age.

a. X-ray abdomen is usually not appropriate.
b. X-ray fluoroscopy upper GI series may be appropriate.
c. US abdomen may be appropriate.
d. Radionuclide gastric motility scan is usually not appropriate.
e. *No ideal imaging exam* is the correct answer.

Solution

The most common cause of nonbilious vomiting in neonates is gastroesophageal reflux. Most children with reflux who are otherwise healthy do not need further diagnostic evaluation. Upper GI series does not reliably confirm or exclude reflux but can assess for anatomic abnormalities that may produce similar symptoms.

A 6-week-old boy with the new onset of nonbilious vomiting.

a. X-ray abdomen
b. X-ray fluoroscopy upper GI series
c. US abdomen
d. Radionuclide gastric motility scan
e. No ideal imaging exam

New onset of nonbilious vomiting in infants up to 3 months of age.

a. X-ray abdomen is usually not appropriate.
b. X-ray fluoroscopy upper GI series may be appropriate.
c. *US abdomen* is the most appropriate.
d. Radionuclide gastric motility scan is usually not appropriate.

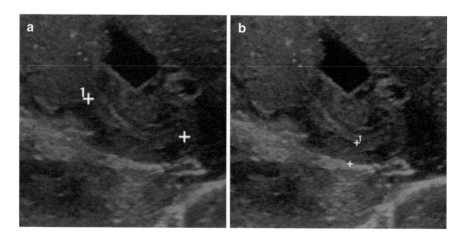

Fig. 8.17 Hypertrophic pyloric stenosis. Abdomen US measures (calipers) the length (**a**) and wall thickness (**b**) of the pylorus which is >2 cm and >4 mm, respectively

Solution
New onset of vomiting in this age group should raise concern for hypertrophic pyloric stenosis. US is the preferred imaging exam for diagnosis and provides real-time assessment of the pyloric muscle and channel.

8.7   Suspected Appendicitis

A 14-year-old girl evaluated for acute appendicitis with low clinical risk.

a. X-ray abdomen
b. US abdomen
c. CT abdomen and pelvis with contrast
d. MRI abdomen and pelvis without and with contrast
e. No ideal imaging exam

A child. Suspected acute appendicitis with low clinical risk.

a. X-ray abdomen is usually not appropriate.
b. US abdomen is usually not appropriate.
c. CT abdomen and pelvis with contrast is usually not appropriate.
d. MRI abdomen and pelvis without and with contrast is usually not appropriate.
e. *No ideal imaging exam* is the correct answer.

Solution

For pediatric patients with low clinical risk, imaging for acute appendicitis is usually not warranted, and alternative causes for the patient's symptoms should be considered.

A 12-year-old boy evaluated for acute appendicitis with intermediate clinical risk.

a. X-ray abdomen
b. US abdomen
c. CT abdomen and pelvis with contrast
d. MRI abdomen and pelvis without and with contrast
e. No ideal imaging exam

A child. Suspected acute appendicitis with intermediate clinical risk.

a. X-ray abdomen may be appropriate.
b. *US abdomen* is the most appropriate.
c. CT abdomen and pelvis with contrast may be appropriate.
d. MRI abdomen and pelvis without and with contrast may be appropriate.

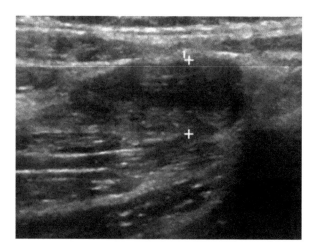

Fig. 8.18 Acute appendicitis. Abdomen US reveals an abnormally thickened blind ending loop of bowel (calipers) measuring 9 mm that does not deform with compression

Solution
Abdominal US is the preferred initial exam for a child with intermediate clinical risk of acute appendicitis. However, the performance characteristics of US are variable and dependent on the availability of operator expertise at the site. CT or MRI is the second-line imaging modality should US prove nondiagnostic.

An 11-year-old girl evaluated for acute appendicitis with high clinical risk.

a. X-ray abdomen
b. US abdomen
c. CT abdomen and pelvis with contrast
d. MRI abdomen and pelvis without and with contrast
e. No ideal imaging exam

A child. Suspected acute appendicitis with high clinical risk.

a. X-ray abdomen is usually not appropriate.
b. US abdomen may be appropriate.
c. CT abdomen and pelvis with contrast may be appropriate.
d. MRI abdomen and pelvis without and with contrast may be appropriate.
e. *No ideal imaging exam* is the correct answer.

Solution

Pediatric patients at high clinical risk of appendicitis may not require imaging before directly proceeding to surgical intervention. However, the management varies with site and surgeon. Imaging is sometimes used to confirm the diagnosis, to exclude other processes that can clinically mimic acute appendicitis, and to evaluate for complications such as perforation.

A 14-year-old boy evaluated for acute appendicitis with nondiagnostic right lower quadrant US. Next imaging exam.

a. X-ray abdomen
b. US pelvis
c. CT abdomen and pelvis with contrast
d. MRI abdomen and pelvis without and with contrast
e. No ideal imaging exam

A child. Suspected acute appendicitis with equivocal or nondiagnostic right lower quadrant US. Next imaging exam.

a. X-ray abdomen is usually not appropriate.
b. US pelvis is usually not appropriate.
c. *CT abdomen and pelvis with contrast* and choice (d) are equally the most appropriate.
d. *MRI abdomen and pelvis without and with contrast* and choice (c) are equally the most appropriate.

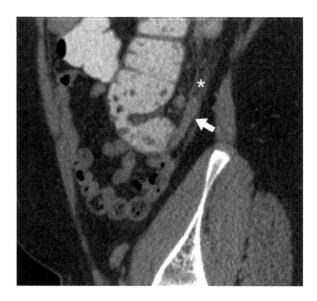

Fig. 8.19 Acute appendicitis. Abdomen and pelvis CT with contrast sagittal reconstruction image shows an enlarged retrocecal appendix (arrow) with adjacent fat stranding (star). The appendix could not be seen by US due to its position posterior to the cecum

Solution
Both CT and MRI are highly accurate for diagnosing acute appendicitis following a nondiagnostic US exam. A repeat US after an initially equivocal result increases sensitivity but is less accurate than CT or MRI.

A 10-year-old girl evaluated for acute appendicitis with right lower quadrant US suspicious for an abscess. Next imaging exam.

a. X-ray abdomen
b. CT abdomen and pelvis without contrast
c. CT abdomen and pelvis with contrast
d. MRI abdomen and pelvis without and with contrast
e. No ideal imaging exam

A child. Suspected acute appendicitis with clinical evaluation or initial imaging suggestive of complication (e.g., abscess, bowel obstruction). Next imaging exam.

a. X-ray abdomen is usually not appropriate.
b. CT abdomen and pelvis without contrast may be appropriate.
c. *CT abdomen and pelvis with contrast* is the most appropriate.
d. MRI abdomen and pelvis without and with contrast may be appropriate.

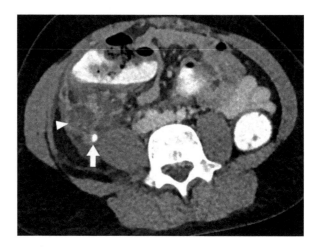

Fig. 8.20 Acute appendicitis with perforation. Abdomen and pelvis CT with contrast shows an appendicolith (arrow) with an adjacent abscess (arrowhead) from a perforated appendix

Solution
CT with contrast is the best exam to assess for complications of acute appendicitis including abscess and bowel obstruction.

8.8   Urinary Tract Infection

A 1-month-old boy with first episode of febrile urinary tract infection.

a. US kidneys and bladder
b. X-ray fluoroscopy voiding cystourethrography
c. Radionuclide cystography
d. Radionuclide renal cortical scintigraphy
e. No ideal imaging exam

Age <2 months, first febrile urinary tract infection.

a. *US kidneys and bladder* is the most appropriate.
b. X-ray fluoroscopy voiding cystourethrography may be appropriate.
c. Radionuclide cystography may be appropriate.
d. Radionuclide renal cortical scintigraphy is usually not appropriate.

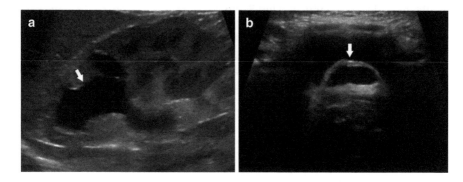

Fig. 8.21 Duplex collecting system, hydronephrosis and ureterocele. Sagittal US image of the right kidney (**a**) shows a duplex collecting system with dilatation of the upper pole (arrow). A transverse image of the bladder (**b**) from the same exam shows an ureterocele (arrow)

Solution

US is used to identify urinary tract anomalies such as hydronephrosis, duplex renal collecting system, hydroureter, and ureterocele. Voiding cystourethrography may be used to assess for vesicoureteral reflux and, in boys, a posterior urethral valve. Radionuclide cystography can also demonstrate reflux but does not demonstrate the urinary tract anomalies.

A 2-year-old girl with first episode of febrile urinary tract infection and good response to treatment.

a. US kidneys and bladder
b. X-ray fluoroscopy voiding cystourethrography
c. Radionuclide cystography
d. Radionuclide renal cortical scintigraphy
e. No ideal imaging exam

Age >2 months and ≤6 years, first febrile urinary tract infection with a good response to treatment.

a. *US kidneys and bladder* is the most appropriate.
b. X-ray fluoroscopy voiding cystourethrography may be appropriate.
c. Radionuclide cystography may be appropriate.
d. Radionuclide renal cortical scintigraphy is usually not appropriate.

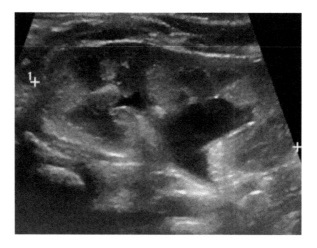

Fig. 8.22 Hydronephrosis. Sagittal US image of the left kidney (calipers) shows a dilated collecting system

Solution

In this age group, US is useful for detecting underlying congenital renal anomalies. Vesicoureteral reflux is better detected with voiding cystourethrography or radionuclide cystography.

A 9-year-old girl with the first episode of febrile urinary tract infection and good response to treatment.

a. US kidneys and bladder
b. X-ray fluoroscopy voiding cystourethrography
c. Radionuclide cystography
d. Radionuclide renal cortical scintigraphy
e. No ideal imaging exam

Age >6 years, first febrile urinary tract infection with good response to treatment.

a. US kidneys and bladder may be appropriate.
b. X-ray fluoroscopy voiding cystourethrography is usually not appropriate.
c. Radionuclide cystography is usually not appropriate.
d. Radionuclide renal cortical scintigraphy is usually not appropriate.
e. *No ideal imaging exam* is the correct answer.

Solution

Imaging is usually not indicated given the low likelihood of detecting unknown underlying renal anomalies in this age group.

A 2-year-old girl with recurrent febrile urinary tract infections.

a. US kidneys and bladder
b. X-ray fluoroscopy voiding cystourethrography
c. Radionuclide cystography
d. Radionuclide renal cortical scintigraphy
e. No ideal imaging exam

Child. Atypical (poor response to antibiotics within 48 h, sepsis, poor urine stream, raised creatinine, or non–*E. coli* organism) or recurrent febrile urinary tract infection.

a. *US kidneys and bladder* and choice (b) are equally the most appropriate.
b. *X-ray fluoroscopy voiding cystourethrography* and choice (a) are equally the most appropriate.
c. Radionuclide cystography is usually appropriate, but there is a better choice here.
d. Radionuclide renal cortical scintigraphy may be appropriate.

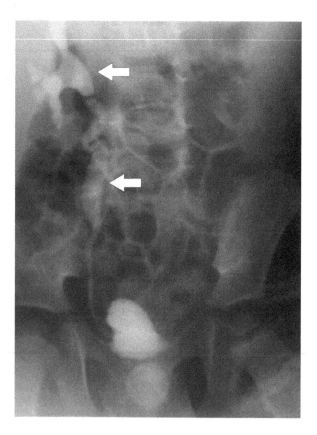

Fig. 8.23 Vesicoureteral reflux. Abdomen X-ray anteroposterior view from a voiding cystoure-throgram demonstrates contrast reflux into the right renal collecting system and ureter (arrows)

Solution
In this setting, US and voiding cystourethrography are complementary exams. US detects hydronephrosis, stones, or complications such as a renal or perirenal abscess. Cystourethrography evaluates for vesicoureteral reflux, which may require prophylactic antibiotic treatment or surgical intervention.

8.9 Hematuria

A 6-year-old boy with isolated episode of nonpainful microscopic hematuria without proteinuria. No history of trauma.

a. X-ray abdomen and pelvis
b. X-ray fluoroscopy voiding cystourethrography
c. US kidneys and bladder
d. CT abdomen and pelvis with contrast
e. No ideal imaging exam

Child. Isolated microscopic hematuria (nonpainful, nontraumatic) without proteinuria.

a. X-ray abdomen and pelvis is usually not appropriate.
b. X-ray fluoroscopy voiding cystourethrography is usually not appropriate.
c. US kidneys and bladder is usually not appropriate.
d. CT abdomen and pelvis with contrast is usually not appropriate.
e. *No ideal imaging exam* is the correct answer.

Solution

Imaging is usually not indicated in this scenario as these patients are unlikely to have clinically significant renal disease.

A 9-year-old boy with isolated episode of nonpainful microscopic hematuria with proteinuria. No history of trauma.

a. X-ray abdomen and pelvis
b. X-ray fluoroscopy voiding cystourethrography
c. US kidneys and bladder
d. CT abdomen and pelvis with contrast
e. No ideal imaging exam

Child. Isolated microscopic hematuria (nonpainful, nontraumatic) with proteinuria.

a. X-ray abdomen and pelvis is usually not appropriate.
b. X-ray fluoroscopy voiding cystourethrography is usually not appropriate.
c. *US kidneys and bladder* is the most appropriate.
d. CT abdomen and pelvis with contrast is usually not appropriate.

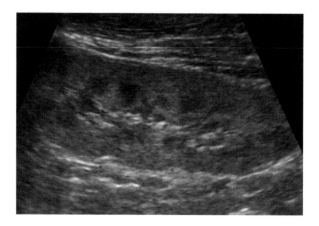

Fig. 8.24 Glomerulonephritis. Sagittal US image of the left kidney shows a diffusely echogenic cortex of normal thickness. Right kidney (not shown) appeared similar

Solution

US evaluates for findings of glomerulonephritis, such as increased echogenicity of the renal cortex. In the acute setting, the kidneys may also be enlarged. In long-standing glomerular disease, the kidneys become atrophic.

A 3-year-old girl with isolated episode of nonpainful macroscopic hematuria. No history of trauma.

a. X-ray abdomen and pelvis
b. X-ray fluoroscopy voiding cystourethrography
c. US kidneys and bladder
d. CT abdomen and pelvis with contrast
e. No ideal imaging exam

Child. Isolated macroscopic hematuria (nonpainful, nontraumatic).

a. X-ray abdomen and pelvis is usually not appropriate.
b. X-ray fluoroscopy voiding cystourethrography is usually not appropriate.
c. *US kidneys and bladder* is the most appropriate.
d. CT abdomen and pelvis with contrast is usually not appropriate.

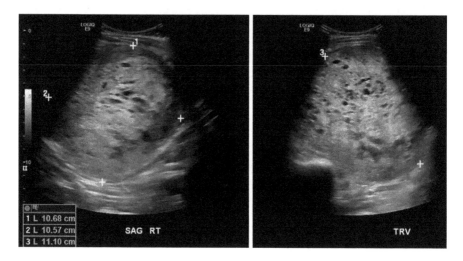

Fig. 8.25 Wilms tumor. Sagittal (left) and transverse (right) US images show a 11 cm predominantly solid mass (calipers) that has replaced much of the right kidney

Solution

US evaluates for nephrolithiasis, underlying urologic abnormalities, and, rarely, renal or bladder tumors as causes of macroscopic hematuria. A renal or bladder mass that is found by US may require additional imaging with CT or MRI.

An 11-year-old girl with painful hematuria and no history of trauma. Urolithiasis is suspected.

a. X-ray abdomen and pelvis
b. US kidneys and bladder
c. CT abdomen and pelvis without contrast
d. CT abdomen and pelvis with contrast
e. No ideal imaging exam

Child. Painful hematuria (nontraumatic). Suspected urolithiasis.

a. X-ray abdomen and pelvis may be appropriate.
b. *US kidneys and bladder* and choice (c) are equally the most appropriate.
c. *CT abdomen and pelvis without contrast* and choice (b) are equally the most appropriate.
d. CT abdomen and pelvis with contrast is usually not appropriate.

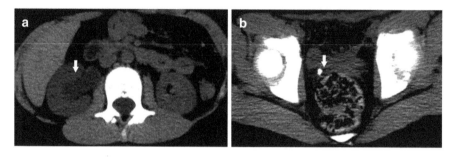

Fig. 8.26 Obstructive urolithiasis. Abdomen and pelvis CT without contrast image of the kidneys (**a**) shows right hydronephrosis (arrow). Image of the bladder (**b**) shows a stone (arrow) at the right ureterovesicle junction

Solution

CT is the most accurate imaging exam for urolithiasis. US is less sensitive than CT but can serve as the initial exam. However, a negative US does not exclude urolithiasis, and CT may still be needed.

A 15-year-old boy with macroscopic hematuria following trauma.

a. X-ray abdomen and pelvis
b. US kidneys and bladder
c. CT abdomen and pelvis without contrast
d. CT abdomen and pelvis with contrast
e. No ideal imaging exam

Child. Traumatic hematuria (macroscopic).

a. X-ray abdomen and pelvis is usually not appropriate.
b. US kidneys and bladder is usually not appropriate.
c. CT abdomen and pelvis without contrast is usually not appropriate.
d. *CT abdomen and pelvis with contrast* is the most appropriate.

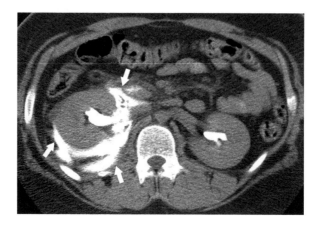

Fig. 8.27 Ureteral injury. Abdomen and pelvis CT with contrast during the excretory phase demonstrates urine leaking (arrows) outside the collecting system

Solution

Contrast-enhanced CT is the best imaging exam to evaluate for renal trauma. If renal injury is found, then delayed post-contrast imaging should be performed to assess the integrity of the urinary collecting system.

A 16-year-old boy with microscopic hematuria following trauma.

a. X-ray abdomen and pelvis
b. US kidneys and bladder
c. CT abdomen and pelvis without contrast
d. CT abdomen and pelvis with contrast
e. No ideal imaging exam

Child. Traumatic hematuria (microscopic).

a. X-ray abdomen and pelvis is usually not appropriate.
b. US kidneys and bladder may be appropriate.
c. CT abdomen and pelvis without contrast is usually not appropriate.
d. *CT abdomen and pelvis with contrast* is the most appropriate.

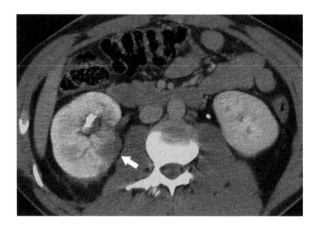

Fig. 8.28 Renal injury. Abdomen and pelvis CT with contrast demonstrates a hematoma in the right renal cortex (arrow)

Solution
In children, the relationship between posttraumatic microscopic hematuria and renal trauma is not well-established. Contrast-enhanced CT is the preferred imaging exam to evaluate for renal trauma. However, its use should be guided by mechanism of injury and clinical exam and not be based on urinalysis alone.

8.10   Developmental Dysplasia of the Hip

A 3-week-old girl with equivocal physical exam findings (Ortolani and Barlow maneuvers).

a. X-ray pelvis
b. US hips
c. CT pelvis without contrast
d. MRI pelvis without contrast
e. No ideal imaging exam

Child younger than 4 weeks of age with equivocal physical findings or risk factors.

a. X-ray pelvis is usually not appropriate.
b. US hips is usually not appropriate.
c. CT pelvis without contrast is usually not appropriate.
d. MRI pelvis without contrast is usually not appropriate.
e. *No ideal imaging exam* is the correct answer.

Solution

In this age group, hip abnormalities may simply reflect physiologic laxity and immaturity. The vast majority will spontaneously normalize. Additionally, a short delay in intervention has no negative impact on outcome, whereas false-positive results may risk overtreatment.

A 2-month-old boy with equivocal physical exam findings (Ortolani and Barlow maneuvers).

a. X-ray pelvis
b. US hips
c. CT pelvis without contrast
d. MRI pelvis without contrast
e. No ideal imaging exam

A child between 4 weeks and 4 months of age with equivocal physical findings or risk factors.

a. X-ray pelvis is usually not appropriate.
b. *US hips* is the most appropriate.
c. CT pelvis without contrast is usually not appropriate.
d. MRI pelvis without contrast is usually not appropriate.

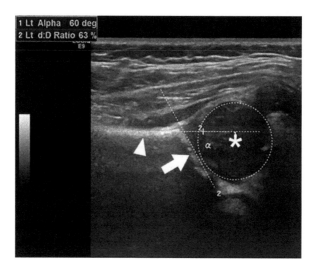

Fig. 8.29 Normal hip. Coronal image from a hip US shows a normal relationship between the femoral head (star), acetabular roof (arrow), and iliac bone (arrowhead)

Solution

In this setting, US assessment for developmental dysplasia of the hip expedites diagnosis and decreases the need for eventual surgical intervention. The US exam includes imaging of the hip joint at stasis according to a morphologic geometric classification scheme and imaging with hip movement to evaluate for femoral head instability.

A 3-month-old girl with suspected developmental dysplasia of the hip. Physical exam findings (Ortolani and Barlow maneuvers) are positive.

a. X-ray pelvis
b. US hips
c. CT pelvis without contrast
d. MRI pelvis without contrast
e. No ideal imaging exam

A child younger than 4 months of age with positive physical exam findings.

a. X-ray pelvis is usually not appropriate.
b. *US hips* is the most appropriate.
c. CT pelvis without contrast is usually not appropriate.
d. MRI pelvis without contrast is usually not appropriate.

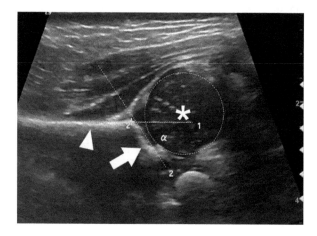

Fig. 8.30 Developmental dysplasia of the hip. Coronal image from a hip US shows insufficient coverage of the femoral head (star) by the acetabular roof (arrow), which has an abnormally shallow angle to the iliac bone (arrowhead)

Solution

In this age group, US is the best imaging exam to confirm a clinically suspected diagnosis and reduce false-positive physical examinations that could lead to overtreatment.

A 11-month-old girl with suspected developmental dysplasia of the hip.

a. X-ray pelvis
b. US hips
c. CT pelvis without contrast
d. MRI pelvis without contrast
e. No ideal imaging exam

A child older than 4 months of age with concern for developmental dysplasia of the hip.

a. *X-ray pelvis* is the most appropriate.
b. US hips may be appropriate between 4 and 6 months of age and is usually not appropriate after 6 months of age.
c. CT pelvis without contrast is usually not appropriate.
d. MRI pelvis without contrast is usually not appropriate.

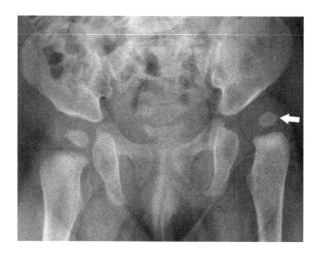

Fig. 8.31 Developmental dysplasia of the hip. Hip X-ray anteroposterior view shows abnormal left acetabular shape and superior and lateral displacement of the left femoral head (arrow)

Solution

US becomes less useful for diagnosis of hip dysplasia after 4 months of age and is not recommended after 6 months. Radiography becomes the preferred imaging exam to image the ossifying femoral head, the proximal femur, and the acetabular morphology.

8.11 Acutely Limping Child Up to Age 5

A 2-year-old girl with a new limp and nonlocalized symptoms. There is no concern for an infection.

a. X-ray femur
b. X-ray tibia and fibula
c. US hips
d. MRI lower extremity without contrast
e. No ideal imaging exam

A child up to age 5. Acute limp. Nonlocalized symptoms. No concern for infection.

a. X-ray femur may be appropriate.
b. *X-ray tibia and fibula* is the most appropriate.
c. US hips is usually not appropriate.
d. MRI lower extremity without contrast is usually not appropriate.

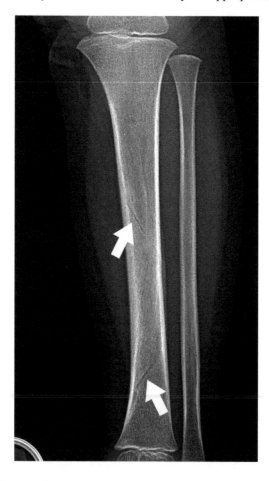

Fig. 8.32 Spiral fracture of the tibia. Tibia and fibula X-ray anteroposterior view shows a spiral fracture (arrows) along the tibia

Solution
The most common cause of acute limping in this age group is minor traumatic injury. Lower extremity radiographs are often normal. When fractures are present, most are spiral fractures of the tibia. Thus, initial imaging should be limited to the tibia and fibula. If this is negative and symptoms persist, then additional imaging elsewhere along the lower extremity may be appropriate.

A 3-year-old boy with a new limp, nonlocalized symptoms, and a fever. There is concern for an infection.

a. X-ray tibia and fibula
b. US hips
c. MRI lower extremity without contrast
d. Tc-99m three-phase bone scan whole body
e. No ideal imaging exam

A child up to age 5. Acute limp. Nonlocalized symptoms. There is concern for infection.

a. X-ray tibia and fibula is usually not appropriate.
b. US hips may be appropriate.
c. *MRI lower extremity without contrast* is the most appropriate.
d. Tc-99m three-phase bone scan whole body may be appropriate.

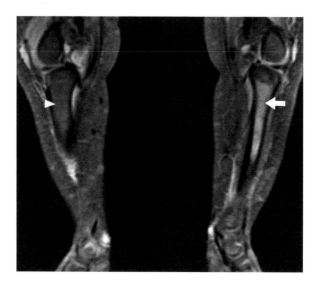

Fig. 8.33 Osteomyelitis. Lower extremity MR coronal T2-weighted image shows abnormal bone marrow signal in the left tibia (arrow), compared to normal marrow signal in the right tibia (arrowhead)

Solution
Imaging helps confirm the diagnosis, localize the site of infection, identify complications that may need surgical intervention, and rule out pathologies that can mimic infection. MRI is the best modality to assess the soft-tissue and bone marrow for pathology. Use of contrast is not necessary but may help better delineate abscesses and, in infants, improve detection of epiphyseal infections.

A 2-year-old boy with a new limp, symptoms that localize to the hip, and a fever. There is concern for an infection.

a. X-ray pelvis
b. US hips
c. CT pelvis without contrast
d. MRI pelvis without contrast
e. No ideal imaging exam

A child up to age 5. Acute limp. Symptoms localized to the hip. There is concern for infection.

a. X-ray pelvis may be appropriate.
b. *US hips* and choice (d) are equally the most appropriate.
c. CT pelvis without contrast is usually not appropriate.
d. *MRI pelvis* without contrast and choice (b) are equally the most appropriate.

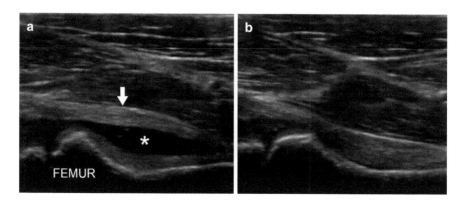

Fig. 8.34 Hip joint effusion. Sagittal oblique US image of the left hip (**a**) shows an effusion (star) within the joint capsule (arrow). A normal right hip (**b**) is shown for comparison

Solution
The primary clinical concern in this scenario is septic arthritis of the hip. US can diagnose hip joint effusions accurately and guide aspiration. MRI can also be used for initial evaluation as it delineates findings of septic arthritis, osteomyelitis, and soft tissue abscess. Analysis of aspirated joint fluid is needed for definitive diagnosis of septic arthritis.

8.12   **Suspected Physical Abuse**

A 1-year-old girl suspected to be a victim of physical abuse with no clinical suspicion for neurological or visceral injury.

a. X-ray skeletal survey
b. CT head without contrast
c. MRI head without contrast
d. Tc-99m bone scan whole body
e. No ideal imaging exam

A child ≤24 months of age. Neurological or visceral injuries are not clinically suspected.

a. *X-ray skeletal survey* is the most appropriate.
b. CT head without contrast may be appropriate.
c. MRI head without contrast may be appropriate.
d. Tc-99m bone scan whole body may be appropriate.

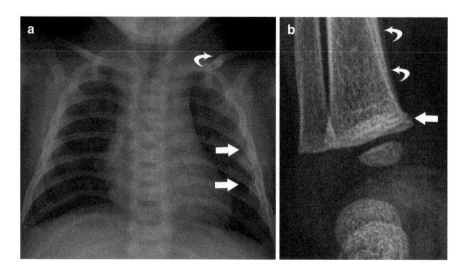

Fig. 8.35 Child abuse. Skeletal survey chest X-ray (**a**) shows healing left rib (straight arrow) and clavicular (curved arrow) fractures. Ankle X-ray (**b**) shows a distal tibial metaphyseal corner fracture (straight arrow) with periosteal reaction (curved arrows)

Solution
Radiographic skeletal surveys are recommended given the high frequency of fractures in physically abused children. Fractures that are highly specific for non-accidental trauma include posterior rib fractures and classic metaphyseal lesions or epiphyseal separation injuries. When there is a high suspicion for abuse and an initial skeletal survey is negative, a more focused skeletal survey should be performed after 2 weeks.

A 1-year-old girl suspected to be a victim of physical abuse with neurologic symptoms.

a. X-ray skeletal survey
b. CT head without contrast
c. MRI head without contrast
d. Tc-99m bone scan whole body
e. No ideal imaging exam

A child with one or more of the following: neurologic signs or symptoms, apnea, complex skull fracture, other fractures, or injuries highly suspicious for child abuse.

a. *X-ray skeletal survey* and choice (b) are equally the most appropriate.
b. *CT head without contrast* and choice (a) are equally the most appropriate.
c. MRI head without contrast is usually appropriate, but there is a better choice here.
d. Tc-99m bone scan whole body may be appropriate.

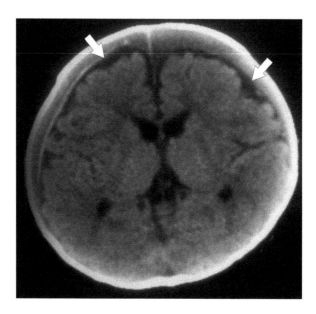

Fig. 8.36 Child abuse. Head CT without contrast demonstrates bilateral subdural hematomas (arrows)

Solution
Although less common than skeletal injuries, most child abuse fatalities are the result of head trauma. Non-contrast head CT should be immediately performed when there is concern for head trauma. Skeletal survey is also recommended for all children <2 years of age.

A 3-year-old girl suspected to be a victim of physical abuse with concern for abdominopelvic injury.

a. X-ray skeletal survey
b. CT abdomen and pelvis without contrast
c. CT abdomen and pelvis with contrast
d. Tc-99m bone scan whole body
e. No ideal imaging exam

A child with suspected thoracic or abdominopelvic injuries (e.g., abdominal skin bruises, distension, tenderness, or elevated liver or pancreatic enzymes).

a. *X-ray skeletal survey* and choice (c) are equally the most appropriate.
b. CT abdomen and pelvis without contrast is usually not appropriate.
c. *CT abdomen and pelvis with contrast* and choice (a) are equally the most appropriate.
d. Tc-99m bone scan whole body may be appropriate.

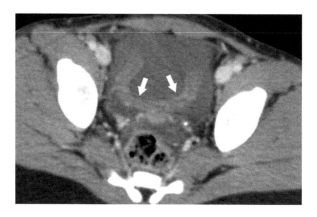

Fig. 8.37 Child abuse. Abdomen and pelvis CT with contrast shows a large hematoma (arrows) in the bladder

Solution
Contrast-enhanced abdominopelvic CT is the best imaging exam for suspected intra-abdominal injuries. Thoracic injury other than rib fractures is uncommon and can be assessed on a concurrent chest CT. Since thoracic or abdominopelvic injury is associated with polytrauma, a skeletal survey is recommended for children <2 years old and should also be considered in older children.

Bibliography

Kuppermann N, et al. Identification of children at very low risk of clinically important brain injuries after head trauma: a prospective cohort study. Lancet. 2009;374(9696):1160–70.

Teasdale G, Jennett B. Assessment of coma and impaired consciousness. Lancet. 1974;2(7872): 81–4.

Vascular Imaging

9

9.1 Penetrating Neck Injury

A 28-year-old man with a penetrating injury to the neck and subcutaneous emphysema.

a. X-ray neck
b. US neck
c. CTA neck
d. Angiography neck
e. No ideal imaging exam

Penetrating neck injury with soft clinical signs of aerodigestive or vascular injury, including non-pulsatile or non-expanding hematoma, venous oozing, dysphagia, dysphonia, and subcutaneous emphysema.

a. X-ray neck is usually appropriate, but there is a better choice here.
b. US neck may be appropriate.
c. *CTA neck* is the most appropriate.
d. Angiography neck may be appropriate.

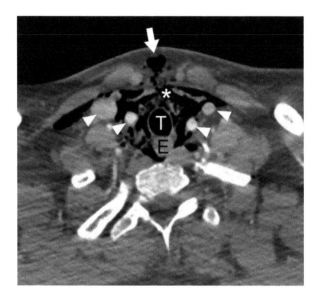

Fig. 9.1 Penetrating neck injury. Neck CTA shows a stab wound (arrow) at anterior midline with air in the soft tissues (star). There is no injury to the major vessels (arrowheads), trachea (T), or esophagus (E)

Solution

Hard clinical signs of vascular or aerodigestive injury such as active hemorrhage, hemodynamic instability, or airway compromise often necessitate immediate surgical exploration. For patients with soft signs, further imaging with CTA of the neck is usually indicated. CTA is highly accurate for the evaluation of vascular, aerodigestive, and extravascular soft tissue injuries.

A 31-year-old woman with a penetrating injury to the neck. CTA is equivocal, and there is a persistent concern for vascular injury.

a. US neck
b. MRA neck without contrast
c. MRA neck without and with contrast
d. Angiography neck
e. No ideal imaging exam

Penetrating neck injury with a normal or equivocal CTA and concern for vascular injury.

a. US neck may be appropriate.
b. MRA neck without contrast may be appropriate.
c. MRA neck without and with contrast may be appropriate.
d. *Angiography neck* is the most appropriate.

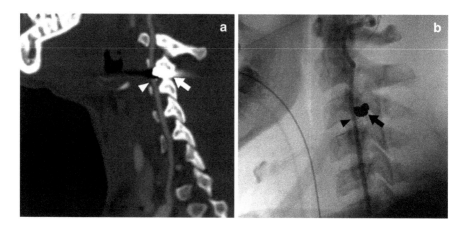

Fig. 9.2 Penetrating neck injury. Neck CTA sagittal reconstruction image (**a**) and neck angiogram sagittal view (**b**) show a bullet fragment (arrow) within the cervical spine. The adjacent vertebral artery (arrowhead) was not well-evaluated by CTA due to beam hardening artifact from the bullet fragment. Angiography shows that it is uninjured

Solution
Catheter angiography is used to evaluate patients with a concerning penetrating foreign body trajectory where the CTA is normal or equivocal or when endovascular therapy is planned. The accuracy of CTA is sometimes limited by beam hardening artifact from metallic foreign bodies.

A 21-year-old woman with a penetrating injury to the neck. CTA is equivocal, and there is persistent concern for aerodigestive injury.

a. X-ray single-contrast esophagram
b. US neck
c. MRI neck without and with contrast
d. Angiography neck
e. No ideal imaging exam

Penetrating neck injury with a normal or equivocal CTA and concern for aerodigestive injury.

a. *X-ray single-contrast esophagram* is the most appropriate.
b. US neck is usually not appropriate.
c. MRI without and with contrast neck may be appropriate.
d. Angiography neck is usually not appropriate.

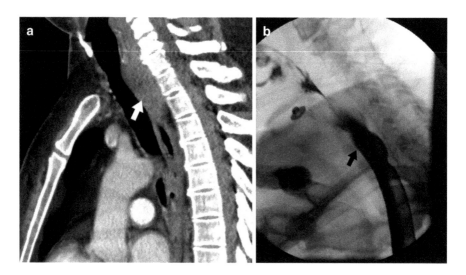

Fig. 9.3 Penetrating neck injury. Neck CTA sagittal reconstruction image (**a**) shows a hematoma
along the upper esophageal wall (arrow) concerning for injury. Single-contrast esophagram (**b**)
shows an intact upper esophagus (arrow)

Solution
Evaluation for aerodigestive injury is best performed with a combination of laryn-
goscopy, bronchoscopy, and esophagoscopy (flexible and rigid). X-ray single-
contrast esophagram may be useful in conjunction with these direct visualization
techniques. Water-soluble contrast is indicated due to risk of extraluminal contrast
extravasation.

9.2   Suspected Pulmonary Arteriovenous Malformation

A 29-year-old woman with clinically suspected pulmonary arteriovenous malformation.

a. X-ray chest
b. US echocardiography transthoracic bubble study
c. CTA chest
d. Angiography pulmonary
e. No ideal imaging exam

Clinically suspected pulmonary arteriovenous malformation.

a. X-ray chest is usually appropriate, but there is a better choice here.
b. *US echocardiography transthoracic bubble study* and choice (c) are equally the most appropriate.
c. *CTA chest* and choice (b) are equally the most appropriate. CTA is often performed after positive transthoracic echocardiography.
d. Angiography pulmonary may be appropriate.

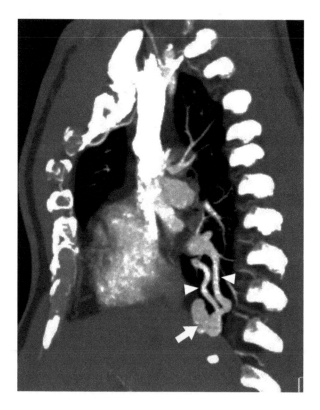

Fig. 9.4 Pulmonary arteriovenous malformation. Chest CTA sagittal MIP image shows the nidus of an arteriovenous malformation (arrow) in the right lower lobe with a feeding artery and draining vein (arrowheads)

Solution
Transthoracic echocardiography bubble study is often used for initial evaluation of or screening for a suspected pulmonary arteriovenous malformation. CTA is usually performed after a positive echocardiogram to obtain detailed anatomic information, such as lesion size and location.

9.3   Thoracic Aortic Aneurysm

A 68-year-old woman suspected with thoracic aortic aneurysm.

a. CT chest without contrast
b. CT chest with contrast
c. CTA chest
d. MRA chest without and with contrast
e. No ideal imaging exam

Thoracic aortic aneurysm is suspected.

a. CT chest without contrast may be appropriate.
b. CT chest with contrast is usually not appropriate.
c. *CTA chest* and choice (d) are equally the most appropriate.
d. *MRA chest without and with contrast* and choice (c) are equally the most appropriate.

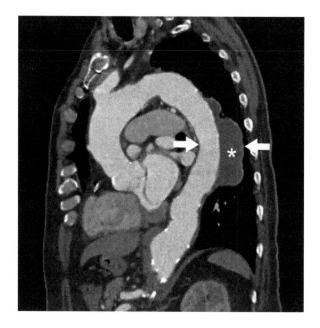

Fig. 9.5 Thoracic aortic aneurysm. Chest CTA sagittal oblique reconstruction image shows an aneurysm of the descending thoracic aorta (between arrows) with a mural thrombus (star)

Solution

CTA and MRA are both equally appropriate for the diagnosis of suspected thoracic aortic aneurysm.

9.4   Pulsatile Abdominal Mass

A 79-year-old man with a pulsatile abdominal mass on physical exam. An abdominal aortic aneurysm is suspected.

a. US abdominal aorta
b. CT abdomen without contrast
c. CTA abdomen
d. MRA abdomen without and with contrast
e. No ideal imaging exam

Abdominal aortic aneurysm is suspected.

a. *US abdominal aorta* is the most appropriate.
b. CT abdomen without contrast is usually appropriate, but there is a better choice here.
c. CTA abdomen is usually appropriate, but there is a better choice here.
d. MRA abdomen without and with contrast is usually appropriate, but there is a better choice here.

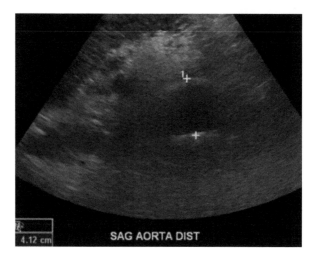

Fig. 9.6 Abdominal aortic aneurysm. Abdomen ultrasound sagittal view of the aorta shows a 4.1 cm infrarenal abdominal aortic aneurysm (calipers)

Solution
Dedicated US evaluation of the abdominal aorta is the preferred initial imaging exam for suspected abdominal aortic aneurysm. Non-contrast CT is an alternative when US imaging is limited by patient body habitus. CTA and MRA are recommended for definitive diagnosis, characterization, and intervention planning.

9.5 Mesenteric Ischemia

A 70-year-old woman with suspected acute mesenteric ischemia.

a. US abdomen with Doppler
b. CTA abdomen and pelvis
c. MRA abdomen and pelvis without and with contrast
d. Angiography abdomen
e. No ideal imaging exam

Acute mesenteric ischemia is suspected.

a. US abdomen with Doppler may be appropriate.
b. *CTA abdomen and pelvis* is the most appropriate.
c. MRA abdomen and pelvis without and with contrast may be appropriate.
d. Angiography abdomen may be appropriate.

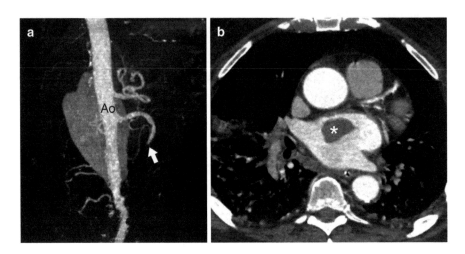

Fig. 9.7 Superior mesenteric artery occlusion. Abdomen CTA sagittal oblique MIP image (**a**) shows an abrupt cut-off of the superior mesenteric artery (arrow) due to embolic occlusion. Chest CTA (**b**) performed at the same time shows a thrombus (star) within the left atrium, the likely source of the embolus. *Ao* abdominal aorta

Solution
CTA enables fast, accurate, and noninvasive evaluation of the bowels and intestinal vasculature and assesses for alternative causes of acute abdominal pain. MRA assesses the vessels but, as it is motion sensitive, offers less detailed evaluation of bowel.

A 72-year-old man with suspected chronic mesenteric ischemia.

a. US abdomen with Doppler
b. CTA abdomen and pelvis
c. MRA abdomen and pelvis without and with contrast
d. Angiography abdomen
e. No ideal imaging exam

Chronic mesenteric ischemia is suspected.

a. US abdomen with Doppler may be appropriate.
b. *CTA abdomen and pelvis* and choice (c) are equally the most appropriate.
c. *MRA abdomen and pelvis without and with contrast* and choice (b) are equally the most appropriate.
d. Angiography abdomen may be appropriate.

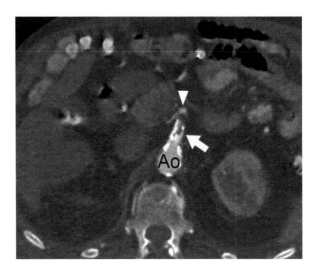

Fig. 9.8 Superior mesenteric artery stenosis. Abdomen CTA shows atherosclerosis with severe stenosis of the superior mesenteric artery (arrow) just distal to its origin. Blood flow is present (arrowhead) beyond the stenotic segment. *Ao* abdominal aorta

Solution

CTA and MRA are both recommended for the evaluation of chronic mesenteric ischemia. CTA is the more accurate of these two exams for grading mesenteric vessel stenosis and can also help assess for other causes of chronic abdominal pain.

9.6   Suspected Upper Extremity Deep Vein Thrombosis

A 48-year-old man with suspected upper extremity deep venous thrombosis.

a. US upper extremity with Doppler
b. CTA upper extremity
c. MRA upper extremity without and with contrast
d. Angiography upper extremity
e. No ideal imaging exam

Suspected upper extremity deep venous thrombosis.

a. *US upper extremity with Doppler* is the most appropriate.
b. CTA upper extremity may be appropriate.
c. MRA upper extremity without and with contrast may be appropriate.
d. Angiography upper extremity is usually not appropriate.

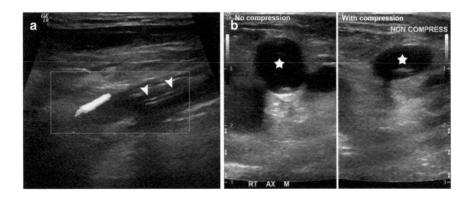

Fig. 9.9 Right arm deep venous thrombosis. Right upper extremity US Doppler image of the subclavian vein (**a**) demonstrates no blood flow and a catheter (arrowheads) in place. Gray scale images (**b**) show a non-compressible right axillary vein (stars) indicating intraluminal thrombus

Solution

US can be performed at the bedside and is well-suited for serial evaluation. On US, thrombosis is identified as echogenic material in the venous lumen, a non-compressible vessel, or abnormal blood flow.

9.7   Suspected Lower Extremity Deep Vein Thrombosis

A 72-year-old woman with suspected lower extremity deep venous thrombosis.

a. US lower extremity with Doppler
b. CTA lower extremity and pelvis
c. MRA lower extremity and pelvis without and with contrast
d. Angiography lower extremity and pelvis
e. No ideal imaging exam

Suspected lower extremity deep venous thrombosis.

a. *US lower extremity with Doppler* is the most appropriate.
b. CTA lower extremity and pelvis may be appropriate.
c. MRA lower extremity and pelvis without and with contrast may be appropriate.
d. Angiography lower extremity and pelvis is usually not appropriate.

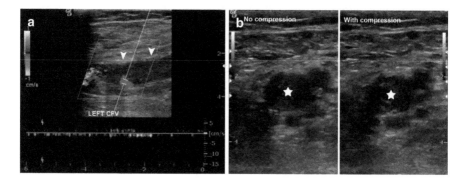

Fig. 9.10 Left leg deep venous thrombosis. Left lower extremity US Doppler image (**a**) demonstrates no blood flow (arrowheads) in the common femoral vein which on gray scale images (**b**) is non-compressible (stars) indicating intraluminal thrombus

Solution

US can be performed at the bedside and is well-suited for serial evaluation. On US, thrombosis is identified as echogenic material in the venous lumen, a non-compressible vessel, or abnormal blood flow. US accuracy is limited above the inguinal canal and below the knee.

9.8   Sudden Onset of Cold, Painful Leg

An 83-year-old woman with a history of left femoral artery stent, now presents with sudden onset of a cold painful leg.

a. US lower extremity with Doppler
b. CTA lower extremity
c. MRA lower extremity without and with contrast
d. Angiography lower extremity
e. No ideal imaging exam

Sudden onset of cold, painful leg.

a. US lower extremity with Doppler may be appropriate.
b. CTA lower extremity is usually appropriate, but there is a better choice here.
c. MRA lower extremity without and with contrast is usually appropriate, but there is a better choice here.
d. *Angiography lower extremity* is the most appropriate.

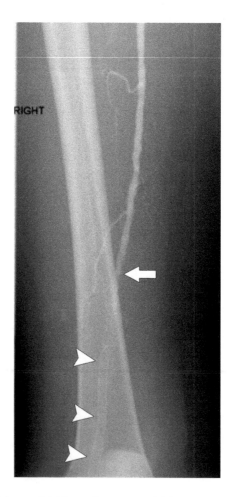

Fig. 9.11 Occluded left superficial femoral artery stent. Right leg angiogram with contrast injection proximal to the stent reveals lack of contrast flow (arrow) into the stent (arrowheads)

Solution
Angiography is the most accurate exam for the detection of peripheral vascular occlusive disease and allows for therapeutic intervention during the same procedure.

9.9   Vascular Claudication

A 73-year-old man with claudication and abnormal noninvasive hemodynamic tests. Assessment for revascularization is needed.

a. US lower extremity with Doppler
b. CTA lower extremity
c. MRA lower extremity without and with contrast
d. Angiography lower extremity
e. No ideal imaging exam

Assessment for revascularization.

a. US lower extremity with Doppler is usually appropriate, but there is a better choice here.
b. *CTA lower extremity* and choice (c) are equally the most appropriate.
c. *MRA lower extremity without and with contrast* and choice (b) are equally the most appropriate.
d. Angiography lower extremity is usually appropriate, but there is a better choice here.

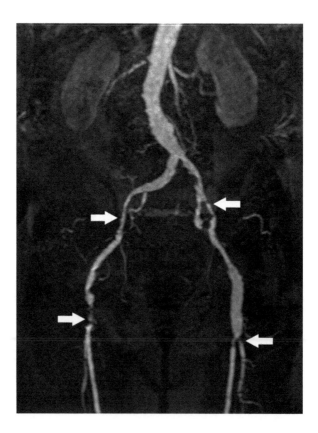

Fig. 9.12 Bilateral lower extremity atherosclerosis. Lower extremity MRA coronal MIP image shows irregular caliber of the iliac and superficial femoral arteries with segments of severe stenosis (arrows)

Solution
Noninvasive hemodynamic tests such as the ankle brachial index, segmental pressures, and pulse volume recordings are used for the initial evaluation of claudication. When these tests are positive, CTA or MRA is performed to characterize lesions and triage patients for medical, percutaneous endovascular, or surgical intervention.

Musculoskeletal Imaging

10

10.1 Suspected Spine Trauma

10.1.1 NEXUS Criteria

Cervical spine imaging is recommended in trauma patients unless they meet all of the following criteria:

- No posterior midline cervical spine tenderness
- No evidence of intoxication
- Normal level of alertness
- No focal neurological deficit
- No clinically apparent painful injuries that might distract from pain of a cervical spine injury

Hoffman et al. 2000

© The Author(s), under exclusive license to Springer Nature
Switzerland AG 2021
G. X. Wang et al., *Choosing the Correct Radiologic Test*,
https://doi.org/10.1007/978-3-030-65185-5_10

10.1.2 Canadian C-Spine Rules (CCR)

For alert (Glasgow Coma Scale Score = 15) and stable trauma patients, imaging for suspected cervical spine injury is not necessary if all of the following three criteria are met:

1. Absence of any of the following high-risk factors:
   a. Age ≥65 years
   b. Dangerous mechanism—fall from an elevation of ≥3 ft or five stairs, axial load to the head (e.g., diving), motor vehicle collision at high speed or with rollover or ejection, collision involving a motorized recreational vehicle, or bicycle collision
   c. Paresthesia in the extremities
2. Presence of any of the following low-risk factors that allow safe assessment of range of motion:
   a. Simple rear-end motor vehicle collision—excludes being pushed into oncoming traffic; being hit by a bus, a large truck, or a high-speed vehicle; or a rollover
   b. Sitting position in emergency department
   c. Ambulatory at any time
   d. Delayed onset of neck pain
   e. No midline cervical spine tenderness
3. Able to actively rotate neck 45° left and right

Stiell et al. 2001

A 23-year-old man with suspected cervical spine trauma after a low-speed motor vehicle collision and complaining of neck pain. There are no other clinically apparent injuries. He is alert and sitting upright and does not appear intoxicated. On exam, no point tenderness over posterior midline of spine or focal neurologic deficit is elicited. He can actively rotate his neck.

a. X-ray cervical spine
b. CT cervical spine without contrast
c. CT cervical spine with contrast
d. MRI cervical spine without contrast
e. No ideal imaging exam

Age ≥ 16 years and less than 65 years. Suspected acute blunt cervical spine trauma; imaging not indicated by NEXUS or CCR clinical decision rules.

a. X-ray cervical spine is usually not appropriate.
b. CT cervical spine without contrast is usually not appropriate.
c. CT cervical spine with contrast is usually not appropriate.
d. MRI cervical spine without contrast is usually not appropriate.
e. *No ideal imaging exam* is the correct answer.

Solution
Trauma patients classified as low risk by NEXUS or CCR clinical decision rules typically do not need imaging of the cervical spine. However, because sensitivity of NEXUS criteria declines in elderly patients, imaging may be considered for all blunt trauma patients 65 years of age or older, including those who would otherwise be classified as low risk.

A 33-year-old man with suspected cervical spine trauma after a high-speed motor vehicle accident complaining of neck pain. On exam, point tenderness over posterior midline of spine is elicited.

a. X-ray cervical spine
b. CT cervical spine without contrast
c. CT cervical spine with contrast
d. MRI cervical spine without contrast
e. No ideal imaging exam

Age ≥16 years. Suspected acute cervical spine blunt trauma. Imaging indicated by either NEXUS or CCR clinical criteria.

a. X-ray cervical spine may be appropriate.
b. *CT cervical spine without contrast* is the most appropriate.
c. CT cervical spine with contrast is usually not appropriate.
d. MRI cervical spine without contrast is usually not appropriate.

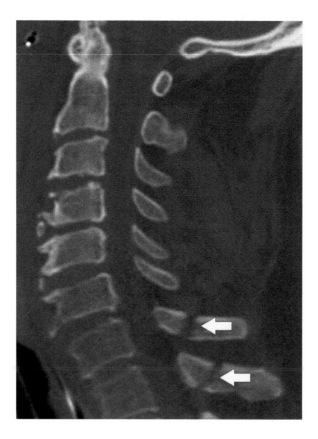

Fig. 10.1 Cervical spine fracture. Cervical spine CT sagittal reconstruction image shows C7 and T1 spinous process fractures (arrows)

Solution

CT is the best imaging exam for identification of cervical spine fractures. Though radiographs have largely been supplanted by CT, a single upright lateral cervical spine radiograph may be useful if the cervical spine CT images are motion degraded. If the region affected by motion is normal on radiography, then repeat CT may not be needed.

A 33-year-old man with cervical spine fracture seen on CT after a high-speed motor vehicle accident and suspected spinal cord injury. Next imaging exam.

a. CTA head and neck
b. CT myelography cervical spine
c. MRI cervical spine without contrast
d. MRI cervical spine without and with contrast
e. No ideal imaging exam

Age ≥16 years. Suspected acute cervical spine blunt trauma. Confirmed or suspected cervical spinal cord or nerve root injury, with or without traumatic injury identified on cervical CT. Next imaging exam.

a. CTA head and neck is usually not appropriate.
b. CT myelography cervical spine may be appropriate.
c. *MRI cervical spine without contrast* is the most appropriate.
d. MRI cervical spine without and with contrast is usually not appropriate.

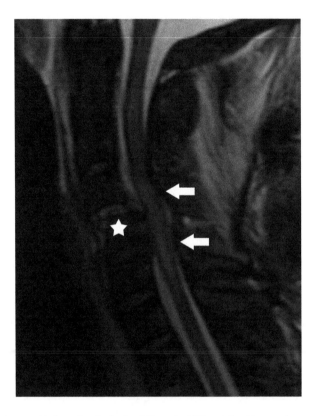

Fig. 10.2 Spinal cord injury. Cervical spine MR sagittal T2-weighted image shows cord compression and edema (arrows) secondary to a C5 fracture (star)

Solution
MRI is the best imaging exam for assessing the cause and extent of spinal cord injury. While CT is the preferred modality for initial assessment of cervical spine injury, it is inferior to MRI for soft tissue pathologies such as spinal cord contusion and nerve root avulsion.

A 47-year-old woman with acute cervical spine injury detected on radiographs after a high-speed motor vehicle accident. Treatment planning for mechanically unstable spine is required.

a. CT cervical spine without contrast
b. CT cervical spine with contrast
c. MRI cervical spine without contrast
d. MRI cervical spine without and with contrast
e. No ideal imaging exam

Age ≥16 years. Acute cervical spine injury detected on radiographs. Treatment planning for mechanically unstable spine.

a. *CT cervical spine without contrast* and choice (c) are equally the most appropriate.
b. CT cervical spine with contrast is usually not appropriate.
c. *MRI cervical spine without contrast* and choice (a) are equally the most appropriate.
d. MRI cervical spine without and with contrast is usually not appropriate.

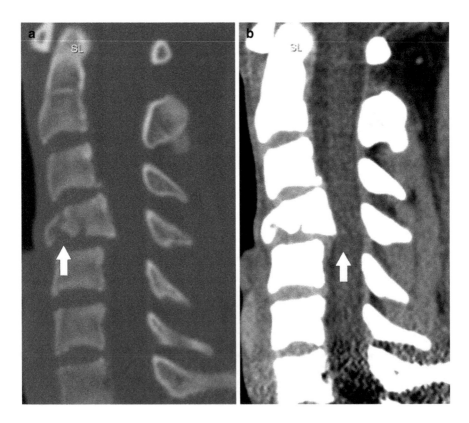

Fig. 10.3 Unstable cervical spine fracture. Cervical spine CT sagittal reconstruction image in bone window (**a**) shows a flexion teardrop-type C4 vertebral body fracture (arrow) and in soft tissue window (**b**) shows a narrowed spinal canal (arrow), concerning for cord compression

Solution
In a patient with an unstable cervical spine injury, CT and MRI are complementary, and both may be performed preoperatively. CT characterizes the bone, and MRI assesses the soft tissues such as the cord, nerve roots, discs, and ligaments.

A 54-year-old man with suspected cervical spine trauma after a motor vehicle accident. Clinical exam and cervical spine CT raise concern for arterial injury.

a. CTA head and neck
b. MRA neck without contrast
c. MRA neck without and with contrast
d. Angiography cervicocerebral
e. No ideal imaging exam

Age ≥16 years. Suspected acute cervical spine blunt trauma. Clinical or imaging findings suggest arterial injury without or with positive cervical spine CT. Next imaging exam.

a. *CTA head and neck* and choice (c) are equally the most appropriate.
b. MRA neck without contrast may be appropriate.
c. *MRA neck without and with contrast* and choice (a) are equally the most appropriate.
d. Angiography cervicocerebral may be appropriate.

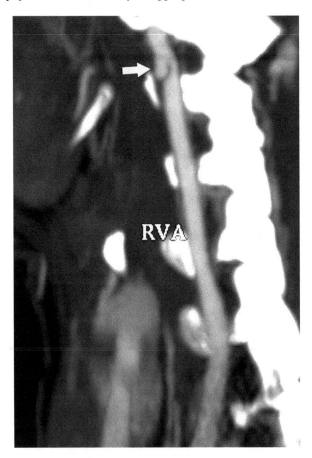

Fig. 10.4 Vertebral artery pseudoaneurysm. Neck CTA sagittal MIP image shows right vertebral artery (RVA) pseudoaneurysm (arrow) at the C2-3 level

Solution
Although angiography is conventionally the standard for diagnosing cervical artery injury, both CTA and MRA can noninvasively detect almost all clinically relevant injuries. CTA and MRA demonstrate similar diagnostic performance for vascular injury from blunt trauma.

A 62-year-old woman with suspected cervical spine trauma after a high-speed motor vehicle accident. She is obtunded without traumatic injury on cervical spine CT.

a. CTA head and neck
b. MRI cervical spine without contrast
c. MRI cervical spine without and with contrast
d. MRA neck without and with contrast
e. No ideal imaging exam

Age ≥16 years. Suspected acute cervical spine blunt trauma. Obtunded patient with no traumatic injury identified on cervical spine CT. Next imaging exam.

a. CTA head and neck is usually not appropriate.
b. *MRI cervical spine without contrast* is the most appropriate.
c. MRI cervical spine without and with contrast is usually not appropriate.
d. MRA neck without and with contrast is usually not appropriate.

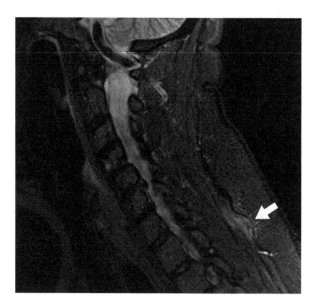

Fig. 10.5 Cervical spine soft tissue trauma. Cervical spine MR sagittal T2-weighted image shows a nuchal ligament injury (arrow) at C7-T1

Solution
Use of MRI in this scenario is controversial. MRI is more sensitive than CT in diagnosing soft tissue injury, such as ligament injury. But injuries detected with MRI in this setting usually do not change management or only extend cervical collar placement. However, in rare cases, patients with unreliable clinical exam and negative CT will have an unstable cervical spinal injury detected on MRI that requires surgical stabilization.

A 32-year-old woman with suspected cervical spine trauma after a motor vehicle accident. Clinical exam and cervical spine CT raise concern for ligamentous injury.

a. CT myelography cervical spine
b. MRI cervical spine without contrast
c. MRI cervical spine without and with contrast
d. MRA neck without and with contrast
e. No ideal imaging exam

Age ≥16 years. Suspected acute cervical spine blunt trauma. Clinical or imaging findings suggest ligamentous injury. Next imaging exam after CT cervical spine without contrast.

a. CT myelography cervical spine is usually not appropriate.
b. *MRI cervical spine without contrast* is the most appropriate.
c. MRI cervical spine without and with contrast is usually not appropriate.
d. MRA neck without and with contrast is usually not appropriate.

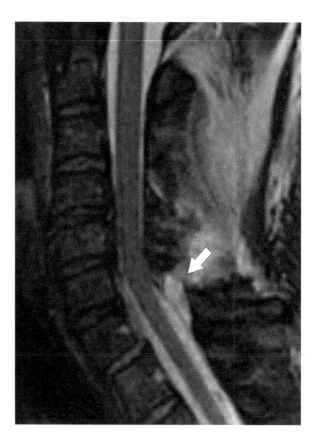

Fig. 10.6 Cervical spine ligamentous injury. Cervical spine MR sagittal T2-weighted image shows disruption of the posterior longitudinal ligament (arrow) at the C7-T1 level

Solution
MRI is the most sensitive imaging exam for the detection of ligament injury. However, ligament injuries that are occult on CT and identified on MRI rarely result in significant changes in clinical management.

A 49-year-old woman with suspected cervical spine trauma after a high-speed motor vehicle accident. Initial CT revealed no unstable injury, but the collar has been left on due to neck pain. Patient now returns for further evaluation. No new neurologic symptoms.

a. X-ray cervical spine
b. CT cervical spine without contrast
c. MRI cervical spine without contrast
d. MRA neck without and with contrast
e. No ideal imaging exam

Age ≥ 16 years. Suspected acute cervical spine blunt trauma. Follow-up imaging on patient with no unstable injury demonstrated initially but kept in collar for neck pain. No new neurologic symptoms. Includes whiplash-associated disorders.

a. X-ray cervical spine may be appropriate.
b. CT cervical spine without contrast may be appropriate.
c. MRI cervical spine without contrast may be appropriate.
d. MRA neck without and with contrast is usually not appropriate.
e. *No ideal imaging exam.*

Solution
Imaging shows little utility in diagnosing and predicting prognosis of whiplash-associated disorders. However, imaging may be appropriate in this population to exclude delayed presentation of a cervical spine instability occult at initial evaluation. This would allow patients to begin exercise and mobilization of the cervical spine.

A 19-year-old woman with suspected thoracolumbar spine trauma following a high-speed motor vehicle accident.

a. X-ray thoracic and lumbar spine
b. CT thoracic and lumbar spine without contrast
c. CT myelography thoracic and lumbar spine
d. MRI thoracic and lumbar spine without contrast
e. No ideal imaging exam

Age ≥16 years. Blunt trauma meeting criteria for thoracic and lumbar imaging. Initial imaging.

a. X-ray thoracic and lumbar spine may be appropriate.
b. *CT thoracic and lumbar spine without contrast* is the most appropriate.
c. CT myelography thoracic and lumbar spine is usually not appropriate.
d. MRI thoracic and lumbar spine without contrast is usually not appropriate.

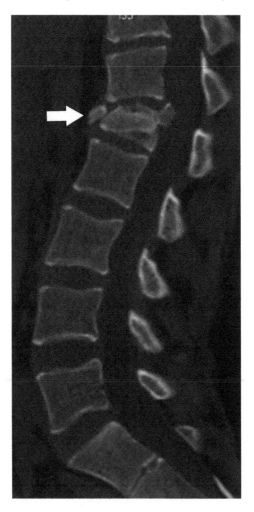

Fig. 10.7 Lumbar spine fracture. Lumbar spine CT sagittal reconstruction image shows a L1 vertebral body fracture (arrow)

Solution
CT is the standard for identifying fractures of the thoracolumbar spine, offering a reported sensitivity of 94–100%. CT is also excellent in identifying the soft tissue injuries of the chest, abdomen, and pelvis that often accompany spinal fractures.

A 35-year-old man with acute lumbar spine trauma detected on non-contrast CT following a high-speed motor vehicle accident. Neurologic abnormalities are present.

a. CT thoracic and lumbar spine with contrast
b. CT myelography thoracic and lumbar spine
c. MRI thoracic and lumbar spine without contrast
d. MRI thoracic and lumbar spine without and with contrast
e. No ideal imaging exam

Age ≥16 years. Acute thoracic or lumbar spine injury detected on radiographs or non-contrast CT. There are neurologic abnormalities. Next imaging exam.

a. CT thoracic and lumbar spine with contrast is usually not appropriate.
b. CT myelography thoracic and lumbar spine may be appropriate.
c. *MRI thoracic and lumbar spine without contrast* is the most appropriate.
d. MRI thoracic and lumbar spine without and with contrast is usually not appropriate.

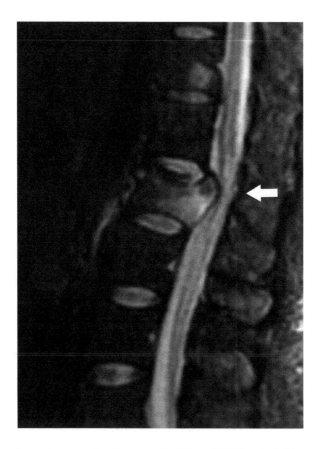

Fig. 10.8 Lumbar cord compression. Lumbar spine MR sagittal T2-weighted image shows an L1 vertebral fracture causing spinal cord compression (arrow)

Solution
MRI is valuable for identifying the causes of myelopathy (e.g., disc protrusion or hematoma) in patients with spinal cord injury. MRI can also be of prognostic value by evaluating the severity of spinal cord injury.

10.2   Traumatic Shoulder Pain

A 20-year-old patient presents with shoulder pain after trauma.

a. X-ray shoulder
b. CT shoulder without contrast
c. CT shoulder with contrast
d. MRI shoulder without contrast
e. No ideal imaging exam

Traumatic shoulder pain. Any etiology. Initial imaging.

a. *X-ray shoulder* is the most appropriate.
b. CT shoulder without contrast is usually not appropriate.
c. CT shoulder with contrast is usually not appropriate.
d. MRI shoulder without contrast is usually not appropriate.

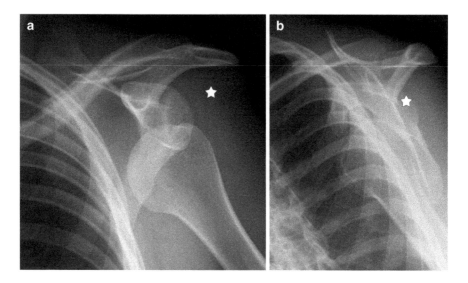

Fig. 10.9 Anterior shoulder dislocation. Shoulder X-ray anteroposterior (**a**) and scapular Y (**b**) views reveal inferior and anterior dislocation of the left humeral head from its expected location (star)

Solution
Radiography is the preferred initial imaging modality in patients presenting with traumatic shoulder pain. It effectively evaluates for fractures and malalignment, the two primary concerns.

A 50-year-old patient presents with shoulder pain after trauma. Radiographs are negative.

a. CT shoulder without contrast
b. CT arthrography shoulder
c. MRI shoulder without contrast
d. MR arthrography shoulder
e. No ideal imaging exam

Traumatic shoulder pain. Nonlocalized shoulder pain. Negative radiographs. Next imaging exam.

a. CT shoulder without contrast is usually not appropriate.
b. CT arthrography shoulder may be appropriate.
c. *MRI shoulder without contrast* is the most appropriate.
d. MR arthrography shoulder may be appropriate.

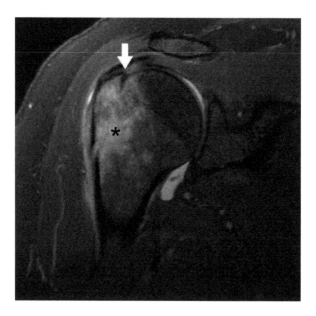

Fig. 10.10 Humeral fracture. Shoulder MR coronal T2-weighted image shows a minimally displaced fracture of the greater tuberosity of the right humerus (arrow) and edema of the underlying bone marrow (star)

Solution
Radiographs can exclude shoulder dislocation, and most displaced fractures as the cause for posttraumatic shoulder pain. When a shoulder X-ray is negative, MRI may be used to diagnose soft tissue injury including rotator cuff and labral tears. MRI also identifies bone contusion and radiographically occult fractures. CT is not appropriate as it does not detect common traumatic soft tissue injuries such as rotator cuff tears.

A 26-year-old patient presents with shoulder pain after trauma. A humeral neck fracture is seen on radiographs.

a. CT shoulder without contrast
b. CT shoulder with contrast
c. CT arthrography shoulder
d. MRI shoulder without contrast
e. MR arthrography shoulder

Traumatic shoulder pain. Radiographs show humeral head or neck fracture. Next imaging exam.

a. *CT shoulder without contrast* is the most appropriate.
b. CT shoulder with contrast is usually not appropriate.
c. CT arthrography shoulder is usually not appropriate.
d. MRI shoulder without contrast is usually not appropriate.
e. MR arthrography shoulder is usually not appropriate.

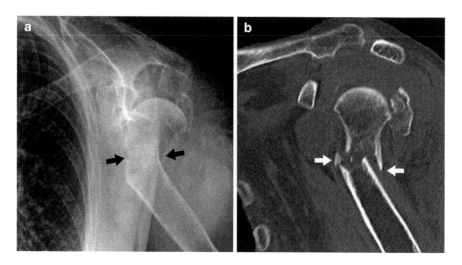

Fig. 10.11 Humeral fracture. Left shoulder X-ray anteroposterior view (**a**) shows a comminuted left humeral neck fracture (arrows) better depicted on a left shoulder CT coronal reconstruction image (**b**)

Solution
Nondisplaced fracture planes and complex bony anatomy can result in underappreciation of the extent of proximal humeral fractures on radiography. CT is the best next imaging exam, since it can accurately characterize fracture patterns and humeral neck angulation.

A 31-year-old patient presents with shoulder pain after trauma. A scapula fracture is seen on radiographs.

a. CT shoulder without contrast
b. CT shoulder with contrast
c. CT arthrography shoulder
d. MRI shoulder without contrast
e. MR arthrography shoulder

Traumatic shoulder pain. Radiographs show scapula fracture. Next imaging exam.

a. *CT shoulder without contrast* is the most appropriate.
b. CT shoulder with contrast is usually not appropriate.
c. CT arthrography shoulder is usually not appropriate.
d. MRI shoulder without contrast is usually not appropriate.
e. MR arthrography shoulder is usually not appropriate.

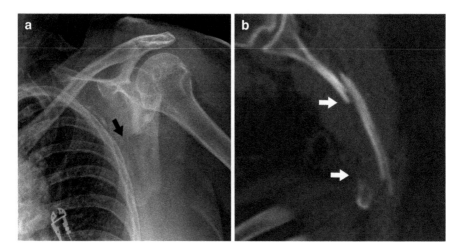

Fig. 10.12 Scapula fracture. Left shoulder X-ray anteroposterior view (**a**) shows a fracture of the scapula body (arrow). Left shoulder CT sagittal reconstruction image (**b**) better depicts the fracture displacement and angulation

Solution
Scapula fractures can be easily missed or underappreciated on radiography due to the scapula's complex morphology and because it overlies the ribs. CT is the best imaging modality for identifying and characterizing scapula fractures.

A 34-year-old patient presents with shoulder pain after trauma. A Bankart lesion is seen on radiographs.

a. CT shoulder without contrast
b. CT shoulder with contrast
c. CT arthrography shoulder
d. MRI shoulder without contrast
e. MR arthrography shoulder

Traumatic shoulder pain. Radiographs show Bankart or Hill–Sachs lesion. Next imaging exam.

a. CT shoulder without contrast may be appropriate.
b. CT shoulder with contrast is usually not appropriate.
c. CT arthrography shoulder may be appropriate.
d. *MRI shoulder without contrast* and choice (e) are equally the most appropriate.
e. *MR arthrography shoulder* and choice (d) are equally the most appropriate.

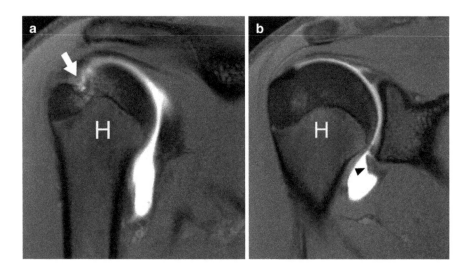

Fig. 10.13 Hill–Sachs and Bankart lesions. Shoulder MR arthrography coronal T1-weighted images show a Hill–Sachs defect (arrow) of the right humeral head (**a**) and an anteroinferior labral tear (arrowhead) consistent with a non-osseous Bankart defect (**b**). *H* humeral head

Solution
Bankart and Hill–Sachs lesions are commonly associated with transient shoulder dislocation and with each other. For both, there are non-osseous types that are occult on radiography and CT. Therefore, MRI or MR arthrography are recommended for further evaluation of these lesions.

A 26-year-old patient presents with shoulder pain after trauma. History and physical exam are consistent with dislocation event or instability. Radiographs are normal.

a. US shoulder
b. CT shoulder without contrast
c. CT arthrography shoulder
d. MRI shoulder without contrast
e. MR arthrography shoulder

Traumatic shoulder pain. Physical examination and history consistent with dislocation event or instability. Negative radiographs. Next imaging exam.

a. US shoulder is usually not appropriate.
b. CT shoulder without contrast may be appropriate.
c. CT arthrography shoulder may be appropriate.
d. *MRI shoulder without contrast* and choice (e) are equally the most appropriate.
e. *MR arthrography shoulder* and choice (d) are equally the most appropriate.

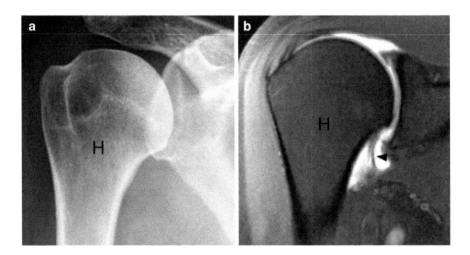

Fig. 10.14 Sequelae of traumatic anterior shoulder dislocation. Shoulder X-ray anteroposterior image (**a**) shows no bony abnormality. MR arthrography coronal T1-weighted image (**b**) shows avulsion of the posterior inferior glenohumeral ligament (arrowhead). *H* humeral head

Solution
With this scenario, labral, ligamentous, and osseous pathologies are all possible. In general, MR arthrography is the preferred exam. In the acute setting, MRI may suffice since a posttraumatic joint effusion may be present to outline the soft tissue structures.

A 37-year-old patient presents with shoulder pain after trauma. Physical exam findings are consistent with a labral tear. Radiographs are normal.

a. CT shoulder without contrast
b. CT arthrography shoulder
c. MRI shoulder without contrast
d. MR arthrography shoulder
e. No ideal imaging exam

Traumatic shoulder pain. Radiographs normal. Physical examination findings consistent with a labral tear. Next imaging exam.

a. CT shoulder without contrast is usually not appropriate.
b. *CT arthrography shoulder* and choices (c) and (d) are equally the most appropriate.
c. *MRI shoulder without contrast* and choices (b) and (d) are equally the most appropriate.
d. *MR arthrography shoulder* and choices (b) and (c) are equally the most appropriate.

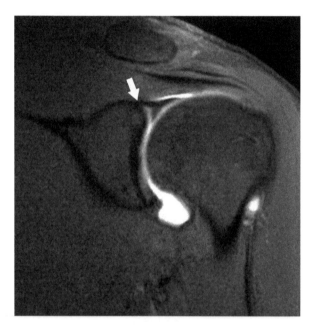

Fig. 10.15 Labral tear. Shoulder MR arthrography coronal T2-weighted image reveals a superior labral tear (arrow)

Solution
MRI may be preferred in the acute setting, as the presence of a posttraumatic joint effusion helps visualize the soft tissues. MR arthrography is more sensitive than MRI for anterior labral and SLAP (superior labral tear from anterior to posterior) tears. CT arthrography demonstrates similar sensitivity and possibly greater specificity in detection of labral lesions and better visualization of the bones.

A 51-year-old patient presents with shoulder pain after trauma, with physical exam findings consistent with rotator cuff tear. Radiographs are normal.

a. US shoulder
b. CT shoulder without contrast
c. CT arthrography shoulder
d. MRI shoulder without contrast
e. MR arthrography shoulder

Traumatic shoulder pain. Radiographs normal. Physical examination findings consistent with rotator cuff tear. Next imaging exam.

a. *US shoulder* and choices (d) and (e) are equally the most appropriate.
b. CT shoulder without contrast is usually not appropriate.
c. CT arthrography shoulder may be appropriate.
d. *MRI shoulder without contrast* and choices (a) and (e) are equally the most appropriate.
e. *MR arthrography shoulder* and choices (a) and (d) are equally the most appropriate.

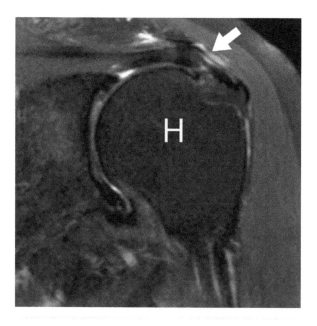

Fig. 10.16 Rotator cuff tear. Shoulder MR coronal T2-weighted image shows a partial thickness tear of the supraspinatus tendon (arrow). *H* humerus

Solution
US, MRI, and MR arthrography have similarly high sensitivity and specificity for full-thickness rotator cuff tears. Compared to arthrography, US and MRI are less sensitive for partial-thickness tears. The decision on the selection of imaging modality is driven by institutional preference.

10.3   Acute Hand and Wrist Trauma

A 57-year-old woman reports wrist pain after trauma.

a. X-ray wrist
b. CT wrist without contrast
c. MRI wrist without contrast
d. Tc-99m bone scan wrist
e. No ideal imaging exam

Wrist trauma, first exam.

a. *X-ray wrist* is the most appropriate.
b. CT wrist without contrast is usually not appropriate.
c. MRI wrist without contrast is usually not appropriate.
d. Tc-99m bone scan wrist is usually not appropriate.

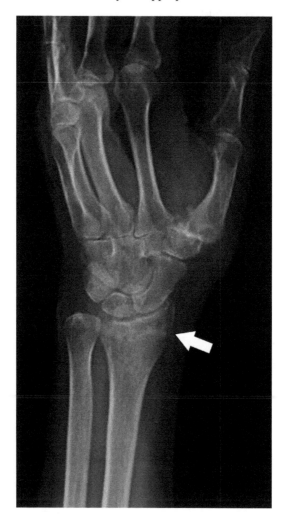

Fig. 10.17 Distal radial fracture. Wrist X-ray semi-pronated oblique view reveals a nondisplaced fracture of the distal radius (arrow)

Solution

Radiography is the preferred initial imaging modality for the evaluation of wrist trauma.

A 31-year-old woman reports wrist pain after trauma. Exam reveals focal tenderness at the distal radius. Radiographs are normal.

a. US wrist
b. CT wrist without contrast
c. MRI wrist without contrast
d. Tc-99m bone scan wrist
e. No ideal imaging exam

Suspect acute fracture. Radiographs normal. Next imaging exam.

a. US wrist is usually not appropriate.
b. *CT wrist without contrast* and choice (c) are equally the most appropriate.
c. *MRI wrist without contrast* and choice (b) are equally the most appropriate. Use if immediate confirmation or exclusion of fracture is required.
d. Tc-99m bone scan wrist is usually not appropriate.

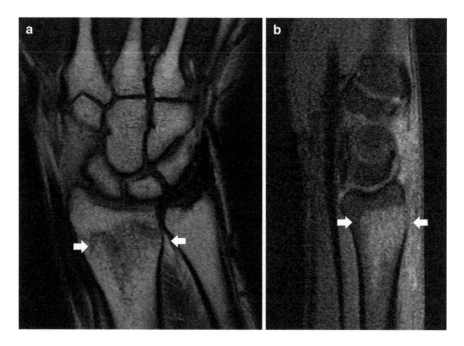

Fig. 10.18 Distal radial fracture. Wrist MR anteroposterior T1-weighted (**a**) and lateral T2-weighted (**b**) images reveal abnormal signal intensity in the distal radius, indicating a fracture

Solution
CT and MRI can both detect radiographically occult fractures and can show intra-articular extension of distal radius fractures better than radiography. Unlike MRI, CT cannot evaluate for associated ligamentous injuries.

A 59-year-old man reports wrist pain after trauma. Radiographs reveal a wrist fracture. Tendon or ligament trauma is suspected.

a. CT wrist without contrast
b. CT arthrography wrist
c. MRI wrist without contrast
d. MR arthrography wrist
e. No ideal imaging exam

Acute wrist fracture on radiographs. Suspect wrist tendon or ligament trauma. Next imaging exam.

a. CT wrist without contrast is usually not appropriate.
b. *CT arthrography wrist* and choices (c) and (d) are equally the most appropriate.
c. *MRI wrist without contrast* and choices (b) and (d) are equally the most appropriate.
d. *MR arthrography wrist* and choices (b) and (c) are equally the most appropriate.

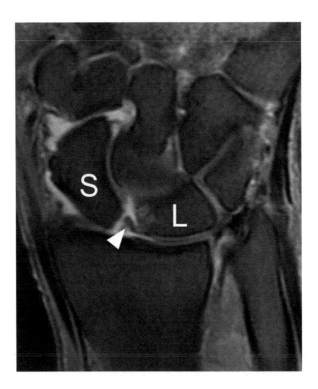

Fig. 10.19 Wrist fracture with a ligament tear. Wrist MR coronal T2-weighted image shows abnormal separation between the scaphoid (S) and lunate (L) with a tear of the scapholunate ligament (arrowhead)

Solution
CT or MR arthrography or MRI can be used to diagnose ligamentous injury in this setting, with CT arthrography being the most accurate. Tendinopathy, tenosynovitis, and tendon rupture can be revealed by MRI.

A 22-year-old man reports thumb pain after trauma. X-ray shows a fracture at the base of the proximal first phalanx. Ligament injury is suspected.

a. US wrist
b. CT wrist without contrast
c. MRI wrist without contrast
d. Tc-99m bone scan wrist
e. No ideal imaging exam

Acute hand fracture on radiographs. Suspect hand tendon or ligament trauma. Next imaging exam.

a. *US hand* and choice (c) are equally the most appropriate.
b. CT wrist without contrast is usually not appropriate.
c. *MRI hand without contrast* and choice (a) are equally the most appropriate.
d. Tc-99m bone scan hand is usually not appropriate.

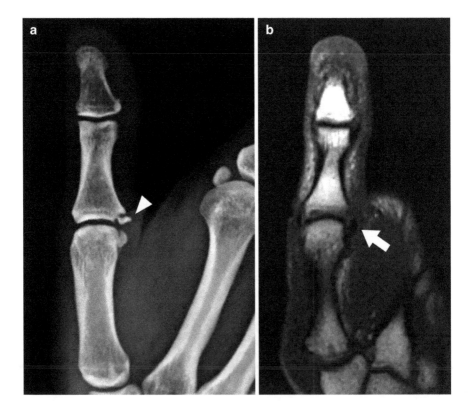

Fig. 10.20 Gamekeeper's thumb fracture. Hand X-ray posteroanterior view (**a**) shows an avulsion fracture at the ulnar side of the base of the first proximal phalanx (arrowhead). Hand MR coronal T1-weighted image (**b**) shows a torn and retracted ulnar collateral ligament (arrow)

Solution
Both US and MRI can diagnose pulley system injuries as well as Stener lesions of the thumb, which can accompany avulsion at the base of the first proximal phalanx. US enables dynamic evaluation of the injury.

A 20-year-old man presents with finger trauma. Radiographs reveal malalignment at the fifth proximal interphalangeal joint without fracture. Tendinous or ligamentous injury is suspected.

a. US hand
b. CT hand without contrast
c. MRI hand without contrast
d. MRI hand without and with contrast
e. No ideal imaging exam

Initial radiographs show metacarpophalangeal or interphalangeal joint malalign-ment without fracture. Next imaging exam.

a. *US hand* and choice (c) are equally the most appropriate.
b. CT hand without contrast is usually not appropriate.
c. *MRI hand without contrast* and choice (a) are equally the most appropriate.
d. MRI hand without and with contrast is usually not appropriate.

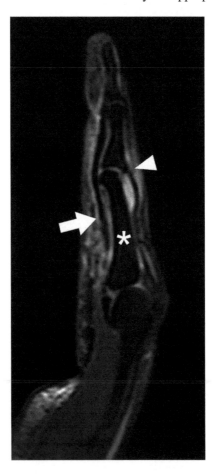

Fig. 10.21 Finger pulley injury. Hand MR sagittal T2-weighted image shows abnormal separa-tion between the flexor tendon (arrow) and the fifth proximal phalanx (star) indicative of an A2 pulley injury and malalignment at the fifth proximal interphalangeal joint (arrowhead)

Solution
Both MRI and US can be used to evaluate for tendon and ligament injuries in this setting, including pulley system injuries. US enables direct real-time visualization of tendon subluxation/dislocation as the patient undergoes maneuvers such as meta-carpophalangeal joint flexion.

A 25-year-old woman reports penetrating injury and a possible splinter in her hand while gardening. Initial radiographs are negative. Next imaging exam.

a. US area of interest
b. CT area of interest without contrast
c. CT area of interest without and with contrast
d. MRI area of interest without contrast
e. No ideal imaging exam

Suspect penetrating trauma with a foreign body in the soft tissues in the hand or wrist. Initial radiographs are negative. Next imaging exam.

a. *US area of interest* and choice (b) are equally the most appropriate.
b. *CT area of interest without contrast* and choice (a) are equally the most appropriate.
c. CT area of interest without and with contrast is usually not appropriate.
d. MRI area of interest without contrast is usually not appropriate.

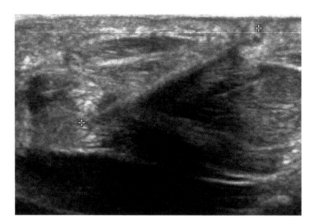

Fig. 10.22 A wooden splinter in soft tissue. Hand US shows a linear foreign object (calipers) within the soft tissues of the palm

Solution
US is superior to radiography for radiolucent foreign bodies such as wood and is the preferred exam when the foreign body is in superficial soft tissue. US can also guide removal of the foreign body. CT is very sensitive for radiopaque foreign bodies (e.g., metal fragments) and is useful when foreign body penetration into deeper tissues or bone is suspected.

10.4   Acute Hip Pain, Suspected Fracture

A 47-year-old patient with acute hip pain after a fall. Hip fracture is suspected.

a. X-ray pelvis and hip
b. CT pelvis and hips without contrast
c. CT pelvis and hips with contrast
d. MRI pelvis and hip
e. No ideal imaging exam

Acute hip pain. Fall or minor trauma. Suspect fracture. Initial imaging.

a. *X-ray pelvis and hip* is the most appropriate.
b. CT pelvis and hips without contrast is usually not appropriate.
c. CT pelvis and hips with contrast is usually not appropriate.
d. MRI pelvis and hip is usually not appropriate.

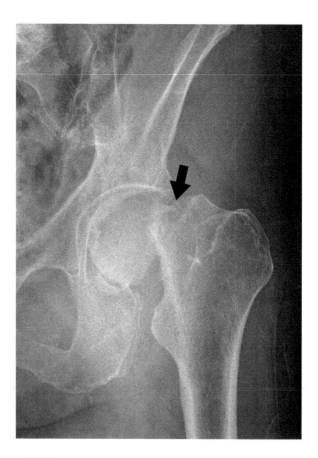

Fig. 10.23   Acute hip fracture. Left hip X-ray anteroposterior view shows an acute impacted and displaced subcapital femoral neck fracture (arrow)

Solution
Patients with clinically suspected proximal femur fracture often have pelvic fractures as well. Thus, radiographs of the pelvis and symptomatic hip are recommended. When a fracture is shown on radiographs, often no additional imaging is needed for treatment planning.

A 72-year-old patient with acute hip pain after a fall. Hip fracture is suspected. Initial radiographs are negative.

a. CT pelvis and hips without contrast
b. CT pelvis and hips with contrast
c. MRI pelvis and hip without contrast
d. MRI pelvis and hip without and with contrast
e. No ideal imaging exam

Acute hip pain following a fall or minor trauma. Negative radiographs. Suspect fracture. Next imaging exam.

a. *CT pelvis and hips without contrast* and choice (c) are equally the most appropriate.
b. CT pelvis and hips with contrast is usually not appropriate.
c. *MRI pelvis and affected hip without contrast* and choice (a) are equally the most appropriate.
d. MRI pelvis and hip without and with contrast is usually not appropriate.

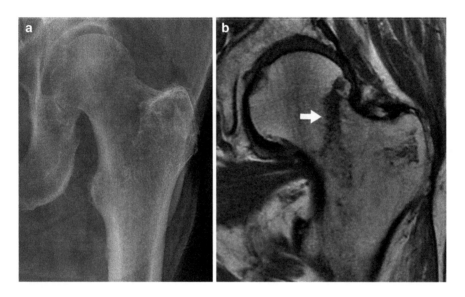

Fig. 10.24 Hip fracture. Hip X-ray anteroposterior view (**a**) is normal. MR coronal T1-weighted image (**b**) shows a fracture line across the left femoral neck (arrow)

Solution

CT and MRI are both appropriate, each with its own advantages. CT is faster and more readily available and is more suitable for patients who cannot cooperate with the exam. MRI is more sensitive for fractures and soft tissue injuries such as hematoma and tendon avulsion. The sensitivity of MRI for proximal femoral fracture is close to 100%.

10.5   Acute Trauma to the Knee

A 35-year-old man reports knee pain after trauma. He is able to walk. Exam reveals no focal tenderness or effusion.

a. X-ray knee
b. US knee
c. CT knee without contrast
d. MRI knee without contrast
e. No ideal imaging exam

584 Musculoskeletal Imaging

Fall or twisting injury with no focal tenderness or effusion. The patient is able to walk.

a. X-ray knee is usually not appropriate.
b. US knee is usually not appropriate.
c. CT knee without contrast is usually not appropriate.
d. MRI knee without contrast is usually not appropriate.
e. *No ideal imaging exam* is the correct answer.

Solution

Well-validated clinical decision rules such as the Ottawa Knee Rule and the Pittsburgh Decision Rule are helpful in identifying patients with acute knee injury who need imaging. Per the Ottawa Knee Rule, patients 18 years of age or older with acute knee pain should have knee radiographs if any of the following criteria are met: 55 years of age or older, tenderness over the head of the fibula, isolated patellar tenderness, cannot flex knee to 90°, cannot weight bear immediately after injury, or cannot walk in the emergency room after taking four steps. However, ultimately, clinical judgment supersedes guideline recommendations.

A 42-year-old man reports knee pain after a fall. Exam reveals he cannot bear weight on the knee.

a. X-ray knee
b. US knee
c. CT knee without contrast
d. CT knee with contrast
e. MRI knee without contrast

Fall or twisting injury with one or more of following: focal tenderness, effusion, or inability to bear weight. Initial exam.

a. *X-ray knee* is the most appropriate.
b. US knee is usually not appropriate.
c. CT knee without contrast is usually not appropriate.
d. CT knee with contrast is usually not appropriate.
e. MRI knee without contrast may be appropriate.

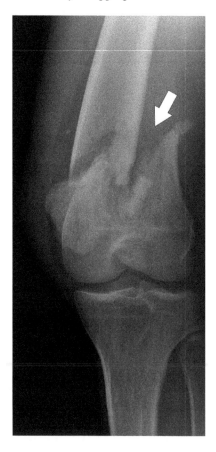

Fig. 10.25 Distal tibial fracture. Knee X-ray anteroposterior view shows a comminuted and displaced tibial fracture (arrow)

Solution
Radiography is the preferred initial exam in this setting. Radiographs are also recommended for patients with gross deformity, palpable mass, penetrating injury, or prosthetic hardware. Imaging should also be performed for patients with an unreliable history or physical exam due to multiple injuries, altered mental status, or neuropathy, or a history suggesting increased fracture risk.

A 34-year-old woman reports trauma to the knee. A Segond fracture is seen on radiography.

a. US knee
b. CT knee without contrast
c. MRI knee without contrast
d. MRI knee without and with contrast
e. No ideal imaging exam

Fall or twisting injury with either no fracture or Segond fracture on initial radiograph. Internal derangement is suspected. Next imaging exam.

a. US knee is usually not appropriate.
b. CT knee without contrast may be appropriate.
c. *MRI knee without contrast* is the most appropriate.
d. MRI knee without and with contrast is usually not appropriate.

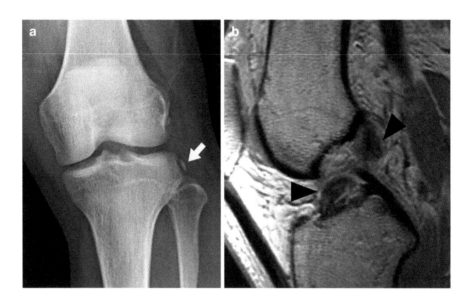

Fig. 10.26 Segond fracture. Knee X-ray anteroposterior view (**a**) shows an avulsion fracture of the lateral tibial plateau or Segond fracture (arrow). MR sagittal proton density-weighted image (**b**) shows complete rupture of the anterior cruciate ligament (arrowheads), which is frequently associated with Segond fractures

Solution
MRI is the optimal imaging modality for identifying meniscal, ligament, chondral, and nondisplaced bone injuries around the knee. Use of contrast is unnecessary.

A 27-year-old woman after a fall, with initial radiographs showing a tibial plateau fracture.

a. US knee
b. CT knee without contrast
c. MRI knee without contrast
d. MRI knee without and with contrast
e. No ideal imaging exam

Fall or twisting injury with a tibial plateau fracture on initial radiographs. Additional bone or soft tissue injury is suspected. Next imaging exam.

a. US knee is usually not appropriate.
b. *CT knee without contrast* is the most appropriate.
c. MRI knee without contrast is usually appropriate, but there is a better choice here.
d. MRI knee without and with contrast is usually not appropriate.

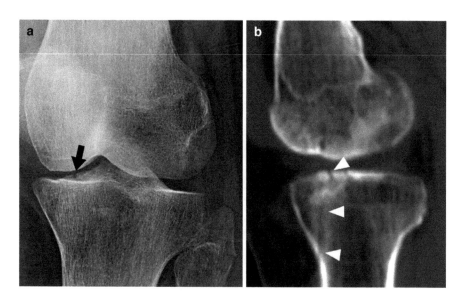

Fig. 10.27 Tibial plateau fracture. Knee X-ray anteroposterior image (**a**) shows a subtle medial tibial plateau fracture (arrow). CT sagittal reconstruction image (**b**) better demonstrates the fracture (arrowheads)

Solution
Some types of tibial plateau fractures can be adequately assessed with radiography alone. CT or MRI can help evaluate and plan surgery for more complex cases. Advantages of CT include good cortical bone depiction, shorter scan time, and greater availability. MRI demonstrates soft tissue injuries better (e.g., meniscal and ligament tears, common in this scenario) while still adequately depicting cortical bone fractures.

A 72-year-old woman reports knee pain after trauma. She is able to walk. Exam reveals knee joint effusion and focal patellar tenderness.

a. X-ray knee
b. US knee
c. CT knee without contrast
d. MRI knee without contrast
e. MRI knee without and with contrast

Injury to knee, mechanism unknown. There is focal patellar tenderness and knee joint effusion. The patient is able to walk.

a. *X-ray knee* is the most appropriate.
b. US knee is usually not appropriate.
c. CT knee without contrast is usually not appropriate.
d. MRI knee without contrast may be appropriate.
e. MRI knee without and with contrast is usually not appropriate.

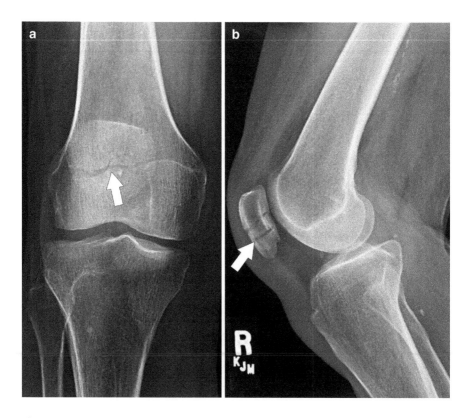

Fig. 10.28 Patellar fracture. Knee X-ray posteroanterior (**a**) and lateral (**b**) views reveal a transverse patellar fracture (arrows)

Solution
Causes for traumatic patellar pain include patellar fracture and transient patellar dislocation. Radiographs may include a dedicated patellar (i.e., sunrise) view.

A 55-year-old man reports knee pain after motor vehicle accident. Knee dislocation is suspected.

a. X-ray knee
b. CT knee without contrast
c. CTA lower extremity
d. MRI knee without contrast
e. MRA knee without and with contrast

Significant trauma to knee from motor vehicle accident. Suspect knee dislocation.

a. *X-ray knee* and choice (d) are equally the most appropriate.
b. CT knee without contrast is usually not appropriate.
c. CTA lower extremity is usually appropriate, but there is a better choice here.
d. *MRI knee without contrast* and choice (a) are equally the most appropriate.
e. MRA knee without and with contrast is usually appropriate but should be performed in conjunction with (d).

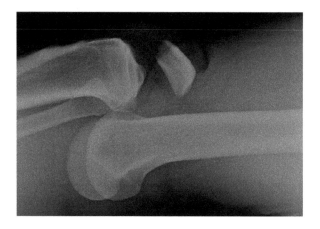

Fig. 10.29 Anterior knee dislocation. Knee X-ray lateral view shows anterior dislocation of the tibia and fibula relative to the femur

Solution

Knee dislocation is an orthopedic emergency due to the risk for nerve or arterial injury. Though radiography is used to assess overall injury, further assessment for vascular or ligament injury is always indicated. Either CTA or MRA is appropriate. MRA is often preferred as it can be performed at the same time as knee MRI to evaluate the ligaments and other soft tissue.

10.6   Acute Trauma to the Ankle

10.6.1 Ottawa Ankle Rules

In a patient with acute ankle injury, radiographs are indicated only if there is pain in the malleolar area and one of the following are present:

1. Bone tenderness along the posterior edge or tip of the lateral malleolus
2. Bone tenderness along the posterior edge or tip of the medial malleolus
3. Inability to bear weight both immediately after injury and in the emergency department

Stiell et al. 1994

A 52-year-old woman with acute ankle injury. The patient is unable to bear weight on the injured ankle.

a. X-ray ankle
b. CT ankle without contrast
c. MRI ankle without contrast
d. Tc-99m bone scan ankle
e. No ideal imaging exam

Adult or child >5 years old and meets criteria for imaging according to the Ottawa Ankle Rules.

a. *X-ray ankle* is the most appropriate.
b. CT ankle without contrast is usually not appropriate.
c. MRI ankle without contrast is usually not appropriate.
d. Tc-99m bone scan ankle is usually not appropriate.

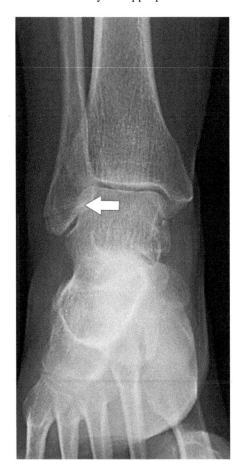

Fig. 10.30 Ankle fracture. Ankle X-ray mortis view shows a fracture through the distal fibula (arrow) with overlying soft tissue swelling

Solution
The Ottawa Ankle Rules criteria identify patients with sufficiently low probability of fracture after ankle trauma that they can safely be treated without imaging. For cases where imaging is indicated, radiography should include anteroposterior, lateral, and mortise views.

A 55-year-old man with acute ankle injury. He does not meet Ottawa Ankle Rules criteria for imaging and is without neurological signs or symptoms on exam.

a. X-ray ankle
b. US ankle
c. CT ankle without contrast
d. MRI ankle without contrast
e. No ideal imaging exam

The patient does not meet the criteria for imaging according to the Ottawa Ankle Rules.

a. X-ray ankle is usually not appropriate.
b. US ankle is usually not appropriate.
c. CT ankle without contrast is usually not appropriate.
d. MRI ankle without contrast is usually not appropriate.
e. *No ideal imaging exam* is the correct answer.

Solution
Patients who do not require imaging by the Ottawa Ankle Rules may be safely treated without it. However, it is important to note that these criteria were validated in children older than 5 years of age. Thus, the Ottawa Ankle Rules should not be used in younger patients or in patients with decreased sensation (e.g., peripheral neuropathy) or inability to communicate.

10.7   Acute Trauma to the Foot

A 25-year-old with acute injury to the foot. There is pain in the midfoot and point tenderness at the base of the fifth metatarsal.

a. X-ray foot
b. US foot
c. CT foot without contrast
d. MRI foot without contrast
e. No ideal imaging exam

Adult or child >5 years old with acute injury to the foot and meets Ottawa Rules criteria for imaging.

a. *X-ray foot* is the most appropriate.
b. US foot is usually not appropriate.
c. CT foot without contrast is usually not appropriate.
d. MRI foot without contrast is usually not appropriate.

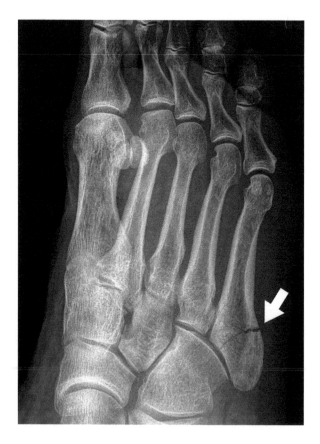

Fig. 10.31 Metatarsal fracture. Foot X-ray oblique view shows a fracture at the base of the fifth metatarsal (arrow)

Solution
Per Ottawa Rules, patients aged >5 years need imaging after foot trauma only if there is midfoot pain and also point tenderness of the navicular or fifth metatarsal base or if they are unable to bear weight both immediately and in the emergency department. Settings where these rules do not apply include pregnancy, skin wound, penetrating trauma, >10 days after trauma, return visit for continued pain, poly-trauma, underlying bone disease, or altered sensorium (Bachmann et al. 2003).

A 22-year-old patient with acute injury to the foot and physical exam concerning for a Lisfranc injury.

a. X-ray foot
b. US foot
c. CT foot without contrast
d. MRI foot without contrast
e. No ideal imaging exam

Adult or child >5 years old with acute injury to the foot. Physical examination is concerning for a Lisfranc injury).

a. *X-ray foot* is the most appropriate.
b. US foot is usually not appropriate.
c. CT foot without contrast is usually not appropriate.
d. MRI foot without contrast is usually not appropriate.

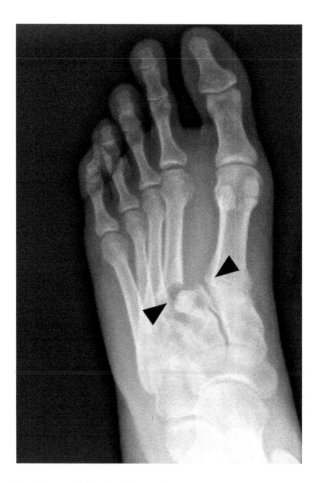

Fig. 10.32 Lisfranc fracture dislocation. Foot radiograph dorsoplantar view shows abnormal widening of the space between the first and second metatarsal base with associated fractures (arrowheads)

Solution
Foot X-ray should be performed when there is clinical concern for Lisfranc fracture. In addition to standard radiographic views, weight-bearing views are added to make it easier to identify Lisfranc injuries.

A 21-year-old patient with acute injury to the foot from penetrating trauma with a metallic foreign object suspected left in the soft tissues.

a. X-ray foot
b. US foot
c. CT foot without contrast
d. MRI foot without contrast
e. No ideal imaging exam

Adult or child >5 years old with acute injury to the foot. Physical examination is concerning for penetrating trauma with a foreign body in the soft tissues.

a. *X-ray foot* is the most appropriate.
b. US foot is usually appropriate, but there is a better choice here. Consider this if the foreign body is known to be radiolucent.
c. CT foot without contrast is usually not appropriate.
d. MRI foot without contrast is usually not appropriate.

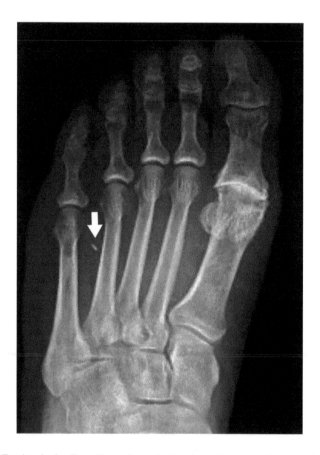

Fig. 10.33 Foreign body. Foot X-ray dorsoplantar view shows a radiopaque foreign object between the fourth and fifth metatarsals (arrow)

Solution

Choice of imaging modality depends on whether the suspected foreign object is radiopaque. For radiopaque foreign objects (e.g., glass, gravel, metal), foot X-ray is the preferred initial exam. For radiolucent foreign bodies (e.g., wood or plastic), US is preferred.

A 17-year-old patient with acute injury to the foot with penetrating trauma. A foreign object is suspected in the soft tissues. Radiographs are negative.

a. US foot
b. CT foot without contrast
c. CT foot with contrast
d. MRI foot without contrast
e. No ideal imaging exam

Adult or child >5 years old with acute injury to the foot. Physical examination is concerning for penetrating trauma with a foreign body in the soft tissues. Radiographs of the foot are negative.

a. *US foot* is the most appropriate.
b. CT foot without contrast may be appropriate.
c. CT foot with contrast is usually not appropriate.
d. MRI foot without contrast may be appropriate.

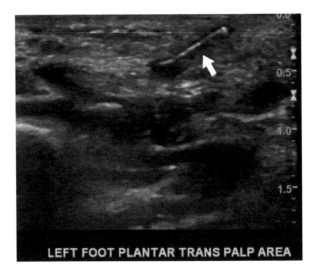

Fig. 10.34 Foreign body in soft tissue. Foot US shows an echogenic linear object (arrow) within the soft tissue of the plantar surface

Solution
When penetrating injury to the foot is suspected and the X-ray is negative, the next imaging exam should be US. It assesses for the presence of a foreign body that is not radiopaque (e.g., wood or plastic).

10.8   Stress (Fatigue or Insufficiency) Fracture

A 51-year-old woman with suspected stress fracture of the hip.

a. X-ray area of interest
b. US area of interest
c. CT area of interest without contrast
d. MRI area of interest without contrast
e. No ideal imaging exam

Suspect stress (fatigue or insufficiency) fracture, excluding vertebrae. Initial imaging.

a. *X-ray area of interest* is the most appropriate.
b. US area of interest is usually not appropriate.
c. CT area of interest without contrast is usually not appropriate.
d. MRI area of interest without contrast is usually not appropriate.

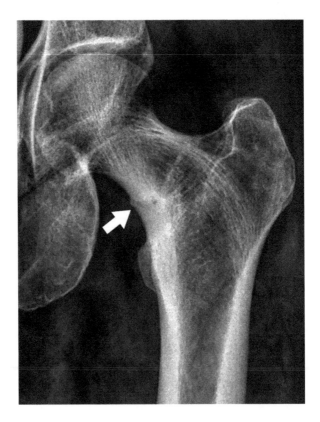

Fig. 10.35 Stress fracture. Hip X-ray anteroposterior view shows a linear lucency extending through an area of focal cortical thickening at the medial left femoral neck (arrow)

Solution
Although stress fractures are often occult on radiography, X-ray remains the most appropriate initial imaging exam because it is widely available. If the findings are conclusive, then no further imaging is needed.

A 55-year-old woman with suspected stress (fatigue) fracture of hip. Radiographs are normal.

a. X-ray area of interest repeated in 10–14 days
b. CT area of interest without contrast
c. MRI area of interest without contrast
d. Tc-99m bone scan with SPECT area of interest
e. No ideal imaging exam

Suspect stress (fatigue) fracture in hip. Radiographs are normal. Next imaging exam.

a. X-ray area of interest repeated in 10–14 days may be appropriate.
b. CT area of interest without contrast may be appropriate.
c. *MRI area of interest without contrast* is the most appropriate.
d. Tc-99m bone scan with SPECT area of interest may be appropriate.

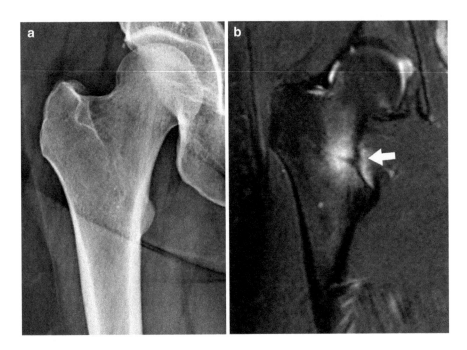

Fig. 10.36 Stress fracture. Hip X-ray anteroposterior image (**a**) is normal. Hip MR coronal T2-weighted image (**b**) shows a fracture line with adjacent edema along the medial right femoral neck (arrow)

Solution
MRI is the preferred exam in this setting and outperforms radiography, CT, and bone scan. MRI is recommended after initial negative radiographs to prevent delayed diagnosis of high-risk fracture types such as those that may progress to avascular necrosis.

A 30-year-old woman with suspected stress (fatigue) fracture of the heel. Radiographs are negative.

a. X-ray area of interest repeated in 10–14 days
b. CT area of interest without contrast
c. MRI area of interest without contrast
d. Tc-99m bone scan with SPECT area of interest
e. No ideal imaging exam

Suspect stress (fatigue) fracture, excluding hip and vertebrae. Radiographs normal.
Next imaging exam.

a. *X-ray area of interest repeated in 10–14 days* is the most appropriate.
b. CT area of interest without contrast may be appropriate.
c. MRI area of interest without contrast is usually appropriate, but there is a better
   choice here. It may be preferred to option (a) in high-risk fracture locations.
d. Tc-99m bone scan with SPECT area of interest may be appropriate.

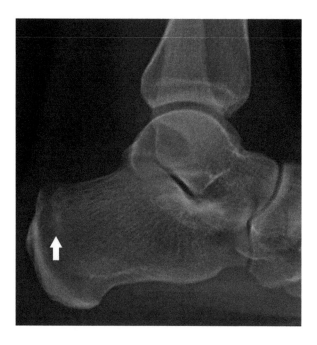

Fig. 10.37   Stress fracture. Ankle X-ray lateral view shows linear sclerosis of the calcaneus (arrow)

Solution
For suspected stress fracture with negative initial radiographs, the choice of subsequent imaging is guided by pain location and likelihood of high-risk injury (i.e.,
stress fractures with increased risk for nonunion or delayed union). When early
diagnosis is not critical, radiographic follow-up can show development of bony
changes at the fracture site.

A 28-year-old man with suspected stress (fatigue) fracture of the tibia. Initial radiographs are negative. Immediate diagnosis is needed.

a. X-ray area of interest
b. CT area of interest without contrast
c. MRI area of interest without contrast
d. Tc-99m bone scan with SPECT area of interest
e. No ideal imaging exam

Suspect stress (fatigue) fracture, excluding vertebrae. Radiographs normal. Immediate "need-to-know" diagnosis. Next imaging exam.

a. X-ray area of interest is usually not appropriate.
b. CT area of interest without contrast may be appropriate.
c. *MRI area of interest without contrast* is the most appropriate.
d. Tc-99m bone scan with SPECT area of interest may be appropriate.

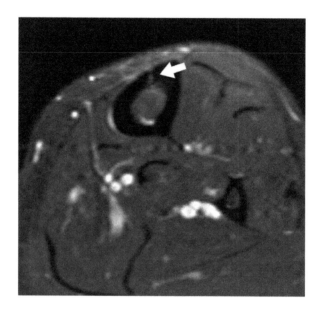

Fig. 10.38 Stress fracture. Tibia and fibula MR axial T2-weighted image shows a fracture along the anterior tibial cortex (arrow)

Solution

Certain stress fractures are at high risk for non-union or delayed union, including those at the anterior tibial diaphysis, lateral femoral neck and head, patella, medial malleolus, navicular, fifth metatarsal base, proximal second metatarsal, tibial hallux sesamoid, and talus. In athletes, stress injuries that are not diagnosed early may progress to more serious fractures. In such cases where there is a need for immediate diagnosis, MRI is recommended due to its high sensitivity and specificity.

A 71-year-old woman with suspected stress (insufficiency) fracture of the pelvis. Radiographs are negative.

a. X-ray area of interest repeated in 10–14 days
b. CT area of interest without contrast
c. MRI area of interest without contrast
d. Tc-99m bone scan with SPECT area of interest
e. No ideal imaging exam

Suspect stress (insufficiency) fracture, pelvis or hip. Radiographs normal. Next imaging exam.

a. X-ray area of interest repeated in 10–14 days may be appropriate.
b. CT area of interest without contrast is usually appropriate, but there is a better choice here.
c. *MRI area of interest without contrast* is the most appropriate.
d. Tc-99m bone scan with SPECT area of interest may be appropriate.

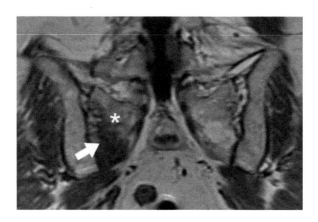

Fig. 10.39 Sacral insufficiency fracture. Pelvic MR coronal T1-weighted image shows a fracture (arrow) along the right sacral ala (star)

Solution
Pelvic and hip insufficiency fractures have varied presentations and often insidious onset. Radiography is used for initial evaluation, but sensitivity is low especially in older or osteoporotic patients. In patients with negative radiography, MRI is recommended due to its high sensitivity and specificity. Bone scan is sensitive but is often non-specific.

A 65-year-old woman with suspected insufficiency fracture of the knee. Radiographs are negative.

a. X-ray area of interest repeated in 10–14 days
b. CT area of interest without contrast
c. MRI area of interest without contrast
d. Tc-99m bone scan with SPECT area of interest
e. No ideal imaging exam

Suspect stress (insufficiency) fracture of lower extremity, excluding pelvis and hip. Negative radiographs. Next imaging exam.

a. X-ray area of interest repeated in 10–14 days is usually appropriate, but there is a better choice here.
b. CT area of interest without contrast may be appropriate.
c. *MRI area of interest without contrast* is the most appropriate.
d. Tc-99m bone scan with SPECT area of interest may be appropriate.

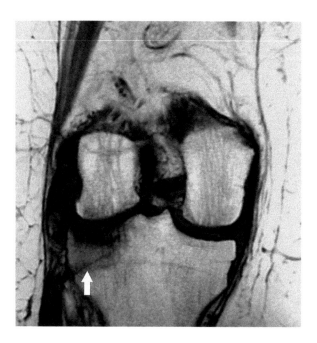

Fig. 10.40 Insufficiency fracture. Knee MR coronal T1-weighted image shows a linear fracture line (arrow) through the lateral tibial plateau

Solution
The high sensitivity and specificity of MRI make it the best exam to provide an immediate diagnosis. If the suspected fracture is not high-risk and a delayed diagnosis is acceptable, then a reasonable alternative is to perform a follow-up X-ray of the area of interest, which is more sensitive than the initial radiographic exam.

A 77-year-old woman with bone scan that shows nonspecific focal tracer uptake in a symptomatic knee, suspicious for stress fracture.

a. X-ray area of interest
b. US area of interest
c. CT area of interest without contrast
d. MRI area of interest without contrast
e. No ideal imaging exam

Follow-up imaging exam for characterizing nonspecific focal uptake on bone scan, suspected to be a stress fracture.

a. *X-ray area of interest* and choice (d) are equally the most appropriate.
b. US area of interest is usually not appropriate.
c. CT area of interest without contrast may be appropriate.
d. *MRI area of interest without contrast* and choice (a) are equally the most appropriate.

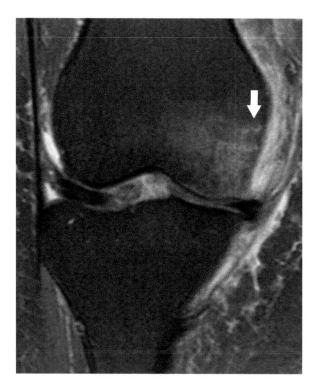

Fig. 10.41 Stress fracture. Knee MR coronal T2-weighted image shows marrow edema in the medial femoral condyle (arrow). There is also edema of the surrounding soft tissues. Radiographs of this area were negative

Solution

Bone scan is sensitive but not specific for stress fractures. Synovitis, arthritis, degenerative joint disease, stress reactions, and tumor may all produce a positive scan. In most cases, additional imaging is needed to provide the diagnosis. While radiography and MRI may both be used, the former may be the preferred immediate next step due to widespread availability.

10.9   Osteoporosis and Bone Mineral Density

A 79-year-old woman with suspected subacute vertebral body fracture and osteoporosis.

a. X-ray spine area of interest
b. CT spine area of interest without contrast
c. CT spine area of interest with contrast
d. MRI spine area of interest without contrast
e. No ideal imaging exam

Suspected fracture of a vertebral body based on acute or subacute symptoms in patient with suspected osteoporosis or treated with corticosteroids >3 months. Initial imaging exam.

a. *X-ray spine area of interest* is the most appropriate.
b. CT spine area of interest without contrast may be appropriate.
c. CT spine area of interest with contrast is usually not appropriate.
d. MRI spine area of interest without contrast is usually not appropriate.

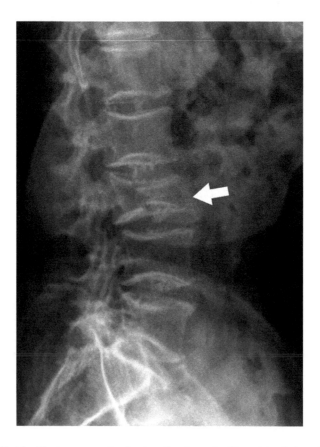

Fig. 10.42 Vertebral body compression fracture. Lumbar spine X-ray lateral view shows a compression fracture of the L3 vertebral body (arrow) and diffuse osteopenia

Solution
Radiography is the first-line imaging exam in this scenario given its widespread availability and favorable radiation profile compared to CT.

An 81-year-old man with suspected subacute vertebral body fracture and osteoporosis. Radiographs are negative.

a. X-ray spine area of interest repeated in 10–14 days
b. CT lumbar spine without contrast
c. CT lumbar spine with contrast
d. MRI lumbar spine without contrast
e. No ideal imaging exam

Suspected fracture of a vertebral body based on acute or subacute symptoms in patient with suspected osteoporosis or treated with corticosteroids >3 months. Initial radiographs are negative.

a. X-ray spine area of interest repeated in 10–14 days is usually not appropriate.
b. CT lumbar spine without contrast is usually appropriate, but there is a better choice here.
c. CT lumbar spine with contrast is usually not appropriate.
d. *MRI lumbar spine* without contrast is the most appropriate.

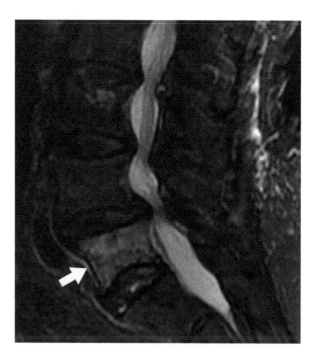

Fig. 10.43 Vertebral body compression fracture. Lumbar spine MR sagittal T2-weighted image shows edema throughout the L5 vertebral body (arrow), consistent with a compression fracture

Solution
MRI is over 99% sensitive for osteoporotic vertebral fractures and therefore is a useful follow-up exam to evaluate for a radiographically occult fracture.

A 69-year-old woman on bisphosphonate treatment for the past 5 years presents with groin pain.

a. X-ray femur
b. CT thigh without contrast
c. CT thigh with contrast
d. MRI thigh without contrast
e. No ideal imaging exam

Patients on long term (3–5 years) of bisphosphonates with thigh or groin pain. Initial imaging exam.

a. *X-ray femur* is the most appropriate.
b. CT thigh without contrast is usually not appropriate.
c. CT thigh with contrast is usually not appropriate.
d. MRI thigh without contrast is usually not appropriate.

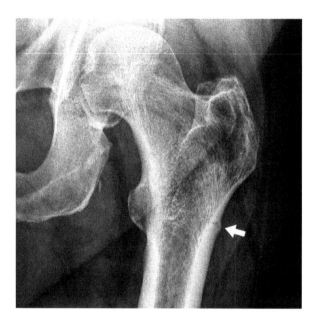

Fig. 10.44 Bisphosphonate-related femoral fracture. Femur X-ray anteroposterior view shows linear lucency with associated cortical thickening of the lateral femoral cortex in the subtrochanteric region (arrow), a location typical for bisphosphonate-related insufficiency fracture

Solution
Atypical subtrochanteric fractures in patients receiving long-term bisphosphates are associated with unique imaging features that differ from typical trauma-related subtrochanteric fractures. Radiography is a reliable first-line exam in this setting. Imaging of the contralateral femur is also recommended due to possible bilateral involvement.

A 71-year-old woman on bisphosphonate treatment for the past 5 years presents with groin pain. Radiographs are negative.

a. CT thigh without contrast bilateral
b. CT thigh with contrast bilateral
c. MRI thigh without contrast bilateral
d. Tc-99m bone scan whole body
e. No ideal imaging exam

Patients on long term (3–5 years) of bisphosphonates with thigh or groin pain. Initial radiographs are negative.

a. CT thigh without contrast bilateral is usually appropriate, but there is a better choice here.
b. CT thigh with contrast bilateral is usually not appropriate.
c. *MRI thigh without contrast bilateral* is the most appropriate.
d. Tc-99m bone scan whole body is usually appropriate, but there is a better choice here.

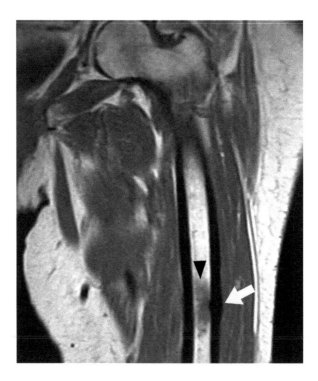

Fig. 10.45 Bisphosphonate-related femoral fracture. Thigh MR coronal T1-weighted image shows cortical thickening along the lateral femoral diaphysis (arrow) and adjacent bone marrow edema (arrowhead), consistent with bisphosphonate-related insufficiency fracture

Solution
MRI can diagnose radiographically occult bisphosphonate-related femoral fractures by detecting marrow signal abnormality and cortical thickening.

10.10 Atraumatic Shoulder Pain

A 61-year-old man with atraumatic shoulder pain.

a. X-ray shoulder
b. US shoulder
c. CT shoulder without contrast
d. MRI shoulder without contrast
e. No ideal imaging exam

Initial evaluation.

a. *X-ray shoulder* is the most appropriate.
b. US shoulder is usually not appropriate.
c. CT shoulder without contrast is usually not appropriate.
d. MRI shoulder without contrast is usually not appropriate.

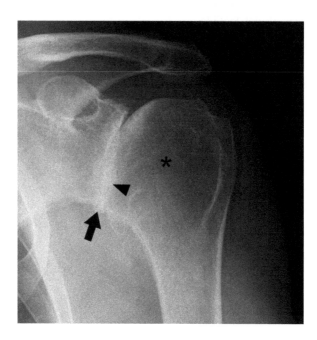

Fig. 10.46 Shoulder osteoarthritis. Shoulder X-ray anteroposterior view shows loss of the gleno-humeral joint space (arrow), subchondral sclerosis (arrowhead), and flattening of the humeral head (star)

Solution

Atraumatic shoulder pain can result from injury to the rotator cuff, glenohumeral articulation, joint capsule, biceps tendon, labrum, or bony structures. Radiography can show a range of pathologies including fracture, evidence of prior shoulder dislocation, osteoarthritis, rheumatoid arthritis, avascular necrosis of the humeral head, and calcific tendonitis.

A 59-year-old woman with atraumatic shoulder pain, with a suspected rotator cuff disorder. Radiographs are negative.

a. US shoulder
b. CT shoulder without contrast
c. MRI shoulder without contrast
d. MR arthrography shoulder
e. No ideal imaging exam

Atraumatic shoulder pain with rotator cuff disorder (e.g., tendinosis, tear, calcific tendinitis) suspected. Initial radiographs normal or inconclusive. Next imaging exam.

a. *US shoulder* and choice (c) are equally the most appropriate.
b. CT shoulder without contrast is usually not appropriate.
c. *MRI shoulder without contrast* and choice (a) are equally the most appropriate.
d. MR arthrography shoulder may be appropriate.

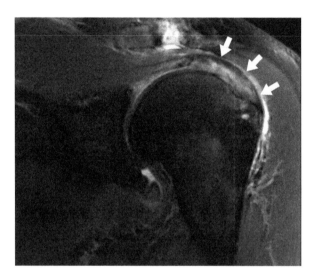

Fig. 10.47 Rotator cuff tear. Shoulder MR coronal T2-weighted image shows a high-grade, subtotal tear of the supraspinatus tendon (arrows) without tendon retraction

Solution
MRI is highly accurate for rotator cuff disease and evaluates for associated findings such as tendon retraction and muscle atrophy that can help guide management (e.g., conservative versus operative repair). US has similar accuracy for rotator cuff disease and can also be used to guide therapeutic interventions such as tenotomy and platelet-rich plasma injections.

A 48-year-old man with atraumatic shoulder pain, with a suspected labral tear. Radiographs are negative.

a. US shoulder
b. CT shoulder without contrast
c. MRI shoulder without contrast
d. MR arthrography shoulder
e. No ideal imaging exam

Atraumatic shoulder pain with labral tear and instability suspected. Initial radiographs normal or inconclusive. Next imaging exam.

a. US shoulder is usually not appropriate.
b. CT shoulder without contrast is usually not appropriate.
c. *MRI shoulder without contrast* and choice (d) are equally the most appropriate.
d. *MR arthrography shoulder* and choice (c) are equally the most appropriate.

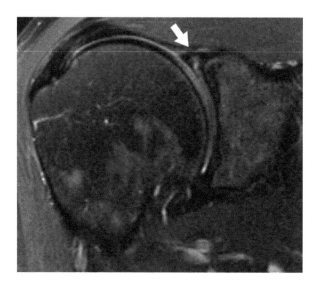

Fig. 10.48 Glenoid labral tear. Shoulder MR coronal T2-weighted image shows a tear of the superior glenoid labrum (arrow)

Solution
Both shoulder MRI and MR arthrography are very sensitive and specific for the evaluation of labral tears. With MR arthrography, provocative positioning maneuvers (e.g., abduction with external rotation) can improve detection of labral pathology.

A 51-year-old man with atraumatic shoulder pain, with suspected bursitis. Radiographs are negative.

a. US shoulder
b. CT shoulder without contrast
c. MRI shoulder without contrast
d. MR arthrography shoulder
e. No ideal imaging exam

Atraumatic shoulder pain with bursitis suspected. Initial radiographs normal or inconclusive. Next imaging exam.

a. *US shoulder* and choice (c) are equally the most appropriate.
b. CT shoulder without contrast is usually not appropriate.
c. *MRI shoulder without contrast* and choice (a) are equally the most appropriate.
d. MR arthrography shoulder is usually not appropriate.

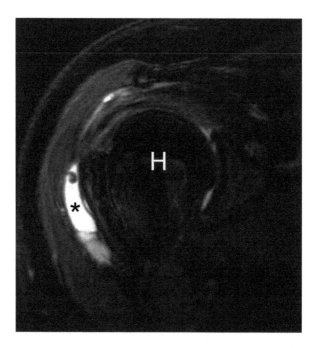

Fig. 10.49 Bursitis. Shoulder MR coronal T2-weighted image shows fluid in the subacromial-subdeltoid bursa (asterisk). *H* humeral head

Solution

Presence of fluid within the bursae around the shoulder is a nonspecific finding and may be seen with rotator cuff tear, inflammatory arthritis, crystal deposition disease, or septic bursitis. Both US and MRI provide excellent evaluation of the bursae. In addition, US can be used to guide aspiration of localized fluid collections.

A 57-year-old woman with atraumatic shoulder pain and suspected adhesive capsulitis. Radiographs are negative.

a. US shoulder
b. CT shoulder without contrast
c. MRI shoulder without contrast
d. MR arthrography shoulder
e. No ideal imaging exam

Atraumatic shoulder pain with suspected adhesive capsulitis. Initial radiographs normal or inconclusive. Next imaging exam.

a. US shoulder may be appropriate.
b. CT shoulder without contrast is usually not appropriate.
c. *MRI shoulder without contrast* is the most appropriate.
d. MR arthrography shoulder is usually not appropriate.

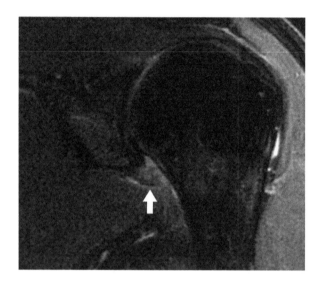

Fig. 10.50 Adhesive capsulitis. Shoulder MR coronal T2-weighted image shows edema and thickening of the axillary pouch and inferior glenohumeral ligament (arrow) with minimal joint fluid

Solution
Radiographs are often negative in adhesive capsulitis and are used mainly to exclude other conditions such as osteoarthritis and calcific tendinitis. MRI findings of adhesive capsulitis include thickening of the capsule, synovium, and ligament around the glenohumeral joint.

A 57-year-old woman with atraumatic shoulder pain, with suspected biceps tendonitis. Radiographs are negative.

a. US shoulder
b. CT shoulder without contrast
c. MRI shoulder without contrast
d. MR arthrography shoulder
e. No ideal imaging exam

Atraumatic shoulder pain with suspect biceps tendinitis, bursitis, dislocation, or tear. Initial radiographs normal or inconclusive. Next imaging exam.

a. *US shoulder* and choice (c) are equally the most appropriate.
b. CT shoulder without contrast is usually not appropriate.
c. *MRI shoulder without contrast* and choice (a) are equally the most appropriate.
d. MR arthrography shoulder may be appropriate.

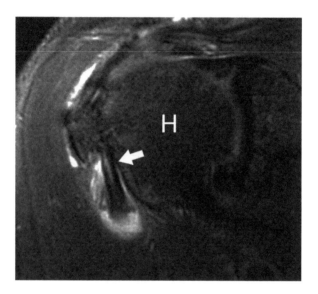

Fig. 10.51 Biceps tendonitis. Shoulder MR coronal T2-weighted image shows thickening, edema, and a partial tear along the biceps tendon (arrow) at the level of the bicipital groove. *H* humeral head

Solution
Either US or MRI can evaluate for tendinosis, tears and rupture, tenosynovitis, subluxation, and dislocation of the biceps tendon. Of note, US allows for use of provocative maneuvers to assess the degree of tendon subluxation in real time. MR arthrography can improve the accuracy of MRI in the detection of long head of the biceps tears.

A 49-year-old man with atraumatic shoulder pain suspected of neurogenic cause (excluding plexopathy). Initial imaging exam.

a. US shoulder
b. CT shoulder without contrast
c. MRI shoulder without contrast
d. MR arthrography shoulder
e. No ideal imaging exam

Atraumatic shoulder pain. Neurogenic pain (excluding plexopathy). Initial imaging.

a. US shoulder may be appropriate.
b. CT shoulder without contrast is usually not appropriate.
c. *MRI shoulder without contrast* is the most appropriate.
d. MR arthrography shoulder is usually not appropriate.

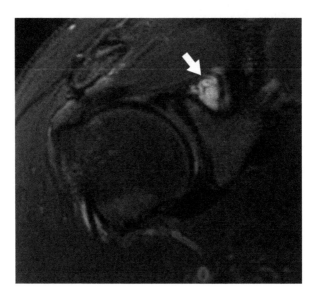

Fig. 10.52 Suprascapular notch cyst. Shoulder MR coronal T2-weighted image shows a multi-loculated cyst (arrow) in the suprascapular notch, where it can compress the suprascapular nerve

Solution
Pain in this scenario is often caused by compression, traction, or inflammation of the suprascapular and/or axillary nerves. MRI can directly visualize the nerves, identify causes of nerve compression, and reveal indirect signs of muscle denervation.

10.11 Chronic Elbow Pain

A 7-year-old boy with chronic elbow pain.

a. X-ray elbow
b. US elbow
c. CT elbow without contrast
d. MRI elbow without contrast
e. No ideal imaging exam

Initial evaluation. Initial imaging exam.

a. *X-ray elbow* is the most appropriate.
b. US elbow is usually not appropriate.
c. CT elbow without contrast is usually not appropriate.
d. MRI elbow without contrast is usually not appropriate.

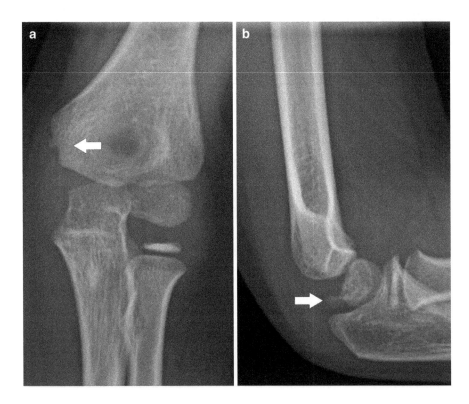

Fig. 10.53 Intra-articular body. Elbow X-ray anteroposterior (**a**) and lateral (**b**) views show a calcified loose body (arrow) in the joint

Solution

Causes for chronic elbow pain diagnosed on radiography include osseocartilaginous intra-articular bodies, osteophytes, heterotopic ossification, and osteochondritis dissecans.

A 24-year-old man with chronic elbow pain and locking, clicking, or limited motion. Intra-articular body or synovial abnormality is suspected. Radiographs are nondiagnostic.

a. US elbow
b. CT elbow without contrast
c. MRI elbow without contrast
d. Tc-99m bone scan elbow
e. No ideal imaging exam

Mechanical symptoms (locking, clicking, limited motion); suspect intra-articular osteo-cartilaginous body or synovial abnormality; radiographs nondiagnostic.

a. US elbow is usually not appropriate.
b. CT elbow without contrast is usually appropriate, but there is a better choice here.
c. *MRI elbow without contrast* is the most appropriate.
d. Tc-99m bone scan elbow is usually not appropriate.

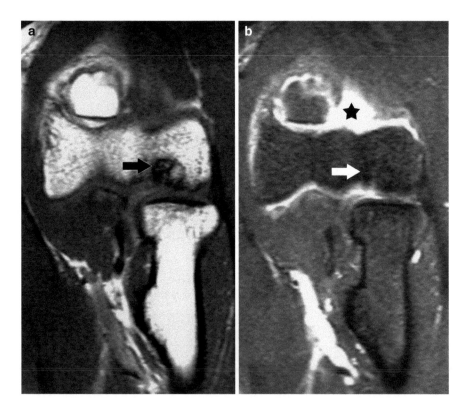

Fig. 10.54 Intra-articular body. Elbow MR coronal T1- (**a**) and T2-weighted (**b**) images show a loose body (arrows) and joint effusion (star)

Solution
Either MRI or MR arthrography are appropriate in this scenario, with selection of the exam dependent on local availability and expertise.

A 14-year-old boy with chronic elbow pain. Radiographs are nondiagnostic. An occult fracture is suspected.

a. CT elbow without contrast
b. CT arthrography elbow
c. MRI elbow without contrast
d. MR arthrography elbow
e. No ideal imaging exam

Occult fracture or other bone abnormality suspected. Radiographs are nondiagnostic.

a. CT elbow without contrast may be appropriate.
b. CT arthrography elbow is usually not appropriate.
c. *MRI elbow without contrast* is the most appropriate.
d. MR arthrography elbow is usually not appropriate.

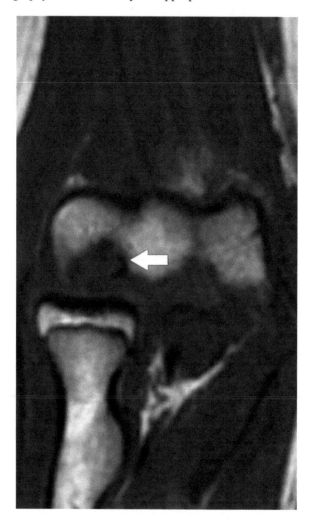

Fig. 10.55 Osteochondral injury. Elbow MR coronal proton density-weighted image reveals an osteochondral injury (arrow) at the capitellum of the humerus

Solution

MRI can demonstrate both traumatic and stress fractures. CT detects acute traumatic fractures but is of limited usefulness in identifying stress fractures at the elbow.

A 41-year-old man with chronic elbow pain and a palpable soft tissue mass. Radiographs are nondiagnostic.

a. US elbow
b. CT elbow with contrast
c. MRI elbow without and with contrast
d. Tc-99m bone scan elbow
e. No ideal imaging exam

Palpable soft tissue mass; radiographs nondiagnostic.

a. US elbow is usually appropriate, but there is a better choice here.
b. CT elbow without contrast is usually not appropriate.
c. *MRI elbow without and with contrast* is the most appropriate.
d. Tc-99m bone scan elbow is usually not appropriate.

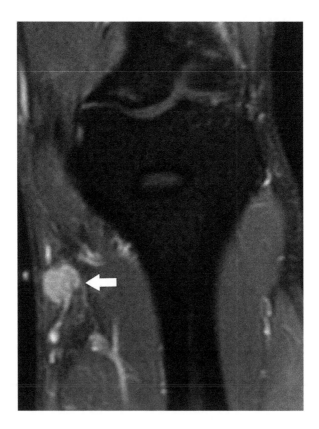

Fig. 10.56 Enlarged lymph node. Elbow MR coronal post-contrast image reveals an enhancing 12 mm soft tissue mass (arrows)

Solution
Use of intravenous contrast with MRI is needed for the evaluation of some, but not all, soft tissue masses. Contrast is usually indicated if a malignancy is suspected. However, a lipoma, for example, can be characterized without the use of contrast.

A 13-year-old boy with chronic elbow pain suspected with epicondylitis and refractory to empiric treatment. Radiographs are nondiagnostic.

a. US elbow
b. CT elbow without contrast
c. CT elbow with contrast
d. MRI elbow without contrast
e. No ideal imaging exam

Chronic epicondylitis suspected. Radiographs are nondiagnostic.

a. US elbow is usually appropriate, but there is a better choice here.
b. CT elbow without contrast is usually not appropriate.
c. CT elbow with contrast is usually not appropriate.
d. *MRI elbow without contrast* is the most appropriate.

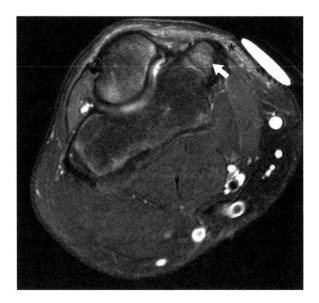

Fig. 10.57 Medial epicondylitis. Elbow MR axial T2-weighted image shows edema in the medial epicondyle (arrow) and in the surrounding soft tissues (star)

Solution
Epicondylitis, caused by degeneration and tearing of the common extensor tendon laterally or common flexor tendon medially, typically does not require imaging for diagnosis. MRI is useful for confirming the diagnosis in refractory cases and to exclude associated tendon and ligament tears.

A 21-year-old man with chronic elbow pain suspicious for collateral ligament tear. Radiographs are nondiagnostic.

a. US elbow
b. CT elbow without contrast
c. CT arthrography elbow
d. MRI elbow without contrast
e. No ideal imaging exam

Collateral ligament tear suspected. Radiographs are nondiagnostic.

a. US elbow may be appropriate.
b. CT elbow without contrast is usually not appropriate.
c. CT arthrography elbow may be appropriate.
d. *MRI elbow without contrast* is the most appropriate.

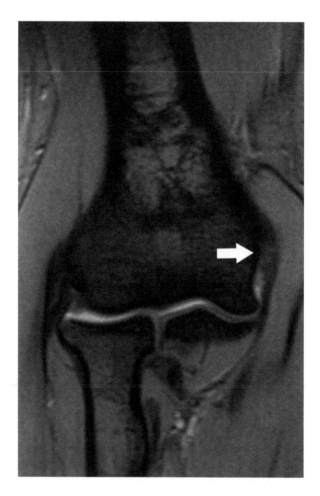

Fig. 10.58 Medial collateral ligament tear. Elbow MR coronal T2-weighted image shows a partial tear (arrow) of the medial collateral ligament at its humeral attachment

Solution
Either MRI or MR arthrography is appropriate in this scenario, with the selection of the imaging exam dependent on local availability and expertise.

A 59-year-old man with chronic elbow pain. Biceps tendon tear is suspected. Radiographs are nondiagnostic.

a. US elbow
b. CT elbow with contrast
c. MRI elbow without contrast
d. MR arthrography elbow
e. No ideal imaging exam

Biceps tendon tear suspected. Radiographs are nondiagnostic.

a. US elbow is usually appropriate, but there is a better choice here.
b. CT elbow with contrast is usually not appropriate.
c. *MRI elbow without contrast* is the most appropriate.
d. MR arthrography elbow is usually not appropriate.

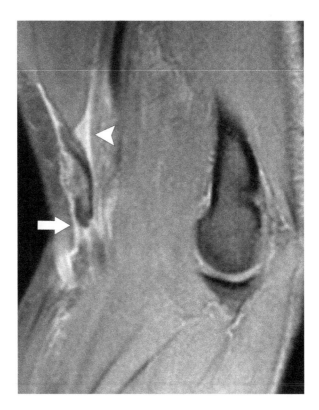

Fig. 10.59 Biceps tendon tear. Elbow MR sagittal T2-weighted image shows a tear (arrow) of the biceps tendon near its radial insertion. Fluid (arrowhead) is seen along the course of the bicipital-radial bursa

Solution
MRI is the preferred modality for this scenario. US can also be used to evaluate for abnormalities of the distal biceps tendon if the necessary operator expertise is available.

A 47-year-old woman with chronic elbow pain suspicious for a nerve abnormality. Radiographs are nondiagnostic.

a. US elbow
b. CT elbow without contrast
c. CT arthrography elbow
d. MRI elbow without contrast
e. MR arthrography elbow

Nerve abnormality suspected. Radiographs are nondiagnostic.

a. US elbow is usually appropriate, but there is a better choice here.
b. CT elbow without contrast is usually not appropriate.
c. CT arthrography elbow is usually not appropriate.
d. *MRI elbow without contrast* is the most appropriate.
e. MR arthrography elbow is usually not appropriate.

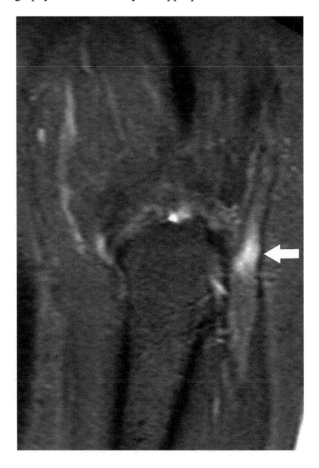

Fig. 10.60 Ulnar neuritis. Elbow MR coronal T2-weighted image shows abnormal signal and thickening of the ulnar nerve (arrow)

Solution
The ulnar nerve is vulnerable to trauma from a direct blow in the region of the cubital tunnel. Anatomic variations of the cubital tunnel retinaculum can also contribute to neuropathy. MRI can demonstrate the size and shape of the nerve as well as signal abnormalities that suggest neuritis. If the necessary operator expertise is available, US is a reasonable alternative.

10.12   Chronic Wrist Pain

A 53-year-old woman presents with chronic wrist pain.

a. X-ray wrist
b. CT wrist without contrast
c. MRI wrist without contrast
d. Tc-99m bone scan wrist
e. No ideal imaging exam

Initial evaluation.

a. *X-ray wrist* is the most appropriate.
b. CT wrist without contrast is usually not appropriate.
c. MRI wrist without contrast is usually not appropriate.
d. Tc-99m bone scan wrist is usually not appropriate.

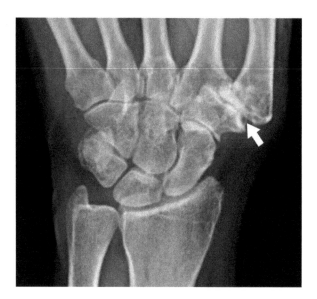

Fig. 10.61 Osteoarthritis. Wrist X-ray anteroposterior view shows findings of severe osteoarthritis at the first carpometacarpal joint (arrow), including severe joint space narrowing, subchondral sclerosis, and subchondral cysts

Solution
Causes of chronic wrist pain that can be diagnosed on radiography include arthritis, complications of injury, infection, bone or soft tissue tumors, impaction syndromes, and static wrist instability. Stress positions and maneuvers can reveal dynamic instability not visible on standard views.

An 18-year-old man with chronic wrist pain, negative radiographs, and persistent symptoms.

a. US wrist
b. CT wrist without contrast
c. MRI wrist without contrast
d. Tc-99m bone scan wrist
e. No ideal imaging exam

Radiographs normal or nonspecific and persistent symptoms.

a. US wrist is usually not appropriate.
b. CT wrist without contrast is usually not appropriate.
c. *MRI wrist without contrast* is the most appropriate.
d. Tc-99m bone scan wrist is usually not appropriate.

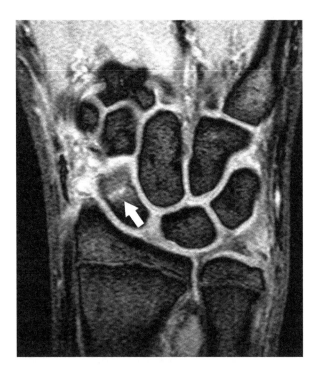

Fig. 10.62 Occult scaphoid fracture. Wrist MR coronal proton density-weighted image shows a nondisplaced scaphoid fracture (arrow)

Solution
In patients with chronic wrist pain when initial radiography does not show a specific diagnosis further imaging is usually not indicated. When additional imaging is needed, MRI is more sensitive for abnormalities of the bones and bone marrow, articular cartilage, intrinsic and extrinsic ligaments, triangular fibrocartilage complex, synovium, tendons, and neurovascular structures.

A 75-year-old man with chronic wrist pain. Radiographs reveal nonspecific arthritis. Infection is a consideration.

a. CT wrist
b. MRI wrist without contrast
c. Tc-99m bone scan wrist
d. Image-guided aspiration of wrist
e. No ideal imaging exam

Radiographs normal or show nonspecific arthritis. Need to exclude infection. Next exam.

a. CT wrist is usually not appropriate.
b. MRI wrist without contrast is usually not appropriate.
c. Tc-99m bone scan wrist is usually not appropriate.
d. *Image-guided aspiration of wrist* is the most appropriate.

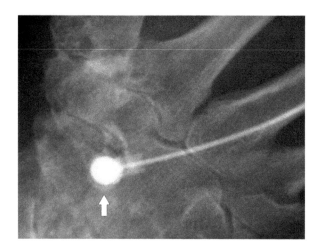

Fig. 10.63   Wrist aspiration. Wrist fluoroscopy anteroposterior view shows a 25G needle (arrow) injecting contrast into a midcarpal joint to confirm needle position for aspiration

Solution
In patients with suspected joint infection, aspiration should not be delayed while awaiting advanced imaging exams. Percutaneous aspiration of the wrist is indicated even when radiography is normal.

A 39-year-old man with chronic wrist pain. Kienbock's disease is suspected. Radiographs are normal.

a. US wrist
b. CT wrist without contrast
c. MRI wrist without contrast
d. Tc-99m bone scan wrist
e. No ideal imaging exam

Radiographs normal or equivocal. Suspect Kienböck's disease. Next exam.

a. US wrist is usually not appropriate.
b. CT wrist without contrast may be appropriate.
c. *MRI wrist without contrast* is the most appropriate.
d. Tc-99m bone scan wrist is usually not appropriate.

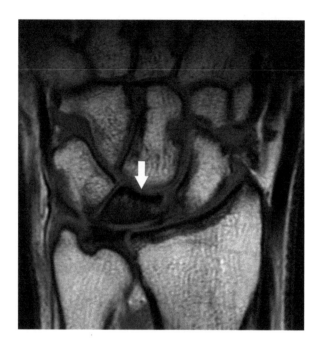

Fig. 10.64 Kienböck's disease. Wrist MR coronal T1-weighted image reveals abnormal bone marrow signal throughout the lunate (arrow) consistent with osteonecrosis

Solution

Suspected Kienböck's disease, or osteonecrosis of the lunate, is most appropriately evaluated with MRI when initial radiographs are normal or equivocal. Of note, in many cases, the radiographic findings are diagnostic and are adequate for treatment planning by depicting the degree of carpal collapse, ulnar variance, and associated osteoarthritis.

A 51-year-old woman with chronic wrist pain with suspected ganglion cyst. Radiographs are normal.

a. US wrist
b. CT wrist with contrast
c. MRI wrist without and with contrast
d. MR arthrography wrist
e. No ideal imaging exam

Palpable mass or suspected occult ganglion cyst. Radiographs normal or nonspecific. Next exam.

a. *US wrist* and choice (c) are equally the most appropriate.
b. CT wrist with contrast is usually not appropriate.
c. *MRI wrist without and with contrast* and choice (a) are equally the most appropriate.
d. MR arthrography wrist is usually not appropriate.

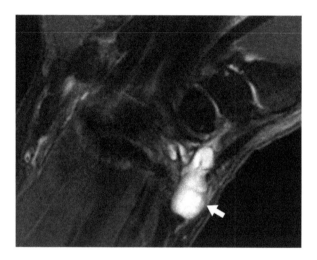

Fig. 10.65 Ganglion cyst. Wrist MR coronal T2-weighted image shows a loculated cyst (arrow) along the radial soft tissues adjacent to the first extensor compartment tendons

Solution
Structures that are well-depicted by wrist MRI include ganglia, cysts, and bursae. Contrast can be helpful to distinguish ganglia from synovitis. When available, US is an alternative with similar accuracy to MRI.

A 32-year-old woman with chronic wrist pain, nondiagnostic radiographs, and suspected occult fracture.

a. US wrist
b. CT wrist without contrast
c. MRI wrist without contrast
d. Tc-99m bone scan wrist
e. No ideal imaging exam

Occult fracture or stress fracture suspected. Radiographs are nondiagnostic. Next exam.

a. US wrist is usually not appropriate.
b. *CT wrist without contrast* and choice (c) are equally the most appropriate.
c. *MRI wrist without contrast* and choice (b) are equally the most appropriate.
d. Tc-99m bone scan wrist may be appropriate.

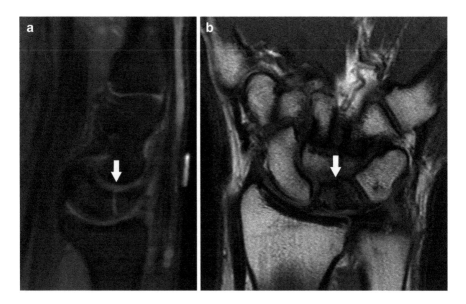

Fig. 10.66 Lunate fracture. Wrist MR sagittal T2-weighted (**a**) and coronal T1-weighted (**b**) images reveal a nondisplaced lunate fracture (arrows) and marrow signal abnormality suggestive of osteonecrosis

Solution
Either CT or MRI is appropriate in this scenario. CT is faster and may be easier to perform in patients who are casted. MRI is more sensitive for marrow abnormalities that accompany occult and stress fractures.

A 47-year-old woman with chronic wrist pain with suspected carpal tunnel syndrome. Radiographs are normal.

a. US wrist
b. CT wrist without contrast
c. MRI wrist without contrast
d. MR arthrography wrist
e. No ideal imaging exam

Suspect carpal tunnel syndrome. Radiographs normal or nonspecific. Next imaging exam.

a. US wrist may be appropriate.
b. CT wrist without contrast is usually not appropriate.
c. MRI wrist without contrast may be appropriate.
d. MR arthrography wrist is usually not appropriate.
e. *No ideal imaging exam.*

Solution
The standard for diagnosing carpal tunnel syndrome is clinical examination combined with electrophysiologic testing. MRI may be used in cases where this initial evaluation is equivocal. US may be used to measure the cross-sectional area of the median nerve or to replace or complement nerve conduction studies.

10.13 Chronic Hip Pain

A 64-year-old woman with chronic hip pain.

a. X-ray pelvis and hip
b. CT hip without contrast
c. MRI hip without contrast
d. Tc-99m bone scan hip
e. No ideal imaging exam

Initial evaluation.

a. *X-ray pelvis and hip* is the most appropriate.
b. CT hip without contrast is usually not appropriate.
c. MRI hip without contrast is usually not appropriate.
d. Tc-99m bone scan hip is usually not appropriate.

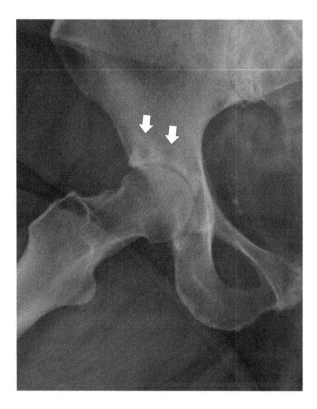

Fig. 10.67 Osteoarthritis. Hip X-ray frog leg lateral view reveals joint space narrowing, osteophytes, and subchondral sclerosis (arrows)

Solution
Initial evaluation of chronic hip pain is with pelvis and hip X-ray, which can demonstrate common causes such as arthritis as well as less common disorders such as primary bone tumors. Including a view of the full pelvis is more useful than limiting evaluation to only the ipsilateral hip.

A 47-year-old woman with chronic hip pain and negative radiographs. An extra-articular non-infectious soft tissue cause of pain, such as tendonitis, is suspected.

a. US hip
b. CT hip without contrast
c. MRI hip without contrast
d. Tc-99m bone scan hip
e. No ideal imaging exam

Radiographs negative, equivocal, or nondiagnostic. Suspect extraarticular noninfectious soft tissue abnormality, such as tendonitis.

a. US hip is usually appropriate, but there is a better choice here.
b. CT hip without contrast is usually not appropriate.
c. *MRI hip without contrast* is the most appropriate.
d. Tc-99m bone scan hip is usually not appropriate.

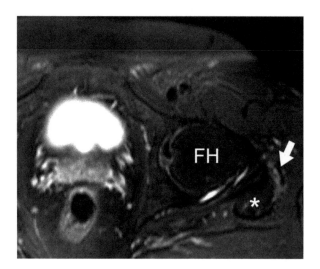

Fig. 10.68 Gluteus minimus tendonitis. Hip MR axial T2-weighted image shows edema along the left gluteus minimus tendon (arrow) adjacent to its attachment site at the left femoral greater trochanter (star). The femoral head (FH) is labeled for reference

Solution
MRI is sensitive and specific for many potential causes of chronic hip pain such as iliopsoas bursitis, athletic pubalgia, abductor tendinosis or tears, tendonitis, and hamstring injuries. US can help localize fluid collections such as paralabral cysts.

A 32-year-old man with chronic hip pain, negative radiographs, and suspected femoroacetabular impingement.

a. US hip
b. CT hip without contrast
c. MRI hip without contrast
d. Tc-99m bone scan hip
e. No ideal imaging exam

Radiographs negative, equivocal, or nondiagnostic. Suspect femoroacetabular impingement.

a. US hip may be appropriate.
b. CT hip without contrast may be appropriate.
c. *MRI hip without contrast* is the most appropriate.
d. Tc-99m bone scan hip is usually not appropriate.

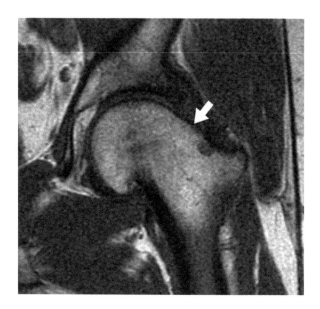

Fig. 10.69 Femoroacetabular impingement. Hip MR coronal T1-weighted image shows overgrowth of the superior left femoral neck (arrow), indicating a cam-type femoroacetabular impingement

Solution
Either CT or MRI can be used to accurately evaluate femoral head and neck morphology to provide a noninvasive assessment of hips at risk for femoroacetabular impingement. MRI offers superior soft tissue characterization compared to CT to look for extra-articular impingement.

A 23-year-old man with chronic hip pain and a suspected labral tear. Radiographs are negative.

a. CT hip without contrast
b. CT arthrography hip
c. MRI hip without contrast
d. MR arthrography hip
e. No ideal imaging exam

Radiographs negative or equivocal. Labral tear suspected with or without clinical findings suggesting femoroacetabular impingement.

a. CT hip without contrast is usually not appropriate.
b. CT arthrography hip is usually appropriate, but there is a better choice here.
c. MRI hip without contrast may be appropriate.
d. *MR arthrography hip* is the most appropriate.

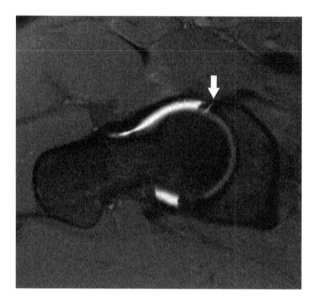

Fig. 10.70 Labral tear. Hip MR arthrography axial T1-weighted image reveals a full-thickness tear (arrow) of the anterolateral acetabular labrum

Solution

MR arthrography using direct intra-articular contrast injection is an established method for the evaluation of labral tears and, in general, is more sensitive than MRI or CT arthrography.

A 31-year-old woman with chronic hip pain. Evaluation of the articular cartilage is needed. Radiography has already been performed.

a. CT hip without contrast
b. CT arthrography hip
c. MRI hip without contrast
d. MRI arthrography hip
e. No ideal imaging exam

Evaluate articular cartilage. Next exam after radiographs.

a. CT hip without contrast is usually not appropriate.
b. CT arthrography hip is usually appropriate, but there is a better choice here.
c. *MRI hip without contrast* and choice (d) are equally the most appropriate.
d. *MR arthrography hip* and choice (c) are equally the most appropriate.

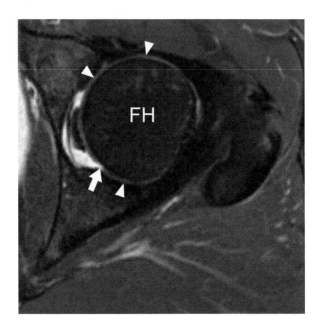

Fig. 10.71 Articular cartilage defect. Hip MR axial T2-weighted image shows a focal defect (arrow) along the cartilage of the left femoral head (FH). Normal cartilage is present elsewhere (arrowheads)

Solution
MRI, MR arthrography, or CT arthrography can provide excellent assessment of articular cartilage. With arthrography, intra-articular injection of anesthetic and/or steroid can be performed at the same time as the contrast injection, which can be both diagnostic and therapeutic.

10.14 Chronic Knee Pain

A 67-year-old woman with chronic knee pain.

a. X-ray knee
b. US knee
c. CT knee without contrast
d. MRI knee without contrast
e. No ideal imaging exam

Initial evaluation.

a. *X-ray knee* is the most appropriate.
b. US knee is usually not appropriate.
c. CT knee without contrast is usually not appropriate.
d. MRI knee without contrast is usually not appropriate.

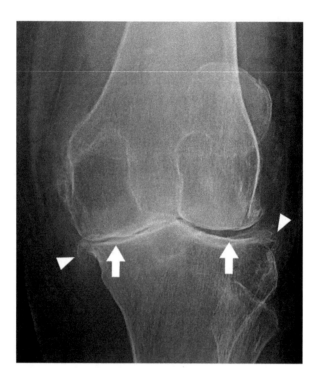

Fig. 10.72 Osteoarthritis. Knee radiograph anteroposterior view shows medial and lateral compartment joint space narrowing (arrows), subchondral sclerosis, and osteophyte formation (arrowheads)

Solution
Radiography is the preferred initial exam for chronic knee pain. In the elderly, osteoarthritis is the most common etiology. Findings of osteoarthritis include joint space narrowing, osteophytes, subchondral cysts, and subarticular sclerosis. Articular cartilage loss is assessed indirectly by visualization of joint space narrowing and changes in subchondral bone.

A 52-year-old woman with chronic knee pain. Radiographs are negative.

a. CT knee without contrast
b. CT arthrography knee
c. MRI knee without contrast
d. MR arthrography knee
e. No ideal imaging exam

Initial knee radiograph negative or demonstrates joint effusion. Next imaging exam.

a. CT knee without contrast may be appropriate.
b. CT arthrography knee may be appropriate.
c. *MRI knee without contrast* is the most appropriate.
d. MR arthrography knee may be appropriate.

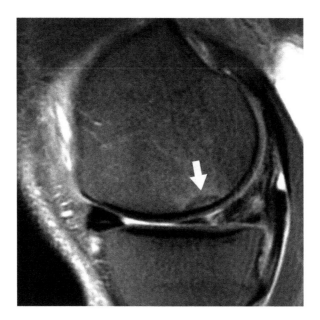

Fig. 10.73 Subchondral insufficiency fracture. Knee MR sagittal T2-weighted image shows a non-displaced subchondral insufficiency fracture (arrow) with adjacent marrow edema along the medial femoral condyle

Solution
MRI depicts numerous etiologies of chronic knee pain including articular cartilage and meniscal abnormalities, bone marrow lesions, subchondral insufficiency fractures, ruptured popliteal cysts, patellar tendinopathy, and iliotibial band syndrome.

10.15   Chronic Ankle Pain

A 28-year-old man with chronic ankle pain.

a. X-ray ankle
b. CT ankle without contrast
c. MRI ankle without contrast
d. Tc-99m bone scan ankle
e. No ideal imaging exam

Initial evaluation.

a. *X-ray ankle* is the most appropriate.
b. CT ankle without contrast is usually not appropriate.
c. MRI ankle without contrast is usually not appropriate.
d. Tc-99m bone scan ankle is usually not appropriate.

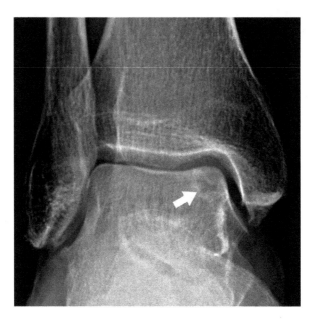

Fig. 10.74 Osteochondral lesion. Ankle radiograph anteroposterior view shows subchondral lucency (arrow) at the medial talar dome

Solution

Radiography can show a range of bone and soft tissue abnormalities that may cause chronic ankle pain, including osteoarthritis, calcified or ossified intra-articular bodies, osteochondral abnormalities, stress fractures, or sequela of prior trauma.

A 46-year-old woman with chronic ankle pain. Osteochondral injury is suspected. Radiographs are normal.

a. CT ankle without contrast
b. CT arthrography ankle
c. MRI ankle without contrast
d. MR arthrography ankle
e. No ideal imaging exam

Normal ankle radiographs normal and suspected osteochondral injury. Next exam.

a. CT ankle without contrast may be appropriate.
b. CT arthrography ankle may be appropriate.
c. *MRI ankle without contrast* is the most appropriate.
d. MR arthrography ankle may be appropriate.

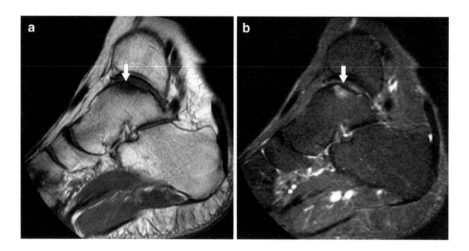

Fig. 10.75 Osteochondral injury. Ankle MR sagittal T1- (**a**) and T2-weighted (**b**) images reveal abnormal signal (arrow) at the articular surface of the talar dome

Solution
Osteochondral injuries usually involve the talar dome or, less commonly, the tibial plafond or the tarsal navicular bone. Radiography often does not show the full extent of the injury and may be initially negative if the injury is limited to the articular hyaline cartilage. MRI is highly sensitive for osteochondral abnormalities and can be used to assess stability and to preoperatively stage osteochondral lesions.

A 53-year-old woman with chronic ankle pain suspicious for tendon abnormality. Radiographs are normal.

a. US ankle
b. CT ankle without contrast
c. CT arthrography ankle
d. MRI ankle without contrast
e. No ideal imaging exam

Normal ankle radiographs and suspected tendon abnormality. Next exam.

a. *US ankle* and choice (d) are equally the most appropriate.
b. CT ankle without contrast is usually not appropriate.
c. CT arthrography ankle is usually not appropriate.
d. *MRI ankle without contrast* and choice (a) are equally the most appropriate.

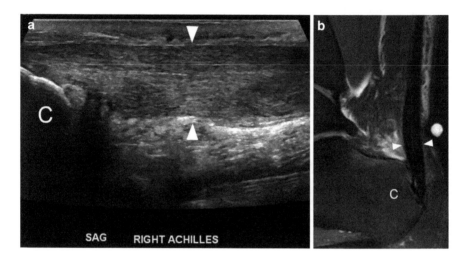

Fig. 10.76 Achilles tendinopathy. Ankle US sagittal image (**a**) and MR sagittal T2-weighted image (**b**) show thickening of the distal Achilles tendon (between arrowheads) with interstitial edema near its attachment at the calcaneus (C)

Solution
Possible tendon abnormalities include tenosynovitis, tendinopathy, partial or complete tear, subluxation, or dislocation. US and MRI are equally appropriate in this scenario, although US requires operator skill and expertise which is not as widely available. US provides the advantage of dynamic assessment for tendon subluxation and dislocation.

A 55-year-old man with chronic ankle pain and instability. Radiographs are negative.

a. US ankle
b. CT ankle without contrast
c. CT arthrography ankle
d. MRI ankle without contrast
e. MR arthrography ankle

Ankle instability with negative radiographs. Next exam.

a. US ankle may be appropriate.
b. CT ankle without contrast is usually not appropriate.
c. CT arthrography ankle may be appropriate.
d. *MRI ankle without contrast* and choice (e) are equally the most appropriate.
e. *MR arthrography ankle* and choice (d) are equally the most appropriate.

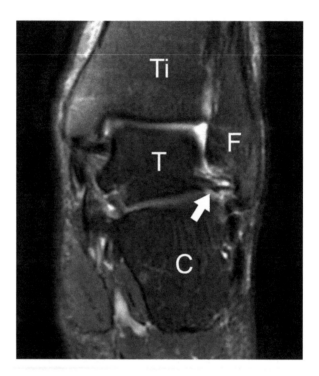

Fig. 10.77 Ankle instability. Ankle MR coronal T2-weighted image shows a partial tear of the posterior talofibular ligament (arrow). The anterior talofibular ligament was also torn (not shown). *C* calcaneus, *F* fibula, *T* talus, *Ti* tibia

Solution
MRI can accurately diagnose injuries to ankle ligaments and evaluate for abnormalities associated with ankle instability such as tenosynovitis, tendinopathy, and osteochondral lesions.

A 50-year-old man with chronic ankle pain suspicious for impingement syndrome. Radiographs are normal.

a. CT ankle without contrast
b. CT arthrography ankle
c. MRI ankle without contrast
d. MR arthrography ankle
e. No ideal imaging exam

Normal ankle radiographs and suspected ankle impingement syndrome. Next imaging exam.

a. CT ankle without contrast may be appropriate.
b. CT arthrography ankle may be appropriate.
c. *MRI ankle without contrast* is the most appropriate.
d. MR arthrography ankle may be appropriate.

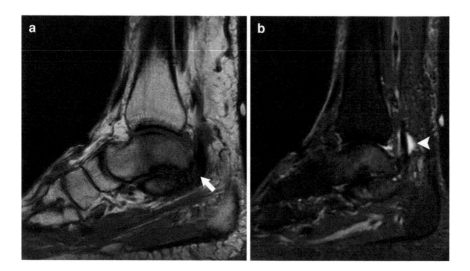

Fig. 10.78 Posterior impingement syndrome. Ankle MR sagittal proton density (**a**) and T2-weighted (**b**) images show an os trigonum (arrow) and fluid (arrowhead) around a thickened flexor hallucis longus tendon

Solution

MRI is useful for diagnosing impingement syndrome and for surgical planning. Additionally, it can help exclude other pathologies that may mimic or coexist with impingement syndromes. However, an accurate diagnosis requires careful correlation of imaging features with clinical findings since MRI findings alone are nonspecific and can be seen in asymptomatic individuals.

10.16 Chronic Foot Pain

A 51-year-old woman with chronic foot pain. Initial imaging exam.

a. X-ray foot
b. US foot
c. CT foot without contrast
d. MRI foot without contrast
e. No ideal imaging exam

Chronic foot pain of unknown etiology. First imaging exam.

a. *X-ray foot* is the most appropriate.
b. US foot is usually not appropriate.
c. CT foot without contrast is usually not appropriate.
d. MRI foot without contrast is usually not appropriate.

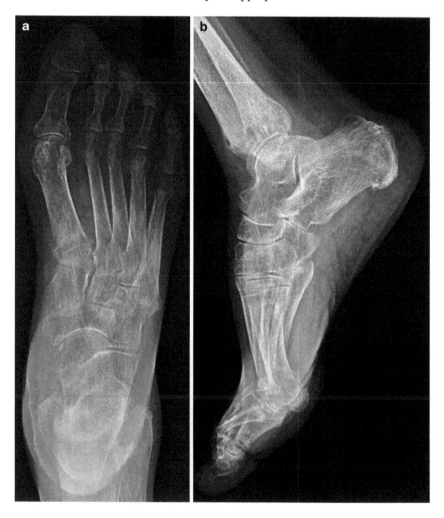

Fig. 10.79 Complex regional pain syndrome type 1. Foot X-ray anteroposterior (**a**) and lateral (**b**) views reveal diffuse osteopenia

Solution

Radiography is the preferred initial exam to evaluate foot pathology. It can reveal a range of etiologies for chronic foot pain including tarsal coalition, avascular necrosis of the metatarsal head, and different types of arthritis.

A 56-year-old woman with chronic foot pain and clinical concern for complex regional pain syndrome type 1. Radiographs are negative.

a. US foot
b. CT foot without contrast
c. MRI foot without contrast
d. Tc-99m three-phase bone scan foot
e. No ideal imaging exam

Clinical concern for complex regional pain syndrome type I. Radiographs are negative or equivocal.

a. US foot is usually not appropriate.
b. CT foot without contrast is usually not appropriate.
c. MRI foot without contrast is usually not appropriate.
d. *Tc-99m three-phase bone scan foot* is the most appropriate.

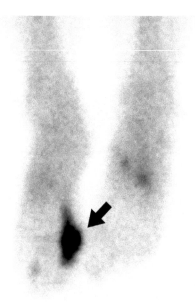

Fig. 10.80 Complex regional pain syndrome type 1. Foot Tc-99m bone scan skeletal phase anteroposterior image shows asymmetrically increased radiotracer uptake at the right great toe base (arrow). Similar increased uptake was present on flow and tissue phase images (not shown)

Solution

Complex regional pain syndrome type I is characterized clinically by pain, tenderness, swelling, diminished motor function, and vasomotor instability. In the majority of patients, radiography shows diffuse osteopenia, which is nonspecific, as it is seen with any disuse of the foot. Three-phase radionuclide bone scans are highly accurate and is used to make the diagnosis.

A 16-year-old boy with chronically painful and rigid flat foot, and clinical concern for tarsal coalition. Radiographs are negative.

a. US foot
b. CT foot without contrast
c. MRI foot without contrast
d. Tc-99m bone scan foot
e. No ideal imaging exam

Adult or child. Painful rigid flat foot and clinical concern for tarsal coalition. Radiographs unremarkable or equivocal.

a. US foot is usually not appropriate.
b. *CT foot without contrast* and choice (c) are equally the most appropriate.
c. *MRI foot without contrast* and choice (b) are equally the most appropriate.
d. Tc-99m bone scan foot is usually not appropriate.

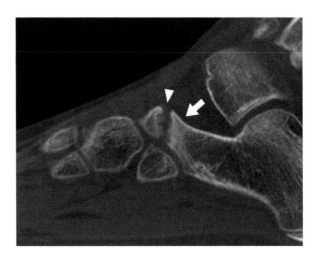

Fig. 10.81 Calcaneonavicular coalition. Foot CT sagittal reconstruction image shows elongation of the anterior process of the calcaneus (arrow) with narrowing and irregularity at the calcaneonavicular joint (arrowhead)

Solution
Tarsal coalition is a congenital fibrous, cartilaginous, or osseous union of two or more tarsal bones. The most common types are calcaneonavicular and talocalcaneal, both readily seen on radiography. When radiographs are negative or equivocal, both CT and MRI are effective and diagnostic.

An 18-year-old girl with chronic pain and tenderness over the second metatarsal head. Freiberg infarction is suspected.

a. X-ray foot
b. CT foot without contrast
c. MRI foot without contrast
d. Tc-99m bone scan foot
e. No ideal imaging exam

Pain and tenderness over head of second metatarsal and clinical concern for Freiberg infarction.

a. *X-ray foot* is the most appropriate.
b. CT foot without contrast is usually not appropriate.
c. MRI foot without contrast is usually not appropriate.
d. Tc-99m bone scan foot is usually not appropriate.

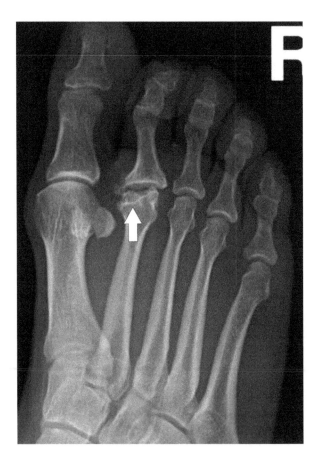

Fig. 10.82 Freiberg infarction. Foot X-ray anteroposterior view reveals flattening and collapse of the second metatarsal head (arrow) consistent with avascular necrosis

Solution
Freiberg infarction is characterized by pain, tenderness, swelling, and limited motion in the affected metatarsophalangeal joint. It most commonly affects the second metatarsal. Radiography can readily show the characteristic findings.

A 52-year-old woman with chronic foot pain and tenderness over the tarsus, unresponsive to conservative therapy. Radiographs show an accessory ossicle.

a. US foot
b. CT foot without contrast
c. MRI foot without contrast
d. Tc-99m bone scan foot
e. No ideal imaging exam

Pain and tenderness over the navicular tuberosity unresponsive to conservative therapy. Radiographs showed accessory navicular.

a. US foot is usually not appropriate.
b. CT foot without contrast is usually not appropriate.
c. *MRI foot without contrast* is the most appropriate.
d. Tc-99m bone scan foot may be appropriate.

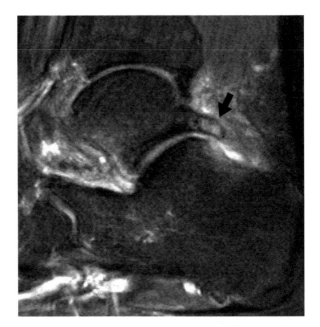

Fig. 10.83 Os trigonum syndrome. Foot MR sagittal T2-weighted image shows edema within the os trigonum at the posterior talus (arrow) and of the surrounding soft tissue

Solution
Potentially painful accessory bones include accessory navicular and os trigonum. Pain is attributed to traumatic or degenerative changes at the synchondrosis or to soft tissue inflammation which can be seen on MRI.

A 55-year-old man with chronic burning pain and paresthesia along the plantar surface of the foot suspicious for tarsal tunnel syndrome. Radiographs are negative.

a. US foot
b. CT foot without contrast
c. MRI foot without contrast
d. Tc-99m bone scan foot
e. No ideal imaging exam

Burning pain and paresthesia along the plantar surface of the foot and clinical concern for tarsal tunnel syndrome. Radiographs are unremarkable or equivocal.

a. US foot may be appropriate.
b. CT foot without contrast is usually not appropriate.
c. *MRI foot without contrast* is the most appropriate.
d. Tc-99m bone scan foot is usually not appropriate.

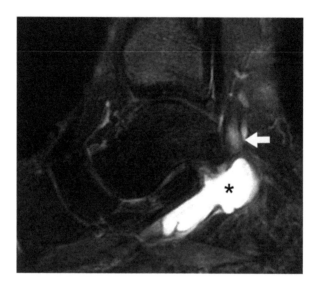

Fig. 10.84 Tarsal tunnel syndrome. Foot MR sagittal T2-weighted image shows a ganglion cyst (star) in the tarsal tunnel with abnormal thickening and edema of the adjacent posterior tibial nerve (arrow)

Solution

Tarsal tunnel syndrome is a neuropathy caused by compression of the posterior tibial nerve or one of its branches. Most commonly, this is caused by inflammatory processes or mass lesions in the tarsal tunnel, which are best evaluated by MRI.

A 47-year-old man with chronic foot pain in the 3–4 web space radiating to the toes. Morton's neuroma is suspected.

a. US foot
b. CT foot without contrast
c. MRI foot without and with contrast
d. Tc-99m bone scan foot
e. No ideal imaging exam

Pain in the 3–4 web space radiating to the toes and clinical concern for Morton's neuroma. Radiographs unremarkable or equivocal.

a. *US foot* and choice (c) are equally the most appropriate.
b. CT foot without contrast is usually not appropriate.
c. *MRI foot without and with contrast* and choice (a) are equally the most appropriate.
d. Tc-99m bone scan foot is usually not appropriate.

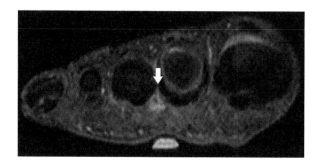

Fig. 10.85 Morton's neuroma. Foot MR axial post-contrast images show a 5 mm enhancing mass (arrow) in the plantar soft tissue underlying the skin marker, indicating the palpable abnormality

Solution
A Morton's neuroma is a perineural fibrous proliferation involving the plantar digital nerve, best seen on MRI. Intravenous contrast improves sensitivity for detection. US is a reasonable alternative when the necessary operator expertise is available and can have similar sensitivity to MRI.

An 18-year-old athlete with chronic foot pain and tenderness over the tarsal navicular. Radiographs are normal.

a. US foot
b. CT foot without contrast
c. MRI foot without contrast
d. Tc-99m bone scan foot
e. No ideal imaging exam

Athlete with pain and tenderness over tarsal navicular and clinical concern for stress injury or occult fracture. Radiographs unremarkable or equivocal.

a. US foot is usually not appropriate.
b. CT foot without contrast may be appropriate.
c. *MRI foot without contrast* is the most appropriate.
d. Tc-99m bone scan foot is usually not appropriate.

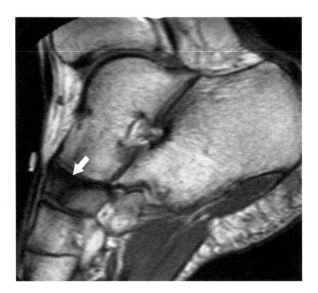

Fig. 10.86 Tarsal navicular fracture. Foot MR sagittal proton density-weighted image shows a nondisplaced fracture of the tarsal navicular (arrow)

Solution
MRI is highly sensitive for stress injury and is the preferred exam for making an early diagnosis. Due to its high specificity, CT may help confirm suspected stress fracture when MRI findings are equivocal.

A 37-year-old man with chronic foot pain with suspected tendinopathy. Radiographs are negative.

a. US foot
b. CT foot without contrast
c. MRI foot without contrast
d. Tc-99m bone scan foot
e. No ideal imaging exam

Radiographs unremarkable or equivocal and persistent clinical concern for tendinopathy.

a. US foot is usually appropriate, but there is a better choice here.
b. CT foot without contrast is usually not appropriate.
c. *MRI foot without contrast* is the most appropriate.
d. Tc-99m bone scan foot is usually not appropriate.

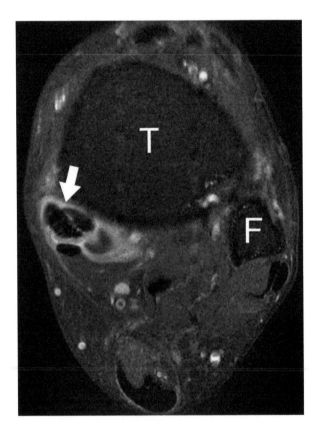

Fig. 10.87 Posterior tibial tendinopathy. Foot MR axial post-contrast image shows enhancement, thickening, and a split-tear of the posterior tibial tendon (arrow). *T* tibia, *F* fibula

Solution
In patients with chronic foot pain with suspected tendinopathy, the most commonly affected structures are the Achilles, posterior tibial, and peroneal tendons. MRI is the preferred exam for depicting tendinopathies ranging from tendinosis to complete tears.

10.17   Chronic Back Pain: Suspected Sacroiliitis/ Spondyloarthropathy

A 35-year-old man with chronic back pain and stiffness, with suspected axial spondyloarthropathy. Initial imaging exam.

a. X-ray spine and sacroiliac joints
b. CT sacroiliac joints without contrast
c. CT spine without contrast
d. MRI spine without contrast
e. No ideal imaging exam

Inflammatory sacroiliac or back symptoms with suspected axial spondyloarthropathy. Initial evaluation.

a. *X-ray spine and sacroiliac joints* is the most appropriate.
b. CT sacroiliac joints without contrast is usually not appropriate.
c. CT spine without contrast is usually not appropriate.
d. MRI spine without contrast is usually not appropriate.

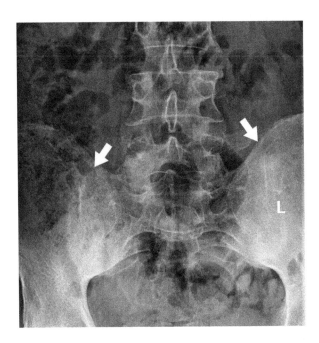

Fig. 10.88 Ankylosing spondylitis. Lumbar spine and sacroiliac joint X-ray anteroposterior view
shows bilateral sacroiliac joint fusion (arrows)

Solution
Imaging evaluation begins with radiography of the sacroiliac joints. Depending on
symptoms, additional views of the cervical, thoracic, and lumbar spine may be warranted. The need for advanced imaging should be guided by initial radiographic
findings and clinical assessment.

A 31-year-old man with symptoms that suggest sacroiliac inflammation with suspected axial spondyloarthropathy. Radiographs are negative.

a. US sacroiliac joints
b. CT sacroiliac joints without contrast
c. MRI sacroiliac joints without and with contrast
d. Tc-99m bone scan with SPECT spine
e. No ideal imaging exam

Inflammatory sacroiliac symptoms and suspected axial spondyloarthropathy. Radiographs negative or equivocal.

a. US sacroiliac joints is usually not appropriate.
b. CT sacroiliac joints without contrast is usually appropriate, but there is a better choice here.
c. *MRI sacroiliac joints without and with contrast* is the most appropriate.
d. Tc-99m bone scan with SPECT spine may be appropriate.

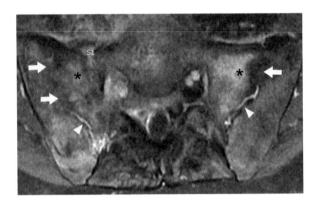

Fig. 10.89 Ankylosing spondylitis. Sacroiliac joint MR axial post-contrast image shows partial fusion of bilateral sacroiliac joints (arrows) and patchy enhancement of the adjacent bone marrow (stars). Arrowheads indicate unfused portions of the sacroiliac joints

Solution
MRI of the sacroiliac joints is the best exam to evaluate for inflammatory changes. Intravenous contrast may help distinguish synovitis from joint effusion but may not improve diagnostic accuracy for sacroiliitis. Thus, it is also appropriate to omit contrast. CT may help identify subtle erosions and soft tissue ossification.

A 41-year-old man with known spine ankyloses, with suspected spinal fracture after a fall.

a. X-ray spine area of interest
b. CT spine area of interest without contrast
c. MRI spine area of interest without contrast
d. Tc-99m bone scan with SPECT spine
e. No ideal imaging exam

Spine ankyloses with suspected spinal fracture.

a. X-ray spine area of interest is usually appropriate, but there is a better choice here.
b. *CT spine area of interest without contrast* is the most appropriate.
c. MRI spine area of interest without contrast is usually appropriate, but there is a better choice here.
d. Tc-99m bone scan with SPECT spine is usually not appropriate.

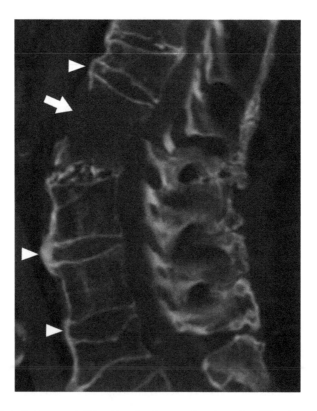

Fig. 10.90 Ankylosing spondylitis with spine fracture. Lumbar spine CT sagittal reconstruction image shows a horizontal fracture through the L2 vertebral body (arrow) and fusion of adjacent vertebrae with flowing syndesmophytes (arrowheads)

Solution
Spinal fractures in the setting of ankylosis are frequently from low-energy mechanisms or without recognizable trauma. They are often unstable with a high rate of associated neurologic injury. Due to the low sensitivity of radiography, CT is needed to exclude spinal fracture in this setting. MRI is indicated if there are neurological symptoms.

10.18 Chronic Extremity Joint Pain: Suspected Inflammatory Arthritis

A 53-year-old woman with chronic hand and wrist pain, with suspected rheumatoid arthritis. Initial imaging exam.

a. X-ray area of interest
b. US area of interest
c. CT area of interest without contrast
d. MRI area of interest without contrast
e. No ideal imaging exam

Chronic extremity joint pain, rheumatoid arthritis suspected. Initial exam.

a. *X-ray area of interest* is the most appropriate.
b. US area of interest is usually appropriate, but there is a better choice here.
c. CT area of interest without contrast may be appropriate.
d. MRI area of interest without contrast is usually appropriate, but there is a better choice here.

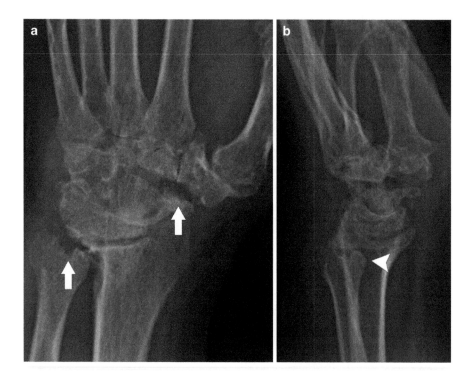

Fig. 10.91   Rheumatoid arthritis. Wrist X-ray oblique (**a**) and lateral (**b**) views show periarticular erosions at the radiocarpal and midcarpal joints (arrows) and subluxation of the ulnocarpal joint (arrowhead)

Solution
Radiography is the preferred initial exam. Findings of rheumatoid arthritis include periarticular osteopenia, uniform joint space narrowing, and osseous erosions. US and MRI can provide additional evaluation of inflammatory changes and structural damage as well as provide prognostic information.

A 45-year-old woman with chronic hand and wrist pain, with suspected psoriatic arthritis. Initial imaging exam.

a. X-ray area of interest
b. US area of interest
c. CT area of interest without contrast
d. MRI area of interest without contrast
e. No ideal imaging exam

Chronic extremity joint pain with suspected seronegative spondyloarthropathy. Initial exam.

a. *X-ray area of interest* is the most appropriate.
b. US area of interest is usually appropriate, but there is a better choice here. This exam completements X-ray.
c. CT area of interest without contrast may be appropriate.
d. MRI area of interest without contrast is usually appropriate, but there is a better choice here. This exam complements X-ray.

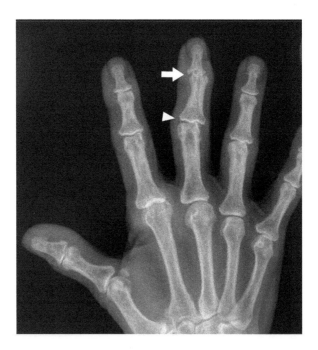

Fig. 10.92 Psoriatic arthritis. Hand X-ray anteroposterior view shows marginal erosion at the third digit distal interphalangeal joint (arrow) and narrowing of the proximal interphalangeal joint space (arrowhead)

Solution
Radiography can readily demonstrate findings of spondyloarthropathy including erosions, enthesitis, and bone proliferation.

A 57-year-old man with chronic foot pain, with suspected gout. Initial imaging exam.

a. X-ray area of interest
b. US area of interest
c. CT area of interest, dual energy without contrast
d. MRI area of interest without contrast
e. No ideal imaging exam

Chronic extremity joint pain with suspected gout. Initial exam.

a. *X-ray area of interest* is the most appropriate.
b. US area of interest is usually appropriate, but there is a better choice here.
c. CT area of interest, dual energy without contrast is usually appropriate, but there is a better choice here.
d. MRI area of interest without contrast may be appropriate.

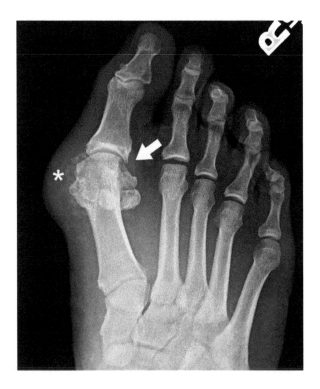

Fig. 10.93 Gout. Foot X-ray anteroposterior view shows marginal erosions with overhanging edges at the first-digit metatarsophalangeal joint (arrow) and soft tissue swelling and mineralization (star) consistent with tophus

Solution
Findings of gout that on radiography include joint effusions, bony erosions, and soft tissue tophi. As with other suspected inflammatory arthritides, radiography is the recommended initial imaging modality to assess for the presence and distribution of lesions.

A 53-year-old woman with chronic wrist pain, with suspected calcium pyrophosphate dihydrate disease (pseudogout).

a. X-ray area of interest
b. US area of interest
c. CT area of interest without contrast
d. MRI area of interest without contrast
e. No ideal imaging exam

Chronic extremity joint pain with suspected calcium pyrophosphate dihydrate disease (pseudogout).

a. *X-ray area of interest* is the most appropriate.
b. US area of interest may be appropriate.
c. CT area of interest without contrast may be appropriate.
d. MRI area of interest without contrast may be appropriate.

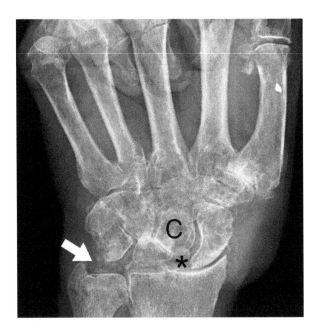

Fig. 10.94 Pseudogout. Wrist X-ray anteroposterior view shows chondrocalcinosis of the triangular fibrocartilaginous complex (arrow), widening of the scapholunate interval (star) with proximal migration of the capitate (C), and diffuse cartilage loss throughout the carpal joints

Solution
Radiography depicts the soft tissue calcifications associated with pseudogout, such as chondrocalcinosis and tendon, ligament, and capsular calcification. Radiography can also show associated arthropathy, typically of the radiocarpal, metacarpophalangeal, and patellofemoral joints.

10.19 Osteonecrosis of the Hip

A 21-year-old woman on chronic steroids with right hip pain. Avascular necrosis is suspected.

a. X-ray pelvis and hips
b. CT hips without contrast
c. MRI hips without contrast
d. Tc-99m bone scan with SPECT hips
e. No ideal imaging exam

Clinically suspected avascular necrosis. Initial imaging exam.

a. *X-ray pelvis and hips* is the most appropriate.
b. CT hips without contrast is usually not appropriate.
c. MRI hips without contrast is usually not appropriate.
d. Tc-99m bone scan with SPECT hips is usually not appropriate.

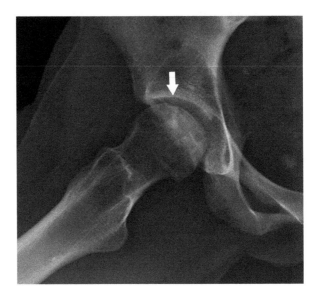

Fig. 10.95 Osteonecrosis of the hip. Hip X-ray frog-leg view reveals sclerosis and subchondral collapse of the right femoral head (arrow)

Solution
Radiography is the recommended initial exam for all patients suspected with osteonecrosis. Anteroposterior view of the pelvis and frog-leg lateral views of the hip should both be obtained, as articular collapse or cortical depression from osteonecrosis may be seen on only one of the projections.

A 37-year-old man with clinically suspected osteonecrosis of the right hip. Radiographs are negative.

a. CT hips without contrast
b. CT hips with contrast
c. MRI hips without contrast
d. Tc-99m bone scan with SPECT hips
e. No ideal imaging exam

Clinically suspected osteonecrosis. Normal or indeterminate radiographs.

a. CT hips without contrast may be appropriate for adults. For children, this exam is usually not appropriate.
b. CT hips with contrast is usually not appropriate.
c. *MRI hips without contrast* is the most appropriate exam for both children and adults.
d. Tc-99m bone scan with SPECT hips may be appropriate for adults. For children, this exam is usually not appropriate.

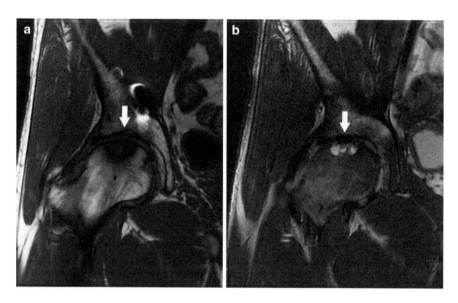

Fig. 10.96 Osteonecrosis of the hip. Hip MR coronal T1-weighted (**a**) and T2-weighted (**b**) images reveal abnormal signal (arrows) on the superior articular surface of the right femoral head

Solution

MRI is the most sensitive and specific imaging modality for osteonecrosis. CT may be useful in adults to assess severity of articular collapse, detect early degenerative joint disease, and aide surgical planning. Bone scan can also identify osteonecrosis but is less sensitive than MRI.

10.20 Suspected Foot Osteomyelitis in Patients with Diabetes Mellitus

A 47-year-old man with diabetes mellitus and suspected foot osteomyelitis. Initial evaluation.

a. X-ray foot
b. CT foot without contrast
c. CT foot with contrast
d. MRI foot with contrast
e. Tc-99m three-phase bone scan foot

Suspected osteomyelitis of the foot in patients with diabetes mellitus. Initial imaging exam.

a. *X-ray foot* is the most appropriate.
b. CT foot without contrast is usually not appropriate.
c. CT foot with contrast is usually not appropriate.
d. MRI foot with contrast is usually not appropriate.
e. Tc-99m three-phase bone scan foot is usually not appropriate.

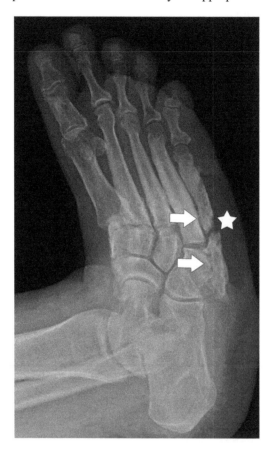

Fig. 10.97 Osteomyelitis. Foot X-ray oblique view reveals bone fragmentation and sclerosis of the proximal fifth metatarsal (arrows) and lucencies in the adjacent soft tissue (star), indicating an ulcer

Solution
Although radiography is insensitive for early osteomyelitis, it is still useful for initial evaluation and can also help identify alternative causes for symptoms. On imaging, early bony changes, including periosteal reaction and osteopenia, are preceded by soft tissue swelling and loss of fat planes.

A 54-year-old woman with diabetes mellitus and soft tissue swelling of the foot without ulcer. Osteomyelitis or early neuropathic arthropathy is suspected. Radiographs have been obtained.

a. US foot
b. CT foot without contrast
c. CT foot with contrast
d. MRI foot without and with contrast
e. In-111 WBC scan foot

Soft tissue swelling without ulcer. Osteomyelitis or early neuropathic arthropathy changes of the foot suspected. Additional imaging following radiographs.

a. US foot is usually not appropriate.
b. CT foot without contrast may be appropriate.
c. CT foot with contrast may be appropriate.
d. *MRI foot without and with contrast* is the most appropriate.
e. In-111 WBC scan foot may be appropriate.

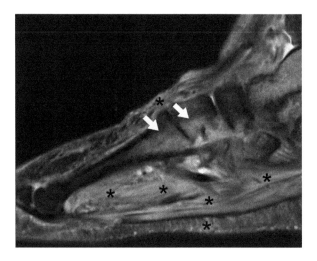

Fig. 10.98 Neuropathic arthropathy. Foot MR sagittal T2-weighted image shows edema within the bones of the midfoot (arrows) and in the surrounding musculature and superficial soft tissues (stars)

Solution
In this scenario, the likelihood of osteomyelitis is low given lack of an associated wound or ulceration. MRI is recommended in this setting to both assess for osteomyelitis and to help identify alternative causes for the clinical findings, such as neuropathic arthropathy and abscess.

A 59-year-old man with diabetes mellitus and soft tissue swelling of the foot with an ulcer. Osteomyelitis is suspected. Radiographs have been obtained.

a. US foot
b. CT foot without contrast
c. CT foot with contrast
d. MRI foot without and with contrast
e. In-111 WBC scan foot

Soft tissue swelling with ulcer. Osteomyelitis with or without neuropathic arthropathy is suspected. Additional imaging following radiographs.

a. US foot is usually not appropriate.
b. CT foot without contrast may be appropriate.
c. CT foot with contrast may be appropriate.
d. *MRI foot without and with contrast* is the most appropriate.
e. In-111 WBC scan foot may be appropriate.

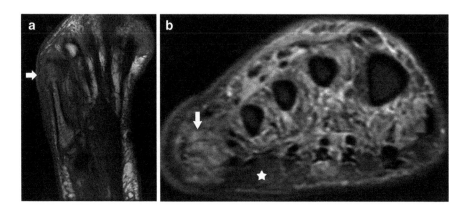

Fig. 10.99 Osteomyelitis. Foot MR axial post-contrast (**a**) and coronal T2-weighted (**b**) images reveal bone destruction of the distal fifth metatarsal (arrow). Also seen is a deep soft tissue ulcer (star) on the plantar surface

Solution
MRI is sensitive and specific for the detection of osteomyelitis. It also guides surgical planning by evaluating the extent of bony involvement and the location and size of drainable fluid collections. The use of intravenous contrast helps identify abscesses, sinus tracts, devitalized regions, and associated fasciitis and myositis.

10.21 Suspected Osteomyelitis, Septic Arthritis, or Soft Tissue Infection (Excluding Spine and Diabetic Foot)

A 21-year-old man with knee pain, suspected with septic arthritis.

a. X-ray area of interest
b. US area of interest
c. CT area of interest
d. MRI area of interest
e. No ideal imaging exam

Suspected osteomyelitis, septic arthritis, or soft tissue infection excluding spine and diabetic foot. Initial exam.

a. *X-ray area of interest* is the most appropriate.
b. US area of interest is usually not appropriate.
c. CT area of interest is usually not appropriate.
d. MRI area of interest is usually not appropriate.

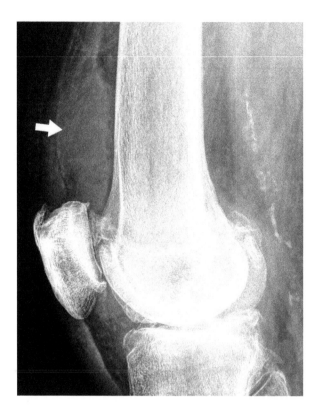

Fig. 10.100 Knee joint effusion. Knee X-ray lateral view shows a large effusion (arrow) in the suprapatellar bursa

Solution
Radiography is the recommended initial imaging modality as it is well tolerated and widely available. Radiographs provide anatomic evaluation of the affected site, depict changes of chronic osteomyelitis, reveal gas or foreign bodies, and suggest alternative diagnoses for suspected musculoskeletal infection such as neuropathic arthropathy or fracture.

A 32-year-old woman with swelling and warmth along the right leg, with suspected soft tissue infection. Radiographs have been performed.

a. US area of interest
b. CT area of interest with contrast
c. MRI area of interest without contrast
d. MRI area of interest without and with contrast
e. No ideal imaging exam

Soft tissue or juxta-articular swelling with suspected soft tissue infection. Additional imaging following radiographs.

a. US area of interest may be appropriate.
b. CT area of interest with contrast may be appropriate.
c. MRI area of interest without contrast is usually appropriate, but there is a better choice here.
d. *MRI area of interest without and with contrast* is the most appropriate.

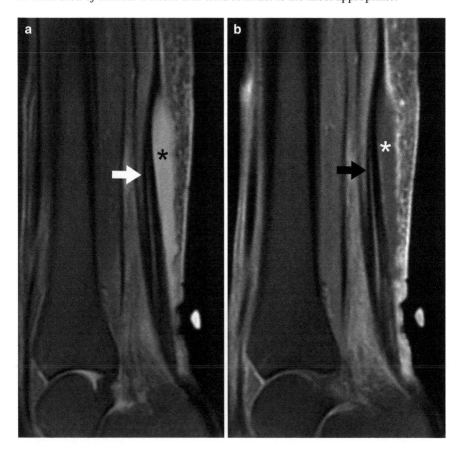

Fig. 10.101 Soft tissue abscess. Leg MR sagittal T2-weighted (**a**) and post-contrast images (**b**) show a fluid collection (star) along the Achilles tendon (arrow) with peripheral enhancement and adjacent edema

Solution

MRI is preferred because it best depicts the extent of soft tissue infections. It is more sensitive than CT for inflammation and associated fasciitis, myositis, and necrosis. Use of intravenous contrast can improve delineation of fluid collections and necrosis.

A 52-year-old man presents with cellulitis and effusion at the elbow following soft tissue trauma. Osteomyelitis is suspected and radiographs have been performed.

a. US area of interest
b. CT area of interest with contrast
c. MRI area of interest without and with contrast
d. Tc-99m three-phase bone scan area of interest
e. No ideal imaging exam

Soft tissue or juxta-articular swelling, cellulitis or a skin lesion, injury, wound, ulcer, or blister. Osteomyelitis suspected. Additional imaging following radiographs.

a. US area of interest is usually not appropriate.
b. CT area of interest with contrast is usually appropriate, but there is a better choice here.
c. *MRI area of interest without and with contrast* is the most appropriate.
d. Tc-99m three-phase bone scan area of interest may be appropriate.

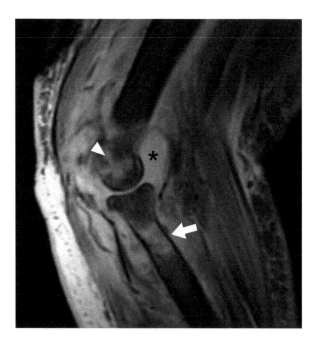

Fig. 10.102 Osteomyelitis. Elbow MR sagittal T2-weighted image shows bone marrow edema in the proximal radius (arrow) and distal humerus (arrowhead), elbow joint effusion (star), and soft tissue edema

Solution
A negative MRI exam excludes acute osteomyelitis. Furthermore, MRI can delineate the extent of osseous and soft tissue involvement, including presence of abscesses. Intravenous contrast helps evaluate for articular and tendon involvement and for areas of necrosis.

A 75-year-old woman with left leg pain, erythema, and crepitus on physical exam.

a. X-ray area of interest
b. US area of interest
c. CT area of interest with contrast
d. MRI area of interest without and with contrast
e. No ideal imaging exam

Clinical exam reveals crepitus and soft tissue gas suspected. First exam.

a. *X-ray area of interest* is the most appropriate.
b. US area of interest is usually not appropriate.
c. CT area of interest with contrast may be appropriate.
d. MRI area of interest without and with contrast is usually not appropriate.

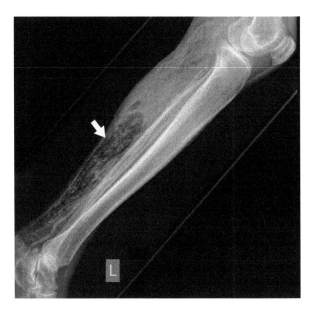

Fig. 10.103 Necrotizing fasciitis. Leg X-ray lateral view shows extensive gas within the soft tissues of the posterior compartment (arrow). Necrotizing fasciitis was confirmed on surgery

Solution
Radiography can evaluate for soft tissue gas but is limited in the evaluation of deep fascial gas. Though radiography is the recommended initial exam, CT is the most sensitive modality for the detection of soft tissue gas and should be performed if there is continued clinical concern following radiography.

A 49-year-old man with crepitus and soft tissue gas seen on radiographs of the left thigh. No puncture wound is seen.

a. US area of interest
b. CT area of interest without contrast
c. CT area of interest with contrast
d. MRI area of interest without and with contrast
e. No ideal imaging exam

Crepitus with soft tissue gas on initial radiographs. There is no puncture wound. Next imaging exam.

a. US area of interest is usually not appropriate.
b. CT area of interest without contrast may be appropriate.
c. CT area of interest with contrast may be appropriate.
d. MRI area of interest without and with contrast may be appropriate.
e. *No ideal imaging exam* is the correct answer.

Solution

In the absence of history of recent surgery, trauma, or puncture wound, soft tissue gas is a reliable indication of infection. In particular, gas in deep fascial planes is a hallmark of necrotizing fasciitis. If radiography shows this, then no additional imaging is needed.

10.22 Soft Tissue Masses

A 32-year-old man with a palpable tender soft tissue mass in the left thigh.

a. X-ray area of interest
b. US area of interest
c. CT area of interest without contrast
d. MRI area of interest without contrast
e. No ideal imaging exam

Soft tissue mass that is superficial or palpable. Initial imaging exam.

a. *X-ray area of interest* and choice (b) are equally the most appropriate.
b. *US area of interest* and choice (a) are equally the most appropriate.
c. CT area of interest without contrast is usually not appropriate.
d. MRI area of interest without contrast may be appropriate.

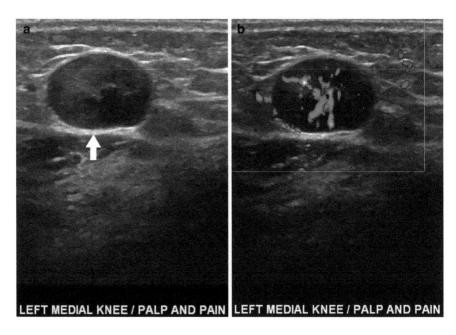

Fig. 10.104 Solid soft tissue mass. Focused US at the site of palpated mass in the medial thigh at the knee (**a**) shows an oval mass (arrow) with interval vascular flow on color Doppler image (**b**). Additional evaluation revealed a schwannoma

Solution
Radiographic features of a soft tissue mass, such as calcifications or bone involvement, can aid in diagnosis. For example, a hemangioma can be diagnosed by visualizing phleboliths. US is most useful for small, superficial lesions such as lipomas, epidermoid cysts, and nerve sheath tumors. It can differentiate solid from cystic lesions and show the relationship of a mass to adjacent neurovascular structures.

A 37-year-old man with a soft tissue mass. Imaging with ultrasound and radiograph are nondiagnostic.

a. CT area of interest without contrast
b. CT area of interest with contrast
c. MRI area of interest without and with contrast
d. FDG-PET/CT area of interest
e. No ideal imaging exam

Soft tissue mass. Nondiagnostic initial evaluation (ultrasound and/or radiography). Next imaging exam.

a. CT area of interest without contrast may be appropriate.
b. CT area of interest with contrast may be appropriate.
c. *MRI area of interest without and with contrast* is the most appropriate.
d. FDG-PET/CT area of interest is usually not appropriate.

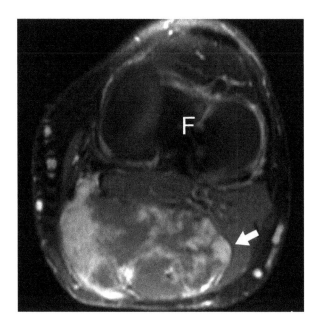

Fig. 10.105 Sarcoma. Leg MR axial post-contrast image shows an enhancing mass (arrow) in the popliteal fossa, which on biopsy was diagnosed as a synovial sarcoma. *F* femur

Solution
With its excellent soft tissue contrast, MRI is the preferred imaging modality for the characterization of soft tissue masses. It is also useful for local staging and identifying neurovascular involvement. Intravenous contrast improves visualization of tumor vascularity and necrosis, reactive changes, and the demarcation of tumor from muscle.

A 52-year-old man with a soft tissue mass. Ultrasound and radiography are nondiagnostic. The patient cannot undergo MRI.

a. CT area of interest without contrast
b. CT area of interest without and with contrast
c. CT area of interest with contrast
d. FDG-PET/CT area of interest
e. No ideal imaging exam

Soft tissue mass and nondiagnostic initial evaluation (ultrasound and/or radiography). The patient has contraindications to MRI. Next imaging exam.

a. CT area of interest without contrast may be appropriate.
b. *CT area of interest without and with contrast* and choice (c) are equally the most appropriate.
c. *CT area of interest with contrast* and choice (b) are equally the most appropriate.
d. FDG-PET/CT area of interest may be appropriate.

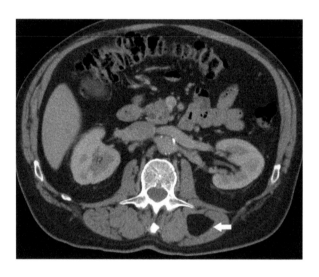

Fig. 10.106 Lipoma. Abdomen CT reveals a fat-density mass (arrow) in the left paraspinal muscles

Solution
In this scenario, CT is the most appropriate imaging modality and can help characterize the mass, such as by showing the presence of calcifications or fat, as well as vascularity and bone involvement. Use of intravenous contrast helps differentiate vascularized from potentially necrotic tissue.

10.23 Primary Bone Tumors

A 50-year-old woman with clinically suspected bone tumor.

a. X-ray area of interest
b. US area of interest
c. CT area of interest without contrast
d. MRI area of interest without contrast
e. No ideal imaging exam

Initial evaluation.

a. *X-ray area of interest* is the most appropriate.
b. US area of interest is usually not appropriate.
c. CT area of interest without contrast is usually not appropriate.
d. MRI area of interest without contrast is usually not appropriate.

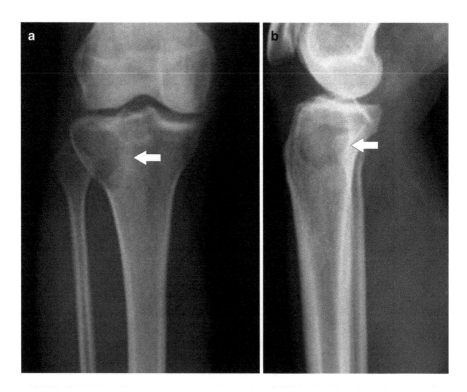

Fig. 10.107 Giant cell tumor. Leg X-ray anteroposterior (**a**) and lateral (**b**) views show a lytic lesion (arrows) in the lateral tibial plateau

Solution

Radiography is the recommended initial exam for evaluating suspected bone tumors. When lesions are characterized as classically nonaggressive on radiography, additional imaging may be unnecessary. If surgical intervention is being considered, additional imaging may be needed.

A 16-year-old boy with persistent symptoms and clinical concern for a bone tumor. Radiographs are negative.

a. US area of interest
b. CT area of interest without contrast
c. MRI area of interest without contrast
d. Tc-99m bone scan whole body
e. No ideal imaging exam

Positive localized or regional symptoms. Radiographs are negative or do not explain the symptoms.

a. US area of interest is usually not appropriate.
b. CT area of interest without contrast may be appropriate.
c. *MRI area of interest without contrast* is the most appropriate.
d. Tc-99m bone scan whole body may be appropriate.

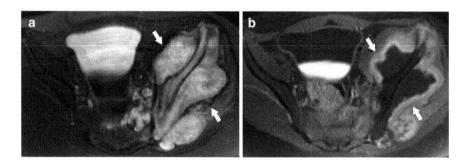

Fig. 10.108 Osteosarcoma. Pelvic MR axial T2-weighted (**a**) and post-contrast (**b**) images reveal a peripherally enhancing soft tissue mass (arrows) centered at the left pelvis

Solution
In general, MRI is the preferred imaging modality in this scenario. It is more sensitive and provides greater anatomic detail than bone scan. MRI is also superior to CT in depicting bone marrow, soft tissue, and neurovascular involvement by tumor. However, CT may be preferred for tumors in certain location, including those located within the periosteal or cortical regions, and along flat bones with thin cortices and little marrow.

A 55-year-old man with bone tumor characterized as definitively benign on radiographs. Osteoid osteoma is not a consideration.

a. US area of interest
b. CT area of interest without contrast
c. MRI area of interest without contrast
d. Tc-99m scan whole body
e. No ideal imaging exam

Definitively benign lesion on radiographs (excluding osteoid osteoma).

a. US area of interest is usually not appropriate.
b. CT area of interest without contrast may be appropriate.
c. MRI area of interest without contrast may be appropriate.
d. Tc-99m scan whole body is usually not appropriate.
e. *No ideal imaging exam* is the correct answer.

Solution
When a lesion is definitively benign on radiography, additional imaging is usually not required unless imaging for surgical planning is needed. Further imaging with CT or MRI may also be appropriate for patients who are symptomatic at the tumor site to evaluate for radiographically occult pathologic fractures.

A 26-year-old man with radiographic and clinical findings that suggest osteoid osteoma.

a. US area of interest
b. CT area of interest without contrast
c. MRI area of interest without contrast
d. Tc-99m bone scan whole body
e. No ideal imaging exam

Radiographic and/or clinical findings suspicious for osteoid osteoma.

a. US area of interest is usually not appropriate.
b. *CT area of interest without contrast* is the most appropriate.
c. MRI area of interest without contrast may be appropriate.
d. Tc-99m bone scan whole body may be appropriate.

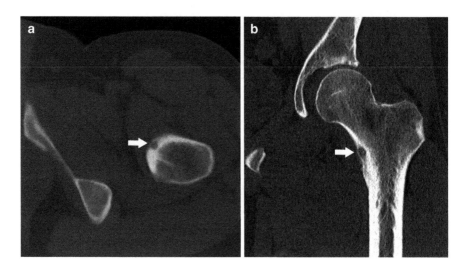

Fig. 10.109 Osteoid osteoma. Hip CT axial (**a**) and coronal reconstruction (**b**) images reveal a well-defined lucent lesion (arrow) in the left femoral neck with adjacent cortical thickening

Solution

The diagnosis of an osteoid osteoma is made by detecting the tumor's characteristic central nidus, which is best seen on CT.

An 18-year-old woman with an aggressive-appearing bone lesion on radiographs. Malignancy is suspected.

a. US area of interest
b. CT area of interest without contrast
c. MRI area of interest without and with contrast
d. Tc-99m bone scan whole body
e. No ideal imaging exam

Aggressive lesion on radiographs, suspicious for malignancy.

a. US area of interest is usually not appropriate.
b. CT area of interest without contrast is usually appropriate, but there is a better choice here.
c. *MRI area of interest without and with contrast* is the most appropriate.
d. Tc-99m bone scan whole body may be appropriate.

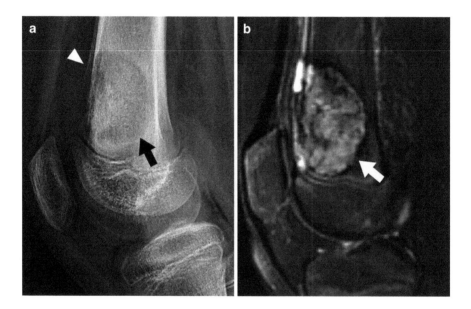

Fig. 10.110 Osteosarcoma. Knee X-ray sagittal view (**a**) shows a lytic lesion (arrow) with aggressive periosteal reaction (arrowhead) in the distal femur. Knee MR T2-weighted sagittal image (**b**) shows a corresponding mass (arrow) that extends through the cortex

Solution
MRI is preferred to evaluate the extent of growth of tumors, e.g. cortical destruction, and joint, soft tissue, and neurovascular involvement. Intravenous contrast helps assess tumor vascularity, vascular invasion, and cystic and/or necrotic areas. CT can help assess for tumor mineralization.

A 52-year-old woman with a pathologic fracture on radiographs.

a. US area of interest
b. CT area of interest without contrast
c. MRI area of interest without and with contrast
d. Tc-99m bone scan whole body
e. No ideal imaging exam

Lesion with pathological fracture on radiographs.

a. US area of interest is usually not appropriate.
b. CT area of interest without contrast may be appropriate.
c. *MRI area of interest without and with contrast* is the most appropriate.
d. Tc-99m bone scan whole body may be appropriate.

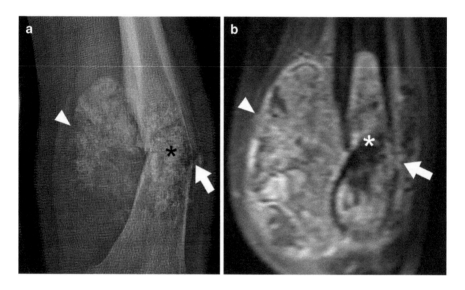

Fig. 10.111 Pathologic fracture. Femur X-ray anteroposterior view (**a**) and MR coronal post-contrast image (**b**) shows a fracture (arrow) through a destructive tumor in the distal femur (star) with extraosseous extension (arrowhead). The tumor was diagnosed on biopsy as osteosarcoma

Solution
Both benign and malignant lesions can present with a pathologic fracture. Hemorrhage and bone resorption secondary to the fracture can lead to a more aggressive appearance, making it difficult to differentiate benign from malignant lesions on radiography. MRI is the preferred modality to characterize the underlying mass.

10.24   Imaging After Shoulder Arthroplasty

A 62-year-old man with symptoms concerning for failed shoulder arthroplasty.

a. X-ray shoulder
b. US shoulder
c. CT shoulder without contrast
d. MRI shoulder without contrast
e. No ideal imaging exam

Symptomatic patient with a primary shoulder arthroplasty. Initial exam.

a. *X-ray shoulder* is the most appropriate.
b. US shoulder is usually not appropriate.
c. CT shoulder without contrast is usually not appropriate.
d. MRI shoulder without contrast is usually not appropriate.

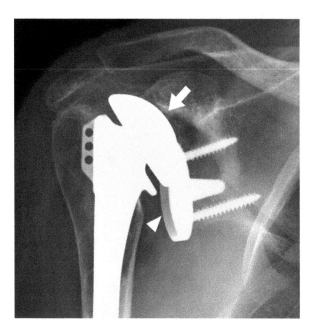

Fig. 10.112 Shoulder arthroplasty complication. Shoulder X-ray anteroposterior view shows superior subluxation of the humeral component of the arthroplasty (arrow) which abuts the superior rim of the glenoid component (arrowhead)

Solution
Radiography is the primary imaging modality for the evaluation of shoulder arthroplasty. Glenoid component loosening is the main cause of failed total shoulder arthroplasty and can manifest as progressive radiolucency around the glenoid component. Evaluation for other potential complications and etiologies for symptoms such as fracture, periprosthetic infection, and rotator cuff tear also starts with radiography.

A 66-year-old woman with a painful shoulder arthroplasty and concern for infection. Radiographs have been performed.

a. US shoulder
b. CT shoulder with contrast
c. MRI shoulder without contrast
d. Aspiration shoulder
e. No ideal imaging exam

A patient with a painful primary shoulder arthroplasty and suspected infection. Additional imaging following radiographs.

a. US shoulder may be appropriate.
b. CT shoulder with contrast may be appropriate.
c. MRI shoulder without contrast may be appropriate.
d. *Aspiration shoulder* is usually appropriate.

Solution

Aspiration should be considered when there is clinical suspicion for an infected shoulder arthroplasty regardless of radiography findings. Aspiration can be performed under fluoroscopic, US, MRI, or CT guidance. CT and MRI can help further assess for the presence of periprosthetic infection, evaluate surrounding soft tissues for abscess, and assist with preoperative planning.

A 62-year-old man with a painful shoulder arthroplasty and concern for fracture. Radiographs have been performed.

a. US shoulder
b. CT shoulder without contrast
c. CT shoulder with contrast
d. MRI shoulder without contrast
e. No ideal imaging exam

Patient with a painful primary total shoulder arthroplasty and suspected fracture. Additional imaging following radiographs.

a. US shoulder is usually not appropriate.
b. *CT shoulder without contrast* is the most appropriate.
c. CT shoulder with contrast is usually not appropriate.
d. MRI shoulder without contrast may be appropriate.

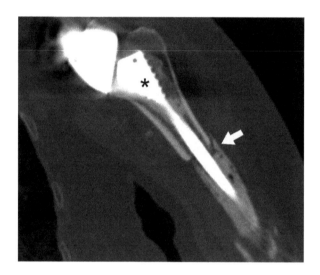

Fig. 10.113 Periprosthetic fracture. Shoulder CT coronal reconstruction image shows a fracture of the proximal humeral shaft and underlying arthroplasty cement (arrow) around the intact humeral component (star) of a total shoulder arthroplasty

Solution
CT without contrast performed with metal reduction protocol can detect clinically suspected, radiographically occult fractures. CT can also characterize periprosthetic fractures seen on radiographs to delineate the extent, degree of displacement, and comminution.

10.25 Imaging After Total Hip Arthroplasty

A 79-year-old woman with a total hip arthroplasty presents for routine follow-up. She is asymptomatic.

a. X-ray hip
b. CT hip without contrast
c. CT hip with contrast
d. MRI hip without contrast
e. No ideal imaging exam

Follow-up of the asymptomatic patient with a total hip arthroplasty.

a. *X-ray hip* is the most appropriate.
b. CT hip without contrast is usually not appropriate.
c. CT hip with contrast is usually not appropriate.
d. MRI hip without contrast is usually not appropriate.

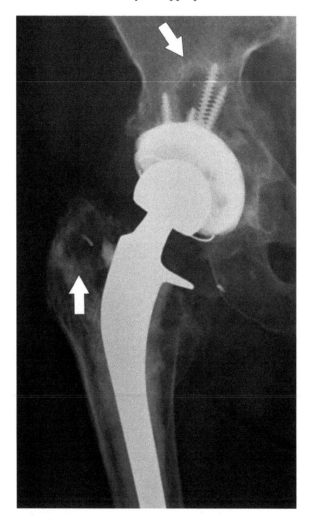

Fig. 10.114 Particle disease. Hip X-ray anteroposterior view shows lucencies (arrows) adjacent to the acetabular and proximal femoral components

Solution
Radiographs obtained shortly after surgery can be used to identify complications such as screw penetration and provide a baseline for future evaluation. Radiography is used to monitor for osteolysis or implant loosening long-term.

A 67-year-old woman with a painful primary total hip arthroplasty. Infection is a consideration.

a. X-ray hip
b. CT hip with contrast
c. MRI hip without and with contrast
d. In-111 white blood cell and Tc-99m sulfur colloid scan hip
e. Aspiration hip

A patient with a painful primary total hip arthroplasty. Infection is a consideration.

a. *X-ray hip* and choice (e) are equally the most appropriate.
b. CT hip with contrast may be appropriate.
c. MRI hip without and with contrast may be appropriate.
d. Indium-111 white blood cell and Tc-99m sulfur colloid scan hip may be appropriate.
e. *Aspiration hip* and choice (a) are equally the most appropriate.

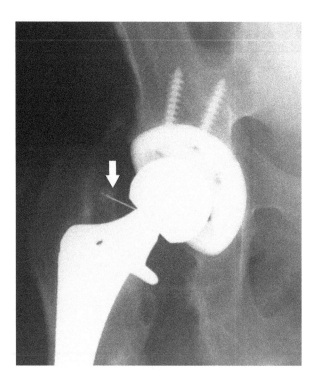

Fig. 10.115 Hip aspiration. Hip aspiration under fluoroscopy demonstrates a 22G needle (arrow) in the hip joint

Solution
Radiography is recommended for initial assessment of hip pain after arthroplasty. However, normal results on radiography does not exclude an infection. Joint aspiration is the definitive test to evaluate for infection.

A 73-year-old man with a total hip arthroplasty. Periprosthetic fracture is suspected.

a. X-ray hip
b. CT hip without contrast
c. CT hip with contrast
d. MRI hip without contrast
e. Tc-99m bone scan hip

Patient with a total hip arthroplasty, with suspected periprosthetic fracture.

a. *X-ray hip* is the most appropriate.
b. CT hip without contrast is usually appropriate, but there is a better choice here.
c. CT hip with contrast is usually not appropriate.
d. MRI hip without contrast may be appropriate.
e. Tc-99m bone scan hip may be appropriate.

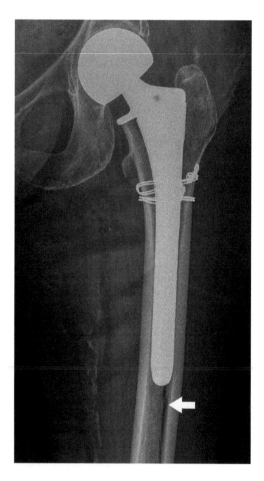

Fig. 10.116 Periprosthetic fracture. Hip X-ray anteroposterior view shows a vertical fracture (arrow) distal to the hip arthroplasty femoral component

Solution
Periprosthetic fractures can usually be detected on radiography. CT is complementary and is used to further delineate known fractures or evaluate for an occult fracture when radiographs are negative.

10.26 Imaging After Total Knee Arthroplasty

A 66-year-old man with a total knee arthroplasty presenting for routine follow-up. He is asymptomatic.

a. X-ray knee
b. Fluoroscopy knee
c. CT knee without contrast
d. MRI knee without contrast
e. No ideal imaging exam

Routine follow-up of an asymptomatic patient with a total knee arthroplasty.

a. *X-ray knee* is the most appropriate.
b. Fluoroscopy knee is usually not appropriate.
c. CT knee without contrast is usually not appropriate.
d. MRI knee without contrast is usually not appropriate.

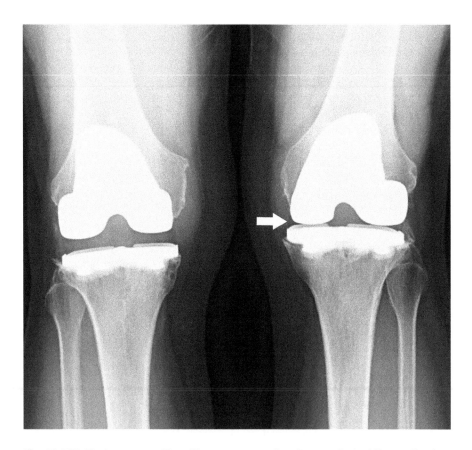

Fig. 10.117 Hardware wear. Knee X-ray anteroposterior view acquired while standing in a patient with bilateral knee arthroplasties reveals narrowing of the space between the left femoral and tibial components (arrow), indicating thinning of the radiolucent polyethylene spacer

Solution
Follow-up radiographs are intended to identify findings of long-term complications. These include abnormal bone or hardware alignment, osteolysis, reactive bone formation, periostitis, fractures, and evidence of polyethylene liner wear.

A 62-year-old man with a total knee arthroplasty presents with pain. Periprosthetic infection is a consideration.

a. X-ray knee
b. US knee
c. CT knee without contrast
d. MRI knee without contrast
e. Aspiration knee

A patient with a painful total knee arthroplasty. Periprosthetic infection is a consideration.

a. X-ray knee is usually appropriate, but there is a better choice here.
b. US knee is usually not appropriate.
c. CT knee without contrast is usually not appropriate.
d. MRI knee without contrast is usually not appropriate.
e. *Aspiration knee* is the most appropriate.

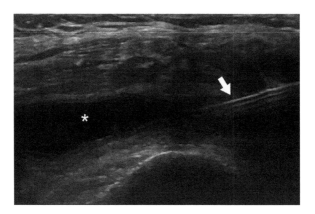

Fig. 10.118 Knee aspiration. Knee US shows a needle (arrow) within a suprapatellar knee joint effusion (asterisk)

Solution
Aspiration is highly sensitive and specific for diagnosing periprosthetic infection. Although less sensitive and specific, radiography is also an integral part of the assessment. Radiographic findings can range from normal to subtle periprosthetic lucency to advanced bone destruction.

A 75-year-old woman with total knee arthroplasty presents with pain. Tests for infection are negative. Osteolysis is suspected. Radiographs have been obtained.

a. CT knee without contrast
b. CT knee with contrast
c. MRI knee without contrast
d. MRI knee without and with contrast
e. Tc-99m bone scan

A patient with a painful total knee arthroplasty, negative tests for infection, and suspected osteolysis. Additional imaging after radiographs.

a. *CT knee without contrast* is the most appropriate.
b. CT knee with contrast is usually not appropriate.
c. MRI knee without contrast may be appropriate.
d. MRI knee without and with contrast is usually not appropriate.
e. Tc-99m bone scan is usually not appropriate.

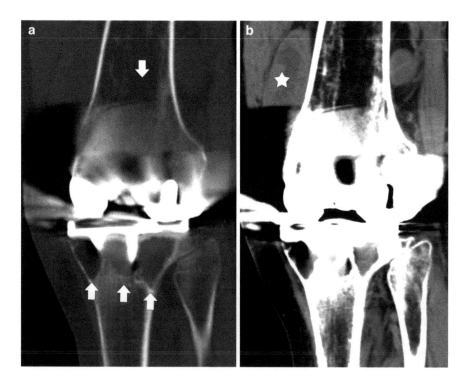

Fig. 10.119 Osteolysis after knee arthroplasty. Knee CT coronal reconstruction images in bone (**a**) and soft tissue (**b**) windows reveal lucencies in bone adjacent to hardware (arrows) and a complex joint effusion (star) which suggests synovitis

Solution
CT is the preferred modality to assess for osteolysis, which results from inflammation caused by debris from polyethylene, cement, or metal. It is the leading cause of late total knee arthroplasty revision.

A 71-year-old woman with a total knee arthroplasty presents with pain. Periprosthetic fracture is suspected.

a. X-ray knee
b. CT knee without contrast
c. CT knee with contrast
d. MRI knee without contrast
e. No ideal imaging exam

A patient with a painful total knee arthroplasty. Periprosthetic fracture is suspected.

a. *X-ray knee* is the most appropriate.
b. CT knee without contrast is usually appropriate, but there is a better choice here.
c. CT knee with contrast is usually not appropriate.
d. MRI knee without contrast may be appropriate.

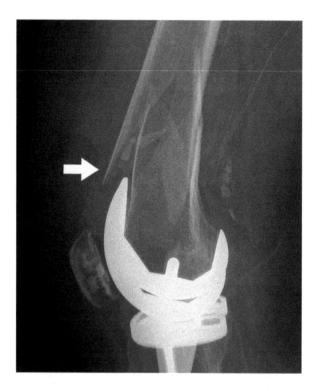

Fig. 10.120 Periprosthetic fracture. Knee X-ray lateral view shows periprosthetic fracture of the distal femur (arrow) proximal to the knee arthroplasty femoral component

Solution
Imaging begins with radiography. CT is also usually appropriate to evaluate for an occult fracture when radiographs are negative or to delineate the extent or complications of the fracture seen on radiography.

Bibliography

Bachmann LM, Kolb E, Koller MT, Steurer J, ter Riet G. Accuracy of Ottawa ankle rules to exclude fractures of the ankle and mid-foot: systematic review. BMJ. 2003;326(7386):417.

Hoffman JR, et al. Validity of a set of clinical criteria to rule out injury to the cervical spine in patients with blunt trauma. National Emergency X-Radiography Utilization Study Group. N Engl J Med. 2000;343:94–9.

Stiell IG, McKnight RD, Greenberg GH, McDowell I, Nair RC, Wells GA, Johns C, Worthington JR. Implementation of the Ottawa ankle rules. JAMA. 1994;271:827–32.

Stiell IG, et al. The Canadian C-spine rule for radiography in alert and stable trauma patients. JAMA. 2001;286:1841–8.

Neurologic Imaging

11

11.1 Head Trauma

11.1.1 Glasgow Coma Scale (GCS)

Eye opening response

- Spontaneous (open with blinking at baseline): 4 points
- To verbal stimuli, command, speech: 3 points
- To pain only (not applied to face): 2 points
- No response: 1 point

Verbal response

- Oriented: 5 points
- Confused conversation, but able to answer questions: 4 points
- Inappropriate words: 3 points
- Incomprehensible speech: 2 points
- No response: 1 point

Motor response

- Obeys commands for movement: 6 points
- Purposeful movement to painful stimulus: 5 points
- Withdraws in response to pain: 4 points
- Flexion in response to pain (decorticate posturing): 3 points
- Extension response in response to pain (decerebrate posturing): 2 points
- No response: 1 point

Teasdale et al. 1974

© The Author(s), under exclusive license to Springer Nature
Switzerland AG 2021
G. X. Wang et al., *Choosing the Correct Radiologic Test*,
https://doi.org/10.1007/978-3-030-65185-5_11

11.1.2 New Orleans Criteria (NOC)

Inclusion criteria

- Age ≥3 years
- Minor head injury (meets all of the following criteria: a witness or the patient reported loss of consciousness or the patient could not remember the traumatic event, normal findings on neurologic examination, GCS score of 15 on emergency department arrival)
- Injury occurred within 24 h

Head CT is not required if *all* of the following are *absent*

- Age >60 years
- Drug or alcohol intoxication
- Deficits in short-term memory
- Headache
- Vomiting
- Seizure
- Any visible evidence of trauma above the clavicles

Haydel et al. 2000

11.1.3 Canadian CT Head Rule (CCHR)

Inclusion criteria

- Blunt head trauma resulting in witnessed loss of consciousness, definite amnesia, or witnessed disorientation
- GCS score ≥13 on emergency department arrival
- Injury occurred within 24 h

Exclusion criteria

- Age <16 years
- Pregnancy
- Has a bleeding disorder or used oral anticoagulants
- Minimal head injury (i.e., no loss of consciousness, amnesia, or disorientation)
- No clear history of trauma as the primary event (e.g., primary seizure or syncope)
- Had seizure before assessment in the emergency department
- Obvious penetrating skull injury or depressed skull fracture
- Acute focal neurological deficit
- Unstable vital signs associated with major trauma
- Returned to emergency department for reassessment of the same head injury

Head CT is not required if *all* of the following are *absent*

- Age ≥65 years
- GCS score <15 at 2 h after injury
- Two or more episodes of vomiting
- Amnesia before impact >30 min
- Suspected open or depressed skull fracture
- Any sign of basilar skull fracture (hemotympanum, "raccoon" eye, cerebrospinal fluid otorrhea or rhinorrhea, Battle's sign)
- Dangerous mechanism (pedestrian struck by motor vehicle, ejection from motor vehicle, fall from height >3 ft or 5 steps)

Stiell et al. 2001

11.1.4 National Emergency X-Radiography Utilization Study (NEXUS-II)

Inclusion criteria

- Acute blunt head trauma
- GCS score of 15

Head CT is not required if *all* of the following are *absent*

- Age ≥65 years
- Evidence of significant skull fracture
- Scalp hematoma
- Neurologic deficit
- Altered level of alertness (including GCS ≤14)
- Abnormal behavior
- Coagulopathy
- Persistent vomiting

Mower et al. 2005

A 30-year-old man with minor acute blunt head injury. The GCS score is 15. Imaging is not indicated by NOC, CCHR, or NEXUS-II clinical decision rules. Initial imaging study.

a. X-ray skull
b. CT head without contrast
c. CT head with contrast
d. MRI head without contrast
e. No ideal imaging exam

Minor acute closed head injury. Imaging is not indicated by NOC, CCHR, or NEXUS-II clinical decision rules. Initial imaging study.

a. X-ray skull is usually not appropriate.
b. CT head without contrast is usually not appropriate.
c. CT head with contrast is usually not appropriate.
d. MRI head without contrast is usually not appropriate.
e. *No ideal imaging exam* is the correct answer.

Solution
The NOC, CCHR, and NEXUS-II clinical decision rules can accurately identify patients with minor acute closed head injury who can safely avoid imaging evaluation. Minor head injury is typically defined as a history of loss of consciousness, disorientation, or amnesia and a GCS score ≥ 13.

A 68-year-old woman with minor acute blunt head injury. The GCS score is 15. Imaging is indicated by NOC, CCHR, or NEXUS-II clinical decision rules.

a. X-ray skull
b. CT head without contrast
c. CT head with contrast
d. MRI head without contrast
e. No ideal imaging exam

Minor acute closed head injury. Imaging is indicated by NOC, CCHR, or NEXUS-II clinical decision rules. Initial imaging.

a. X-ray skull is usually not appropriate.
b. *CT head without contrast* is the most appropriate.
c. CT head with contrast is usually not appropriate.
d. MRI head without contrast may be appropriate. This exam may be considered in an outpatient setting.

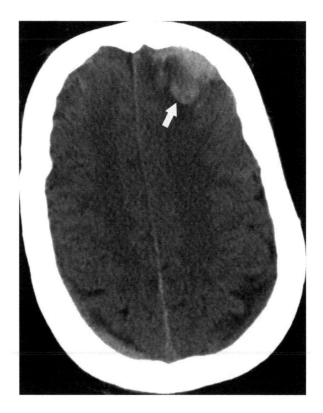

Fig. 11.1 Hemorrhagic contusion. Head CT without contrast shows intraparenchymal blood in the left frontal lobe (arrow)

Solution

Head CT without contrast has a high negative predictive value among patients with minor acute closed head injuries. Use of intravenous contrast is unnecessary as it offers no significant advantages in nonvascular imaging of head trauma. Minor head injury is typically defined as a history of loss of consciousness, disorientation, or amnesia and a GCS score ≥ 13.

A 21-year-old man with severe acute closed head injury. GCS is 7.

a. X-ray skull
b. CT head without contrast
c. CT head with contrast
d. MRI head without contrast
e. No ideal imaging exam

Moderate or severe acute closed head injury (GCS <13).

a. X-ray skull is usually not appropriate.
b. *CT head without contrast* is the most appropriate.
c. CT head with contrast is usually not appropriate.
d. MRI head without contrast is usually not appropriate.

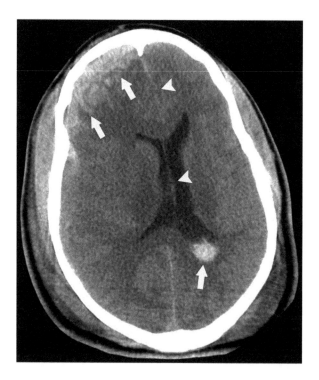

Fig. 11.2 Intracranial hemorrhage with mass effect. Head CT without contrast shows subarachnoid and intraventricular blood (arrows) and leftward midline shift (arrowheads)

Solution
Head CT is highly accurate for identifying bony injuries, acute intracranial hemorrhage, intracranial mass effect, and abnormalities in ventricular size and configuration. Additional advantages of CT are its widespread availability, rapid acquisition time, and compatibility with other medical and life-support devices.

A 27-year-old woman presents for follow-up of acute traumatic brain injury. There has been no interval neurologic deterioration.

a. X-ray skull
b. CT head without contrast
c. CT head with contrast
d. MRI head without contrast
e. No ideal imaging exam

Short-term follow-up of acute traumatic brain injury. No interval neurologic deterioration.

a. X-ray skull is usually not appropriate.
b. CT head without contrast may be appropriate.
c. CT head with contrast is usually not appropriate.
d. MRI head without contrast is usually not appropriate.
e. *No ideal imaging exam* is the correct answer.

Solution

In general, the value of a repeat head CT is low among patients with a stable neurologic examination and a negative initial CT. When the initial head CT is abnormal, the yield of repeat CT for a neurologically stable patient is also low unless the patient is anticoagulated, is over 65 years of age, or had an initial CT that showed intracranial hemorrhage with a volume >10 mL or subfrontal or temporal intraparenchymal contusions.

A 22-year-old man presents for follow-up of acute traumatic brain injury. Clinical evaluation demonstrates persistent, unexplained neurologic deficits.

a. X-ray skull
b. CT head without contrast
c. CT head with contrast
d. MRI head without contrast
e. No ideal imaging exam

Short-term imaging follow-up of acute traumatic brain injury. Neurologic deterioration, delayed recovery, or persistent unexplained deficits.

a. X-ray skull is usually not appropriate.
b. *CT head without contrast* is the most appropriate.
c. CT head with contrast may be appropriate.
d. MRI head without contrast is usually appropriate, but there is a better choice here.

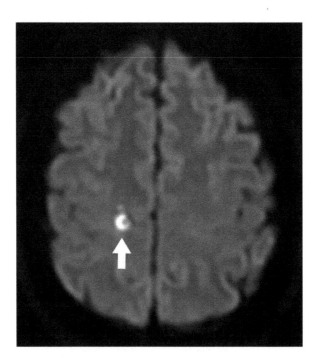

Fig. 11.3 Traumatic axonal injury. Brain MR axial diffusion-weighted image shows focal diffusion restriction (arrow) in the right frontal lobe subcortical white matter after recent head trauma consistent with traumatic axonal injury. The accompanying head CT was normal

Solution

Head CT is the most appropriate initial study. However, MRI is recommended if the patient has ongoing or progressive unexplained neurologic symptoms. Compared to CT, MRI is more sensitive for intracranial injuries such as contusions, axonal injury, and extra-axial hemorrhage.

A 64-year-old man with subacute traumatic brain injury. Exam reveals new neuro-logic deficits.

a. X-ray skull
b. CT head without contrast
c. CT head with contrast
d. MRI head without contrast
e. No ideal imaging exam

Subacute or chronic traumatic brain injury with new cognitive and/or neurologic deficit(s).

a. X-ray skull is usually not appropriate.
b. CT head without contrast is usually appropriate, but there is a better choice here.
c. CT head with contrast is usually not appropriate.
d. *MRI head without contrast* is the most appropriate.

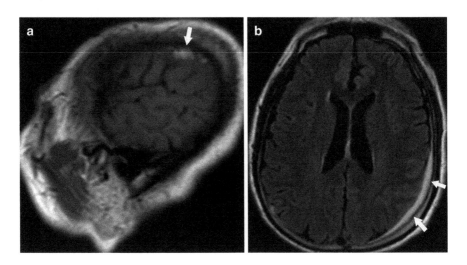

Fig. 11.4 Chronic subdural hemorrhage. Head MR sagittal T1-weighted (**a**) and axial T2-weighted (**b**) images reveal a left subdural collection (arrows) with signal intensity of old blood

Solution
MRI is the preferred imaging exam to detect and characterize brain atrophy and hemorrhage in the subacute and chronic setting.

A 36-year-old woman with suspected traumatic intracranial arterial injury.

a. CT head with contrast
b. CTA head and neck
c. MRA head and neck without and with contrast
d. Angiography cervicocerebral
e. No ideal imaging exam

Suspected intracranial arterial injury.

a. CT head with contrast is usually not appropriate.
b. *CTA head and neck* and choice (c) are equally the most appropriate.
c. *MRA head and neck without and with contrast* and choice (b) are equally the most appropriate.
d. Angiography cervicocerebral may be appropriate.

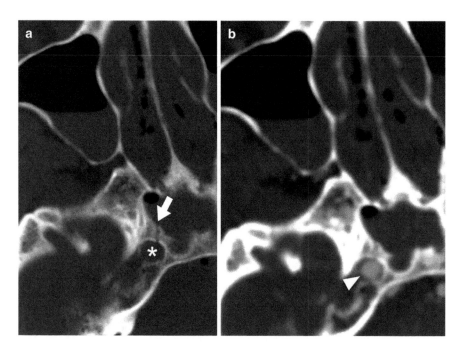

Fig. 11.5 Carotid artery evaluation in skull base fracture. Head CTA pre-contrast bone window (**a**) and post-contrast soft tissue window (**b**) images show a skull base fracture (arrow) extending to the right carotid canal (star) without associated injury to the right internal carotid artery (arrowhead)

Solution

CTA and MRA are highly accurate and noninvasive, so is preferred over catheter angiography. The choice of CTA or MRA depends on institutional preference and availability.

A 47-year-old man with suspected traumatic intracranial venous injury.

a. X-ray skull
b. CT head with contrast
c. CTA head
d. MRA head
e. Angiography cervicocerebral

Suspected intracranial venous injury.

a. X-ray skull is usually not appropriate.
b. CT head with contrast is usually not appropriate.
c. *CTA head* and choice (d) are equally the most appropriate.
d. *MRA head* and choice (c) are equally the most appropriate.
e. Angiography cervicocerebral may be appropriate.

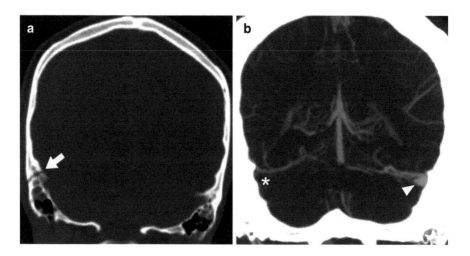

Fig. 11.6 Dural venous sinus thrombosis. Head CTA pre-contrast coronal reconstruction image (**a**) and post-contrast coronal MIP image (**b**) show a right temporal bone fracture (arrow) with non-opacified right transverse sinus (star) indicating thrombosis, compared to a normal left transverse sinus (arrowhead)

Solution
CTA and MRA perform comparably in the diagnosis of traumatic venous sinus thrombosis, which can occur with fractures extending to a dural sinus or jugular foramen. CTA requires intravenous contrast, while MRA may be performed with or without contrast. The choice of CT or MRI depends on institutional preference and availability.

11.2   Cerebrovascular Disease

A 64-year-old man without symptoms of cerebrovascular disease and a cervical bruit detected on physical examination.

a. US carotid with Doppler
b. CT head without and with contrast
c. MRI head without and with contrast
d. Angiography cervicocerebral
e. No ideal imaging exam

Asymptomatic. Carotid artery stenosis suggested by physical exam (cervical bruit) and/or risk factors for atherosclerotic disease.

a. *US carotid with Doppler* is the most appropriate.
b. CT head without and with contrast is usually not appropriate.
c. MRI head without and with contrast may be appropriate.
d. Angiography cervicocerebral is usually not appropriate.

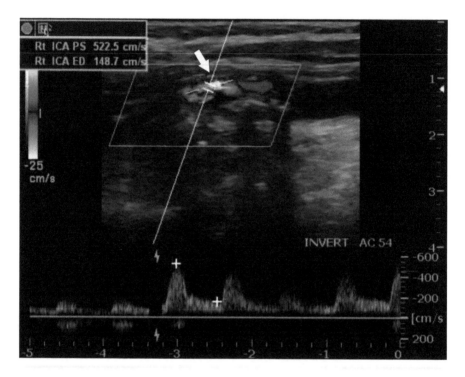

Fig. 11.7 Carotid artery stenosis. Carotid artery US with Doppler shows turbulent flow (arrow) with high velocity on spectral imaging (below) indicating narrowing

Solution

US with Doppler is an effective initial screen for carotid artery stenosis. However, accurate assessment requires operator experience, and it may be limited by artifacts from calcified plaques. CTA and MRA is used if US is inconclusive or positive.

A 56-year-old man with transient ischemic attack in the carotid territory.

a. US carotid with Doppler
b. CT head without and with contrast
c. MRI head and MRA head and neck
d. Angiography cervicocerebral
e. No ideal imaging exam

Carotid territory or vertebrobasilar transient ischemic attack, initial imaging.

a. US carotid with Doppler may be appropriate.
b. CT head without and with contrast is usually not appropriate.
c. *MRI head and MRA head and neck* is the most appropriate.
d. Angiography cervicocerebral is usually not appropriate.

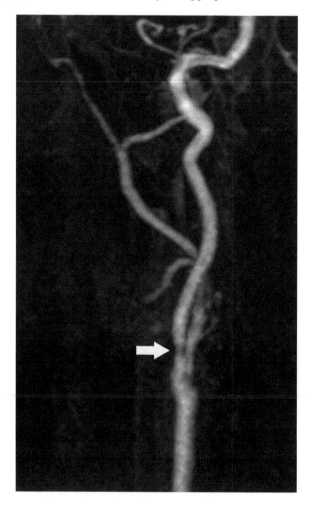

Fig. 11.8 Internal carotid artery stenosis. Neck MRA 3D reconstruction image shows narrowing (arrow) at the origin of the internal carotid artery

Solution
Evaluation of carotid or vertebrobasilar transient ischemic attacks includes both imaging of the brain parenchyma and vascular imaging of the head and neck. A combination of MRI and MRA allows for identification of vascular lesions and detection and characterization of infarcts.

A 71-year-old man with a new focal fixed neurologic deficit that started 3 h ago. A stroke is suspected.

a. US carotid with Doppler
b. CT head without contrast
c. MRI head and MRA head and neck
d. Angiography cervicocerebral
e. No ideal imaging exam

New focal neurologic defect (fixed or worsening) for less than 6 h. Suspected stroke.

a. US carotid with Doppler is usually not appropriate.
b. *CT head without contrast* is the most appropriate.
c. MRI head and MRA head and neck are usually appropriate, but there is a better choice here.
d. Angiography cervicocerebral may be appropriate.

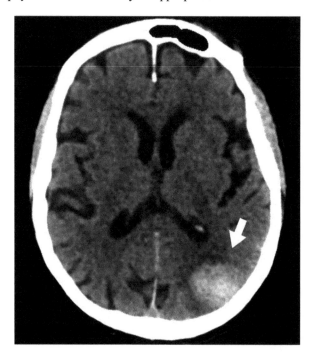

Fig. 11.9 Hemorrhagic stroke. Head CT without contrast shows acute intraparenchymal hemorrhage in the left parieto-occipital lobe (arrow)

Solution
Non-contrast head CT is the preferred initial imaging study in patients presenting with stroke symptoms due to its high sensitivity for acute intracranial hemorrhage, wide availability, high acquisition speed, lack of absolute contraindications, and ease of patient monitoring. Intracranial hemorrhage needs to be excluded before the patient can be considered for intravenous tissue plasminogen activator therapy.

A 74-year-old woman with new focal fixed neurologic deficit that started 12 h ago. A stroke is suspected.

a. US carotid with Doppler
b. CT head without contrast
c. MRI head and MRA head and neck
d. Angiography cervicocerebral
e. No ideal imaging exam

New focal neurologic defect (fixed or worsening) for longer than 6 h. Suspected stroke.

a. US carotid with Doppler is usually not appropriate.
b. *CT head without contrast* and choice (c) are equally the most appropriate.
c. *MRI head and MRA head and neck* and choice (b) are equally the most appropriate.
d. Angiography cervicocerebral may be appropriate.

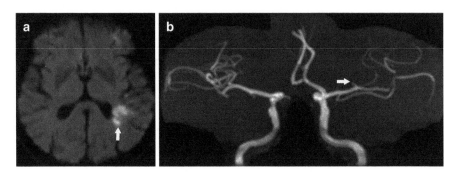

Fig. 11.10 Left hemispheric stroke. Head MR axial diffusion-weighted image (**a**) shows a focus of restricted diffusion in the left parietal lobe (arrow). Concurrent head MRA 3D reconstruction image (**b**) shows occlusion of a branch of the left middle cerebral artery (arrow)

Solution

Non-contrast head CT is the preferred initial imaging exam in patients with stroke symptoms to assess for hemorrhage before tissue plasminogen activator therapy. When the patient is outside of the 6-hour window since symptom onset, combined MRI and MRA is also appropriate to identify vascular lesions and to detect and characterize the age of infarcts.

A 45-year-old woman with multiple first-degree relatives with a history of sub-arachnoid hemorrhage presents for intracranial aneurysm screening.

a. CT head with contrast
b. CTA head
c. MRA head without contrast
d. Angiography cervicocerebral
e. No ideal imaging exam

Risk of unruptured aneurysm, including patients with polycystic kidney disease, at least two first-degree relatives with subarachnoid hemorrhage, or with previously ruptured and treated aneurysms.

a. CT head with contrast is usually not appropriate.
b. CTA head is usually appropriate, but there is a better choice here.
c. *MRA head without contrast* is the most appropriate.
d. Angiography cervicocerebral is not rated in appropriateness.

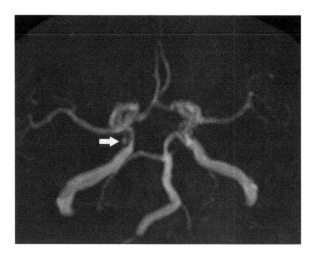

Fig. 11.11 Intracranial aneurysm. Head MRA 3D reconstruction image shows a small aneurysm (arrow) arising along the circle of Willis

Solution
MRA and CTA have comparable sensitivity for intracranial aneurysms. MRA is preferred for screening due to its lack of ionizing radiation or need for intravenous contrast. Though CTA is more specific than MRA, its use of ionizing radiation and intravenous contrast make it less suitable for screening.

A 31-year-old woman with clinically suspected acute subarachnoid hemorrhage.

a. CT head without contrast
b. CTA head
c. MRI head without contrast
d. MRA head
e. No ideal imaging exam

Acute subarachnoid hemorrhage clinically suspected.

a. *CT head without contrast* is the most appropriate.
b. CTA head may be appropriate.
c. MRI head without contrast may be appropriate.
d. MRA head may be appropriate.

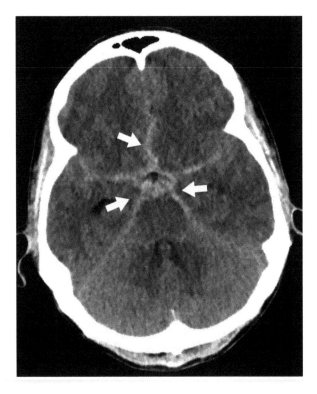

Fig. 11.12 Subarachnoid hemorrhage. Head CT without contrast reveals high-density blood in the basal cisterns (arrows)

Solution
Non-contrast head CT is the preferred initial imaging exam due to its high sensitivity for acute hemorrhage, rapid image acquisition, wide availability, lack of absolute contraindications, and ease of patient monitoring.

A 31-year-old woman with subarachnoid hemorrhage diagnosed on non-contrast head CT. Next imaging exam.

a. CTA head
b. MRI head without contrast
c. MRA head
d. Angiography cervicocerebral
e. No ideal imaging exam

Proven subarachnoid hemorrhage by lumbar puncture or imaging.

a. CTA head is usually appropriate, but there is a better choice here.
b. MRI head without contrast may be appropriate.
c. MRA head is usually appropriate, but there is a better choice here.
d. *Angiography cervicocerebral* is the most appropriate.

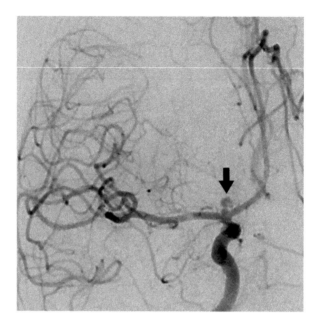

Fig. 11.13 Intracranial aneurysm. Cerebral angiogram coronal view shows an irregularly shaped, multilobulated 3 mm aneurysm (arrow) at the terminus of the right internal carotid artery. This presumed source of an acute subarachnoid hemorrhage underwent coil embolization

Solution
The majority of non-traumatic subarachnoid hemorrhages are caused by aneurysm rupture, and the primary aim of imaging is to identify the culprit lesion. Although CTA and MRA are highly sensitive for aneurysms in general, neither are sensitive for those smaller than 3 mm, which accounts for a significant fraction of ruptured aneurysms. Thus, catheter angiography remains the preferred exam in this setting.

A 43-year-old woman with known subarachnoid hemorrhage. Cause of hemorrhage was not identified on initial catheter angiography. Next imaging exam.

a. US transcranial with Doppler
b. CT head without contrast
c. MRA head
d. Repeat angiography cervicocerebral at 1–2 weeks
e. No ideal imaging exam

Proven subarachnoid hemorrhage. Next imaging exam following negative catheter angiography.

a. US transcranial with Doppler may be appropriate.
b. CT head without contrast may be appropriate.
c. *MRA head* and choice (d) are equally the most appropriate.
d. *Repeat angiography cervicocerebral at 1–2 weeks* and choice (c) are equally the most appropriate.

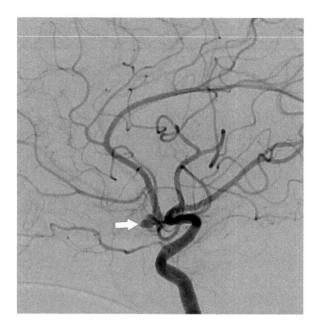

Fig. 11.14 Intracranial aneurysm. Cerebral angiogram lateral view shows an aneurysm (arrow) along the anterior communicating artery

Solution
Initial catheter angiography can be negative in 10–20% of aneurysmal subarachnoid hemorrhage cases. Noninvasive imaging with either MRA or CTA is recommended if not already performed. If both angiography and CTA or MRA are negative, repeat catheter angiography in 1–2 weeks is recommended.

A 68-year-old woman with suspected intraparenchymal hemorrhage.

a. CT head without contrast
b. CTA head
c. MRI head without contrast
d. Angiography cervicocerebral
e. No ideal imaging exam

Clinically suspected intraparenchymal hemorrhage (hematoma).

a. *CT head without contrast* is the most appropriate.
b. CTA head may be appropriate.
c. MRI head without contrast is usually appropriate, but there is a better choice here.
d. Angiography cervicocerebral is not rated in appropriateness.

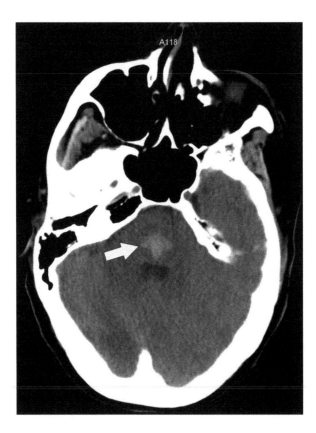

Fig. 11.15 Intraparenchymal hemorrhage. Head CT without contrast shows blood in the brainstem (arrow)

Solution
Non-contrast head CT is highly sensitive for acute intracranial hemorrhage. MRI with susceptibility weighted sequences may have similar sensitivity but is subject to the patient's ability to cooperate and is less readily available.

A 56-year-old woman with known intraparenchymal hemorrhage. Next imaging exam.

a. CT head without contrast
b. CT head without and with contrast
c. MRI head without and with contrast
d. Angiography cervicocerebral
e. No ideal imaging exam

Proven parenchymal hemorrhage (hematoma).

a. CT head without contrast is usually appropriate, but there is a better choice here.
b. CT head without and with contrast may be appropriate.
c. *MRI head without and with contrast* is the most appropriate.
d. Angiography cervicocerebral may be appropriate.

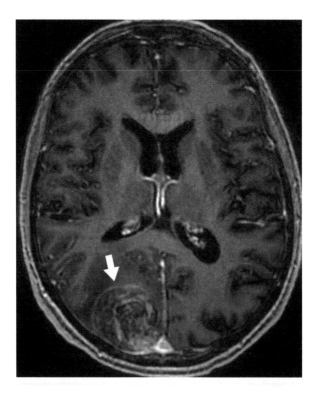

Fig. 11.16 Glioblastoma. Head MR axial post-contrast image shows an enhancing, hemorrhagic right occipital lobe mass (arrow)

Solution
In patients with parenchymal brain hemorrhage, MRI is the preferred exam to evaluate for the underlying cause, which includes amyloid angiopathy, cavernous malformation, neoplasm, venous thrombosis, and dural arteriovenous fistula. However, if initial head CT and clinical history strongly suggest a hypertensive cause, then imaging may be limited to follow-up with serial non-contrast head CT.

A 51-year-old woman with suspected dural venous sinus thrombosis.

a. CT head without contrast
b. CTA head
c. MRA head without and with contrast
d. Angiography cervicocerebral
e. No ideal imaging exam

Suspected dural venous sinus thrombosis.

a. CT head without contrast is usually appropriate, but there is a better choice here.
b. CTA head is usually appropriate, but there is a better choice here.
c. *MRA head without and with contrast* is the most appropriate.
d. Angiography cervicocerebral may be appropriate.

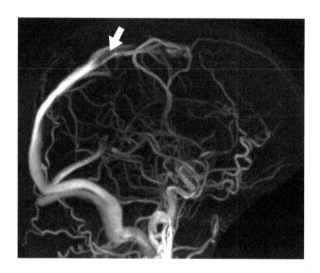

Fig. 11.17 Dural venous sinus thrombosis. Head MRA sagittal MIP image shows thrombosis (arrow) within the superior sagittal sinus

Solution
MRA is performed along with brain MRI to allow for the evaluation of both venous sinus thrombosis and related complications including venous infarction, hemorrhage, and edema. Though use of contrast is preferred for optimum accuracy, MRA can be performed without contrast if necessary.

11.3   Acute Mental Status Change, Delirium, and New-Onset Psychosis

A 74-year-old man with acute mental status change. He is anticoagulated.

a. CT head without contrast
b. CT head with contrast
c. MRI head without contrast
d. MRI head without and with contrast
e. No ideal imaging exam

Acute mental status change. Increased risk for intracranial bleeding (i.e., anticoagulated, coagulopathy), hypertensive emergency, or clinical suspicious for intracranial
infection, mass, or elevated intracranial pressure. Initial imaging.

a. *CT head without contrast* is the most appropriate.
b. CT head with contrast is usually not appropriate.
c. MRI head without contrast is usually appropriate, but there is a better choice here.
d. MRI head without and with contrast may be appropriate.

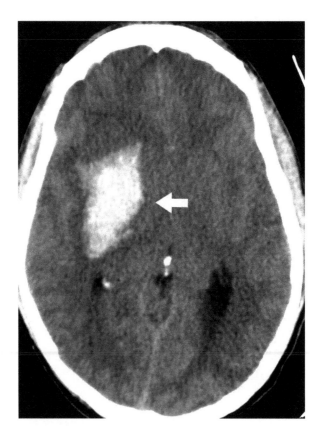

Fig. 11.18 Intraparenchymal hemorrhage. Head CT without contrast shows hemorrhage centered
in the right basal ganglia (arrow)

Solution
Non-contrast head CT is preferred and can be performed safely and rapidly in all
patients with acute change in mental status. MRI has higher sensitivity for ischemia,
encephalitis, and subtle subarachnoid hemorrhage and may be useful if initial head
CT is negative. In settings such as known malignancy, HIV, or endocarditis, MRI
may be the first-line exam.

An 81-year-old woman with known intracranial hemorrhage and acutely worsening mental status.

a. CT head without contrast
b. CT head with contrast
c. MRI head without contrast
d. MRI head without and with contrast
e. No ideal imaging exam

Acute or progressively worsening mental status change in patient with known intra-cranial process (e.g., mass, infection, recent hemorrhage or infarct).

a. *CT head without contrast* and choices (c) and (d) are equally the most appropriate.
b. CT head with contrast may be appropriate.
c. *MRI head without contrast* and choices (a) and (d) are equally the most appropriate.
d. *MRI head without and with contrast* and choices (a) and (c) are equally the most appropriate.

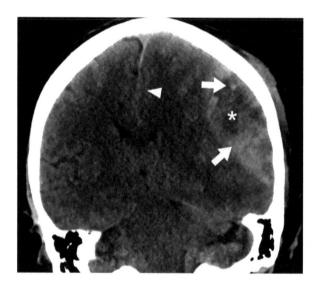

Fig. 11.19 Epidural hematoma. Head CT without contrast coronal reconstruction image shows mixed-density hematoma (star) with hyperdensities (arrows) that suggest ongoing bleed. There is a rightward midline shift (arrowhead)

Solution
Both non-contrast head CT and MRI are used for the evaluation of worsening hemorrhage, mass effect, or hydrocephalus. MRI is more appropriate in the setting of infection and ischemia, and contrast can help evaluate for underlying masses or complications of infection (e.g., abscess).

A 34-year-old woman with acute mental status change, attributed to hypoglycemia based on initial clinical and lab assessment.

a. CT head without contrast
b. CT head with contrast
c. MRI head without contrast
d. MRI head without and with contrast
e. No ideal imaging exam

Acute mental status change. Suspected causes(s) found on initial clinical or lab assessment (e.g., intoxication, medication-related, hypoglycemia, sepsis). Low clinical suspicion for trauma, intracranial hemorrhage, stroke, mass, or intracranial infection.

a. CT head without contrast may be appropriate.
b. CT head with contrast is usually not appropriate.
c. MRI head without contrast may be appropriate.
d. MRI head without and with contrast may be appropriate.
e. *No ideal imaging exam* is the correct answer.

Solution

Imaging can be deferred when there is low clinical suspicion for acute intracranial pathology as the etiology for acute mental status change.

11.4   Seizures and Epilepsy

A 9-year-old girl with medically refractory epilepsy being evaluated for surgical management.

a. CT head without contrast
b. CT head with contrast
c. MRI head without and with contrast
d. MRI functional (fMRI) head without contrast
e. No ideal imaging exam

Medically refractory epilepsy. Surgical candidate or surgical planning.

a. CT head without contrast may be appropriate.
b. CT head with contrast may be appropriate.
c. *MRI head without and with contrast* is the most appropriate.
d. MRI functional (fMRI) head without contrast may be appropriate.

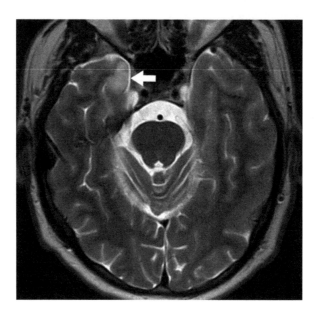

Fig. 11.20 Focal cortical dysplasia. Head MR axial T2-weighted image shows a lobulated lesion (arrow) within the cortex and juxtacortical white matter of the anterior right temporal lobe

Solution
MRI is preferred for detecting structural lesions that may induce seizures. Intravenous contrast can be useful particularly when there is suspicion for infection, tumor, or an inflammatory or vascular lesion. Functional imaging techniques may also help localize the seizure focus when no detectable structural lesions are seen.

A 32-year-old man with new-onset seizure and no history of trauma.

a. CT head without contrast
b. CT head with contrast
c. MRI head without and with contrast
d. Magnetoencephalography
e. No ideal imaging exam

New-onset seizure unrelated to trauma. Age 18 years or older.

a. CT head without contrast is usually appropriate, but there is a better choice here.
b. CT head with contrast may be appropriate.
c. *MRI head without and with contrast* is the most appropriate. However, in the acute or emergency setting, if MRI is not readily available, choice (a) may be the most appropriate.
d. Magnetoencephalography is usually not appropriate.

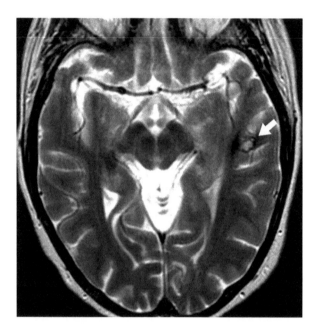

Fig. 11.21 Cavernous malformation. Head MR axial T2-weighted image shows a lobulated lesion (arrow) in the left temporal lobe that is internally hyperintense with a hypointense rim

Solution

MRI is the preferred imaging exam to identify a cause for new-onset seizure. Intravenous contrast should be used if infection, tumor, an inflammatory lesion, or a vascular pathology is suspected.

A 55-year-old woman with new-onset seizure and no history of trauma. Clinical exam reveals a focal neurological deficit.

a. CT head without contrast
b. CT head with contrast
c. MRI head without and with contrast
d. FDG-PET/CT head
e. No ideal imaging exam

New-onset seizure unrelated to trauma. Focal neurological deficit on exam.

a. CT head without contrast is usually appropriate, but there is a better choice here.
b. CT head with contrast is usually appropriate, but there is a better choice here.
c. *MRI head without and with contrast* is the most appropriate. However, in the acute or emergency setting if MRI is not readily available, choices (a) or (b) may be the most appropriate.
d. FDG-PET/CT head is usually not appropriate.

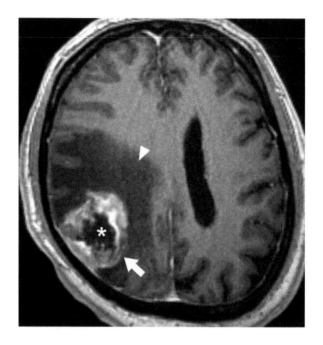

Fig. 11.22 Glioblastoma multiforme. Head MR axial post-contrast image shows an enhancing mass (arrow) with central necrosis (star) and low signal in the adjacent white matter, indicating edema (arrowhead)

Solution
The presence of focal neurological deficit in the setting of new-onset seizure increases the likelihood of having imaging abnormalities. Causes of seizures with focal neurological deficit include primary neoplasm, metastasis, intracranial hemorrhage, infarct, and toxoplasmosis.

A 37-year-old man with new-onset seizure following mild head trauma that occurred 3 days ago.

a. CT head without contrast
b. CT head with contrast
c. MRI head without and with contrast
d. FDG-PET/CT head
e. No ideal imaging exam

New-onset acute posttraumatic seizure.

a. *CT head without contrast* is the most appropriate.
b. CT head with contrast may be appropriate.
c. MRI head without and with contrast is usually appropriate, but there is a better choice here.
d. FDG-PET/CT head is usually not appropriate.

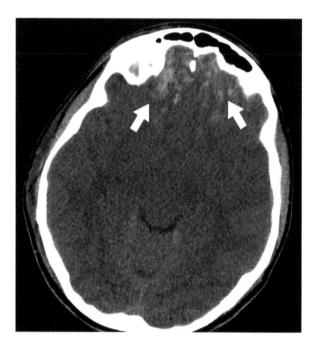

Fig. 11.23 Cerebral contusions. Head CT without contrast following head trauma shows intraparenchymal hemorrhage (arrows) in bilateral frontal lobes adjacent to the frontal bones

Solution

Acute or early posttraumatic seizures are defined to occur within 1 week of head trauma. Non-contrast head CT is recommended to evaluate for intracranial hemorrhage, which is commonly found in this setting. When seizure presents more than a week after head trauma, MRI is preferred due to its higher sensitivity for detecting hemosiderin deposition from more remote intracranial hemorrhage.

11.5   Headache

A 72-year-old man with sudden onset of the "worst headache of his life."

a. CT head without contrast
b. CTA head
c. MRA head
d. Angiography cervicocerebral
e. No ideal imaging exam

Sudden, severe headache or "worst headache of one's life." Initial exam.

   a. *CT head without contrast* is the most appropriate.
   b. CTA head may be appropriate.
   c. MRA head is usually not appropriate.
   d. Angiography cervicocerebral is usually not appropriate.

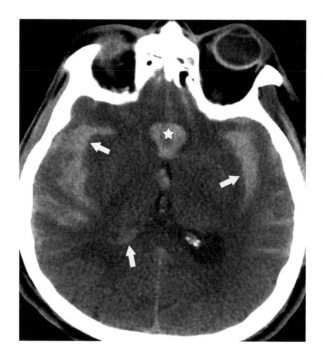

Fig. 11.24 Subarachnoid hemorrhage from aneurysm rupture. Head CT without contrast shows blood bilaterally in the sulci and in the right lateral ventricle (arrows). A rounded high-density collection (star) is the ruptured aneurysm representing the bleeding source

Solution
Imaging is indicated to evaluate for acute intracranial hemorrhage such as subarachnoid hemorrhage from aneurysm rupture. Non-contrast head CT is the preferred initial exam, with sensitivity approaching 100% when performed within 6 h of symptom onset.

A 38-year-old woman with new headache and optic disc edema on exam.

a. CT head without contrast
b. CTA head
c. MRI head
d. MRA head
e. No ideal imaging exam

New headache with optic disc edema on exam.

a. *CT head without contrast* and choice (c) are equally the most appropriate.
b. CTA head may be appropriate.
c. *MRI head* and choice (a) are equally the most appropriate.
d. MRA head may be appropriate.

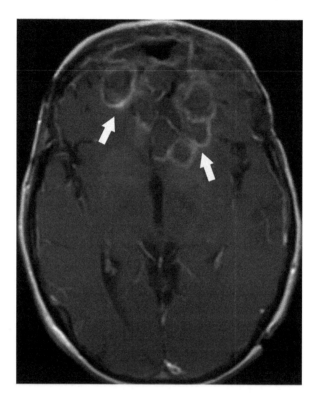

Fig. 11.25 Intracranial abscess. Head MR axial post-contrast image shows a multiloculated rim enhancing collection (arrows) involving bilateral frontal lobes

Solution
Bilateral optic disc edema is an indicator of increased intracranial pressure. CT and MRI are equivalent alternatives to evaluate for etiologies, including intracranial abscess, tumor, hemorrhage, cerebral edema, hydrocephalus, and pseudotumor cerebri. CT or MR angiography can assess for cerebral venous thrombosis as a potential cause.

A 53-year-old woman with known diagnosis of human immunodeficiency virus presents with a new headache.

a. CT head without contrast
b. CTA head
c. MRI head
d. MRA head
e. No ideal imaging exam

New or worsening headache with "red flags" (i.e., ≥50 years of age, pregnant, post-traumatic, neurological deficit, known or suspected cancer, immunocompromised, or related to exertion, position, or sexual activity).

a. *CT head without contrast* and choice (c) are equally the most appropriate.
b. CTA head is usually not appropriate.
c. *MRI head* and choice (a) are equally the most appropriate.
d. MRA head is usually not appropriate.

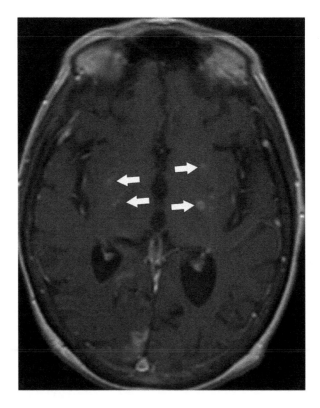

Fig. 11.26 Cryptococcal abscesses. Head MR axial post-contrast image shows enhancing foci in the bilateral basal ganglia (arrows)

Solution
Both CT and MRI are appropriate exams when imaging is indicated due to the presence of a "red flag." Non-contrast head CT is able to rule out mass effect, hemorrhage, or hydrocephalus. MRI is an appropriate alternative. In the setting of malignancy or immunocompromised state, use of intravenous contrast with MRI is warranted.

A 27-year-old woman with new tension-type headache. Neurologic exam is normal.

a. CT head without contrast
b. CTA head
c. MRI head without and with contrast
d. MRA head
e. No ideal imaging exam

New headache. Classic migraine or tension-type primary headache. Normal neurologic examination.

a. CT head without contrast is usually not appropriate.
b. CTA head is usually not appropriate.
c. MRI head without and with contrast is usually not appropriate.
d. MRA head is usually not appropriate.
e. *No ideal imaging exam* is the correct answer.

Solution
Imaging is not indicated for patients who meet criteria for a primary headache syndrome, i.e., no "red flags" and a normal neurologic examination.

A 40-year-old man with chronic headaches. There are no new features and no neurologic deficit.

a. CT head without contrast
b. CTA head
c. MRI head without and with contrast
d. MRA head
e. No ideal imaging exam

Chronic headache with no new features and no neurologic deficit.

a. CT head without contrast is usually not appropriate.
b. CTA head is usually not appropriate.
c. MRI head without and with contrast is usually not appropriate.
d. MRA head is usually not appropriate.
e. *No ideal imaging exam* is the correct answer.

Solution
Imaging is not indicated for chronic headaches without new features or neurologic deficits. In this setting, the diagnostic yield is low.

A 47-year-old woman with chronic headaches that have recently increased in frequency and intensity.

a. CT head without contrast
b. CTA head
c. MRI head without and with contrast
d. MRA head
e. No ideal imaging exam

Chronic headache with new features or increasing frequency.

a. CT head without contrast may be appropriate.
b. CTA head is usually not appropriate.
c. *MRI head without and with contrast* is the most appropriate.
d. MRA head is usually not appropriate.

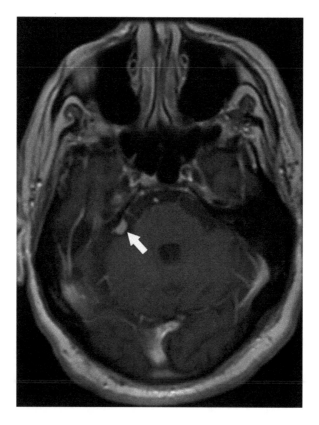

Fig. 11.27 Meningioma. Head MR axial post-contrast image shows an enhancing extra-axial mass (arrow) at the right cerebellopontine angle

Solution
Imaging is indicated when there is a change in the frequency, severity, or character of a chronic headache. MRI is preferred over CT to assess for intracranial pathology including tumors. Intravenous contrast aides in the evaluation of suspected mass or infection.

11.6   Dementia

A 67-year-old man with cognitive decline. Alzheimer disease is suspected.

a. CT head without contrast
b. MRI head without contrast
c. F-18 amyloid PET/CT brain
d. FDG-PET/CT brain
e. No ideal imaging exam

Cognitive decline. Suspected Alzheimer disease.

a. *CT head without contrast* and choice (b) are equally the most appropriate.
b. *MRI head without contrast* and choice (a) are equally the most appropriate.
c. F-18 amyloid PET/CT brain may be appropriate.
d. FDG-PET/CT brain may be appropriate.

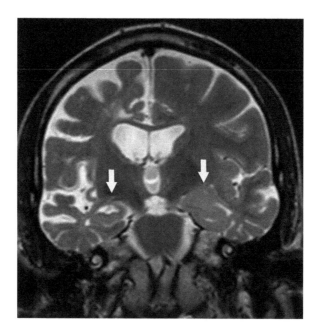

Fig. 11.28 Alzheimer disease. Head MR coronal T2-weighted image shows bilateral hippocampal atrophy (arrows), right greater than left

Solution

A primary role of imaging in the evaluation of suspected Alzheimer disease is to exclude other intracranial pathologies. Both CT and MRI can identify treatable lesions such as a mass or subdural hematoma. MRI can also help in the diagnosis of Alzheimer disease by demonstrating structural changes in the brain such as hippocampal atrophy.

A 62-year-old man with suspected frontotemporal dementia.

a. CT head without contrast
b. MRI head without contrast
c. F-18 amyloid PET/CT brain
d. FDG-PET/CT brain
e. No ideal imaging exam

Suspected frontotemporal dementia.

a. *CT head without contrast* and choice (b) are equally the most appropriate.
b. *MRI head without contrast* and choice (a) are equally the most appropriate.
c. F-18 amyloid PET/CT brain is usually not appropriate.
d. FDG-PET/CT brain may be appropriate.

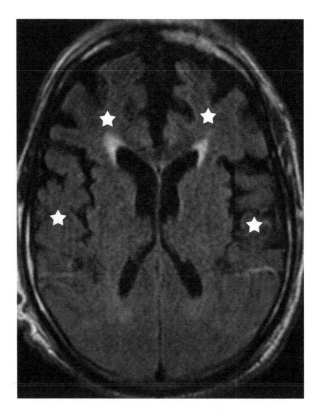

Fig. 11.29 Frontotemporal atrophy. Head MR axial T2-weighted image shows bilateral atrophy of the frontal and temporal lobes (stars)

Solution
Imaging with CT or MRI is used to exclude other structural brain abnormalities that could resemble frontotemporal dementia, differentiate this from other neurodegenerative disorders such as Alzheimer disease, and classify the subtype of this disorder.

A 60-year-old man with suspected dementia with Lewy bodies.

a. CT head without contrast
b. MRI head without contrast
c. F-18 amyloid PET/CT brain
d. FDG-PET/CT brain
e. No ideal imaging exam

Suspected dementia with Lewy bodies.

a. *CT head without contrast* and choice (b) are equally the most appropriate.
b. *MRI head without contrast* and choice (a) are equally the most appropriate.
c. F-18 amyloid PET/CT brain is usually not appropriate.
d. FDG-PET/CT brain may be appropriate.

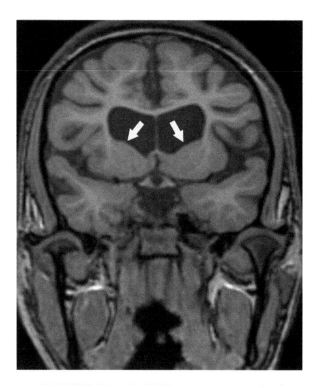

Fig. 11.30 Basal ganglia atrophy. Head MR coronal T1-weighted image shows atrophy of the caudate nucleus bilaterally (arrows)

Solution
CT and MRI help exclude other causes of dementia and can improve the diagnostic accuracy for dementia with Lewy bodies. On MRI, patients with this form of dementia when compared to those with Alzheimer disease show relative preservation of medial temporal lobe structures including the hippocampus and have relatively greater atrophy of subcortical structures such as the thalamus, caudate, and midbrain.

A 65-year-old man with dementia suspected to be of vascular etiology.

a. CT head without contrast
b. CTA head
c. MRI head without contrast
d. MRA head
e. No ideal imaging exam

Suspected vascular dementia.

a. *CT head without contrast* and choice (c) are equally the most appropriate.
b. CTA head is usually not appropriate
c. *MRI head without contrast* and choice (a) are equally the most appropriate.
d. MRA head is usually not appropriate.

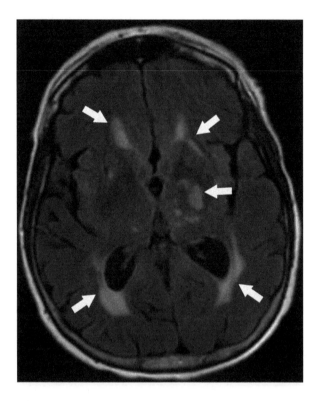

Fig. 11.31 Multifocal small vessel infarcts. Head MR axial T2-weighted image shows ischemic changes (arrows) in the basal ganglia and periventricular white matter

Solution

Vascular dementia can be caused by large or small vessel disease. Both CT and MRI can assess the presence and severity of white matter changes from prior stroke or hemorrhage, with MRI being more sensitive. Vascular imaging with CTA or MRA is not needed as the diagnosis relies on clinical criteria and evidence of end organ damage to the brain.

A 58-year-old woman with dementia and suspected idiopathic normal pressure hydrocephalus.

a. CT head without contrast
b. MRI head without contrast
c. MRI spectroscopy head
d. In-111 DTPA cisternography
e. No ideal imaging exam

Suspected idiopathic normal pressure hydrocephalus.

a. *CT head without contrast* and choice (b) are equally the most appropriate.
b. *MRI head without contrast* and choice (a) are equally the most appropriate.
c. MRI spectroscopy head is usually not appropriate.
d. In-111 DTPA cisternography may be appropriate.

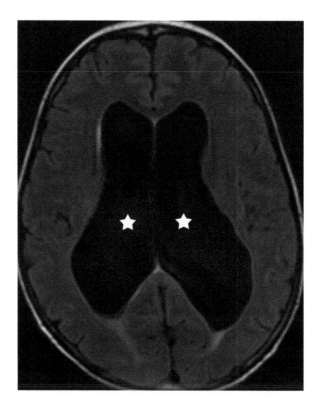

Fig. 11.32 Normal pressure hydrocephalus. Head MR axial T2-weighted image shows enlargement of the lateral ventricles bilaterally (stars) with minimal cortical atrophy

Solution
Findings on CT or MRI include communicating hydrocephalus, enlargement of the ventricles disproportionate to the degree of cortical atrophy, and transependymal flow of cerebrospinal fluid.

11.7 Movement Disorders and Neurodegenerative Diseases

A 55-year-old man with suspected Creutzfeldt–Jakob disease.

a. CT head without contrast
b. MRI head without contrast
c. MR spectroscopy head
d. FDG-PET/CT brain
e. No ideal imaging exam

Rapidly progressive dementia. Creutzfeldt–Jakob disease is suspected.

a. CT head without contrast may be appropriate.
b. *MRI head without contrast* is the most appropriate.
c. MR spectroscopy head is usually not appropriate.
d. FDG-PET/CT brain may be appropriate.

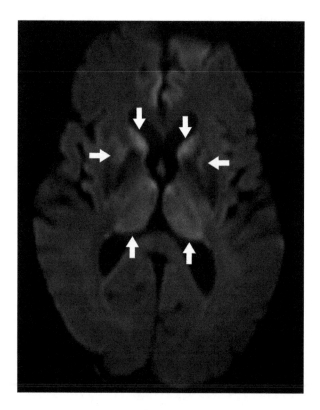

Fig. 11.33 Creutzfeldt–Jakob disease. Head MR axial diffusion weighted image shows restricted diffusion within bilateral basal ganglia and thalami (arrows)

Solution
Rapidly progressive dementias are those with symptom onset over weeks to months, with Creutzfeldt–Jakob disease being the prototypical example. Others include potentially reversible cases such as autoimmune and infectious processes. MRI is the preferred exam as it can show typical features of Creutzfeldt–Jakob disease (e.g., signal abnormalities in the basal ganglia and thalami) and also evaluate for other causes of dementia.

A 39-year-old woman with movement disorder. Huntington's disease is suspected.

a. CT head without contrast
b. MRI head without contrast
c. MR spectroscopy head
d. FDG-PET/CT brain
e. No ideal imaging exam

Chorea. Suspected Huntington's disease.

a. CT head without contrast may be appropriate.
b. *MRI head without contrast* is the most appropriate.
c. MR spectroscopy head is usually not appropriate.
d. FDG-PET/CT brain is usually not appropriate.

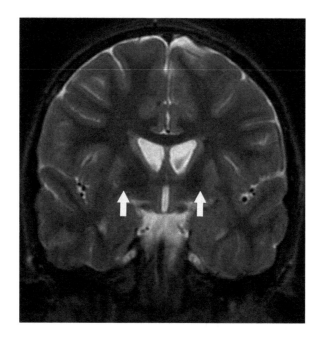

Fig. 11.34 Huntington's disease. Head MR coronal T2-weighted image shows atrophy of the putamen bilaterally (arrows)

Solution
Huntington's disease has characteristic imaging features on MRI, including progressive degeneration and atrophy of the caudate nucleus and the putamen. CT is less useful in making this diagnosis but may help exclude other causes of chorea such as cerebrovascular disease and infectious or inflammatory processes.

A 69-year-old woman with parkinsonian syndrome.

a. CT head without contrast
b. MRI head without contrast
c. MR spectroscopy head
d. FDG-PET/CT brain
e. No ideal imaging exam

Parkinsonian syndromes.

a. CT head without contrast may be appropriate.
b. *MRI head without contrast* is the most appropriate.
c. MR spectroscopy head is usually not appropriate.
d. FDG-PET/CT brain may be appropriate.

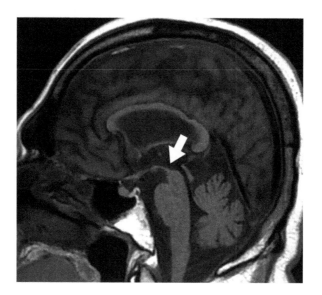

Fig. 11.35 Progressive supranuclear palsy. Head MR sagittal T1-weighted image shows atrophy of the midbrain with relative preservation of the pons (arrow), creating the appearance of the "hummingbird sign" associated with progressive supranuclear palsy

Solution
Parkinsonian syndromes include Parkinson disease and other entities such as progressive supranuclear palsy and multi-system atrophy. These syndromes have characteristic changes, such as midbrain atrophy seen with progressive supranuclear palsy. MRI is the preferred exam to detect these changes in the brain parenchyma and can also demonstrate iron deposition.

A 25-year-old man with movement disorder suspected to be from neurodegeneration with brain iron accumulation.

a. CT head without contrast
b. MRI head without contrast
c. MR spectroscopy head
d. FDG-PET/CT brain
e. No ideal imaging exam

Suspected neurodegeneration with brain iron accumulation.

a. CT head without contrast may be appropriate.
b. *MRI head without contrast* is the most appropriate.
c. MR spectroscopy head is usually not appropriate.
d. FDG-PET/CT brain is usually not appropriate.

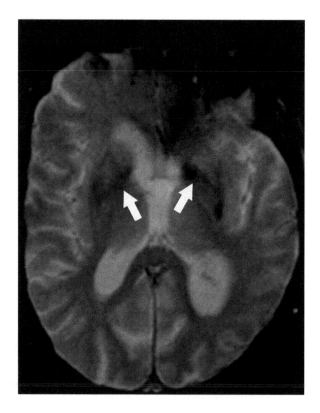

Fig. 11.36 Neurodegeneration with brain iron accumulation. Head MR axial T2-weighted image shows hypointense signal with susceptibility artifact (arrows) consistent with iron deposition in the basal ganglia

Solution
Neurodegeneration with brain iron accumulation is characterized by excess basal ganglia iron deposition. MRI is the preferred imaging exam due to its sensitivity for iron, seen as "susceptibility artifact."

A 51-year-old woman with movement disorder suspected to be degenerative motor neuron disease.

a. CT head without contrast
b. MRI head without contrast
c. MR spectroscopy head
d. FDG-PET/CT brain
e. No ideal imaging exam

Suspected motor neuron disease.

a. CT head without contrast may be appropriate.
b. *MRI head without contrast* is the most appropriate.
c. MR spectroscopy head is usually not appropriate.
d. FDG-PET/CT brain is usually not appropriate.

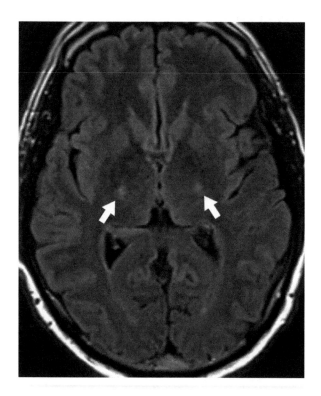

Fig. 11.37 Amyotrophic lateral sclerosis. Head MR axial T2-weighted image shows hyperintense signal along the posterior limb of the internal capsule bilaterally (arrows)

Solution
MRI can show characteristic findings of amyotrophic lateral sclerosis. The most common is abnormal signal within the corticospinal tracts from subcortical white matter to the pons, most frequently seen in the posterior limb of the internal capsule and the cerebral peduncles.

11.8   Ataxia

A 68-year-old woman presents with acute ataxia following head trauma.

a. CT head without contrast
b. CTA head and neck
c. MRI head without contrast
d. MRA head and neck
e. No ideal imaging exam

Acute ataxia following recent head trauma.

a. *CT head without contrast* is the most appropriate.
b. CTA head and neck may be appropriate.
c. MRI head without contrast may be appropriate.
d. MRA head and neck may be appropriate.

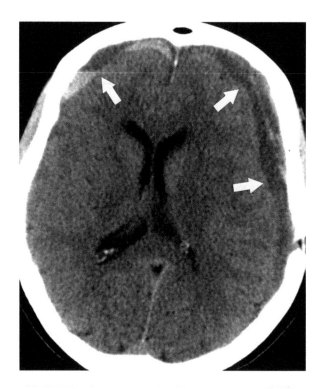

Fig. 11.38 Subdural hemorrhage. Head CT shows subdural collections bilaterally (arrows) with both high- and low high-density material indicating ongoing episodes of bleeding

Solution

In the setting of a new neurologic deficit after head trauma, non-contrast head CT is the preferred initial exam. Posttraumatic gait disturbance may be due to cyst or hematoma expansion anywhere from the frontal lobe along the frontopontocerebellar tract to the cerebellum. Ataxia can also result from traumatic vertebral artery dissection. If vascular injury is suspected, then either CTA or MRA can be performed.

A 45-year-old man with acute onset ataxia and no history of recent trauma. An intracranial etiology is suspected. Intervention for stroke is not being considered.

a. CT head without contrast
b. CTA head and neck
c. MRI head without and with contrast
d. MRA head and neck
e. No ideal imaging exam

Ataxia. No history of trauma. Suspected intracranial process. Stroke intervention not a consideration.

a. CT head without contrast may be appropriate.
b. CTA head and neck is usually not appropriate.
c. *MRI head without and with contrast* is the most appropriate.
d. MRA head and neck is usually not appropriate.

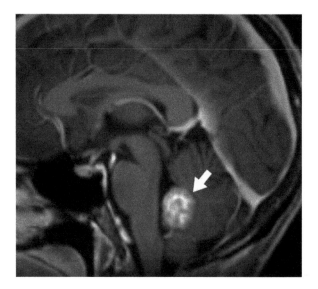

Fig. 11.39 Medulloblastoma. Head MR sagittal post-contrast image shows an enhancing mass (arrow) centered in the fourth ventricle, diagnosed as a medulloblastoma on surgical resection

Solution
MRI is the preferred exam as it can reveal many of the potential causes of ataxia, including posterior fossa mass, cerebellitis, neurodegeneration, siderosis, and congenital malformations. While MRI is superior to CT for soft tissue characterization in general, it particularly outperforms CT for the evaluation of the posterior fossa.

11.9   Orbits, Vision, and Visual Loss

A 53-year-old man with head injury and vision loss.

a. CT head and/or orbits without contrast
b. CTA head and neck
c. MRI head and/or orbits without contrast
d. MRA head and neck
e. No ideal imaging exam

Traumatic visual defect. Suspect orbital injury. Initial imaging.

a. *CT head and/or orbits without contrast* is the most appropriate.
b. CTA head and neck may be appropriate.
c. MRI head and/or orbits without contrast may be appropriate.
d. MRA head and neck may be appropriate.

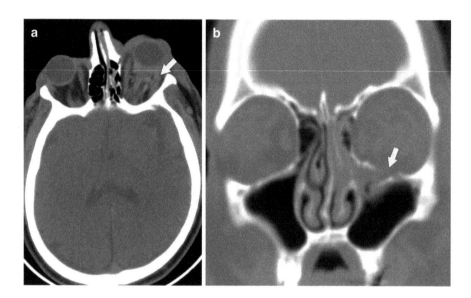

Fig. 11.40 Orbital fracture. Head CT without contrast (**a**) shows retrobulbar hemorrhage (arrow) resulting in left proptosis. Coronal reconstruction image (**b**) reveals a fracture (arrow) of the left orbital floor

Solution
Orbit CT accurately identifies fractures, displaced fracture fragments, optic canal narrowing, intra-orbital foreign bodies, hematomas, and extra-ocular muscle injury. Intravenous contrast is not needed. In patients with more severe trauma, head CT may also be needed for concurrent assessment of intracranial injury.

A 41-year-old woman presents with left exophthalmos.

a. CT orbits with contrast
b. CTA head and neck
c. MRI orbits without and with contrast
d. MRA head and neck
e. No ideal imaging exam

Nontraumatic orbital asymmetry, exophthalmos, or enophthalmos.

a. *CT orbits with contrast* and choice (c) are equally the most appropriate.
b. CTA head and neck may be appropriate.
c. *MRI orbits without and with contrast* and choice (a) are equally the most appropriate.
d. MRA head and neck may be appropriate.

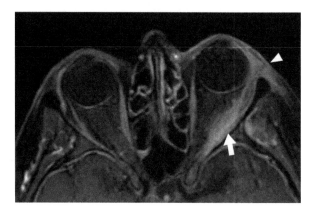

Fig. 11.41 Orbital pseudotumor. Orbit MR axial post-contrast image shows abnormal enhancement of the left lateral rectus muscle (arrow) and periorbital soft tissues (arrowhead) and left exophthalmos

Solution
Both CT and MRI can diagnose a range of causes including orbital inflammatory conditions and underlying mass lesions, with the inherent tissue contrast provided by orbital fat allowing for excellent anatomic definition. CT or MR angiography may be used if a vascular cause, such as carotid-cavernous fistula, is suspected.

A 40-year-old man with uveitis, scleritis, and vision loss in one eye.

a. CT orbits with contrast
b. CTA head and neck
c. MRI orbits without and with contrast
d. MRA head and neck
e. No ideal imaging exam

Suspected orbital cellulitis, uveitis, or scleritis.

a. *CT orbits with contrast* and choice (c) are equally the most appropriate.
b. CTA head and neck may be appropriate.
c. *MRI orbits without and with contrast* and choice (a) are equally the most appropriate.
d. MRA head and neck may be appropriate.

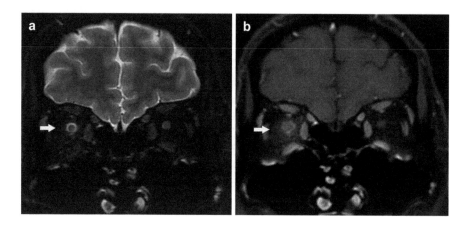

Fig. 11.42 Orbital infection. Head MR coronal T2-weighted (**a**) and post-contrast (**b**) images show edema and abnormal enhancement of the right optic nerve and orbital fat (arrows)

Solution
Imaging is indicated to assess for complications of orbital infection such as intra-orbital abscess and intracranial involvement. CT and MRI are complementary. CT is preferred for the assessment of foreign bodies and bone erosion from an infectious process. CT also evaluates the paranasal sinuses, which are often the source of the infection. MRI provides better evaluation of the intra-orbital spread of infection due to superior soft tissue contrast.

A 37-year-old woman presents with vision loss and eye pain. Optic neuritis is suspected.

a. CT head and/or orbits
b. CTA head and neck
c. MRI head and orbits without and with contrast
d. MRA head and neck
e. No ideal imaging exam

Suspected optic neuritis.

a. CT head and/or orbits is usually not appropriate.
b. CTA head and neck is usually not appropriate.
c. *MRI head and orbits without and with contrast* is the most appropriate.
d. MRA head and neck is usually not appropriate.

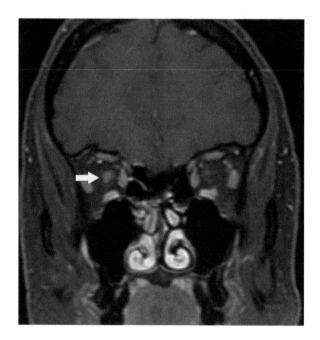

Fig. 11.43 Optic neuritis. Head MR coronal post-contrast image shows a thickened, abnormally enhancing right optic nerve (arrow)

Solution
Optic neuritis is often a manifestation of multiple sclerosis. Therefore, both orbital and head MRI are indicated in order to assess for abnormalities within the optic nerve as well as demyelinating lesions in the brain.

A 42-year-old man presents with visual loss. An intraocular mass is suspected.

a. CT orbits with contrast
b. CTA head and neck
c. MRI orbits
d. MRA head and neck
e. No ideal imaging exam

Visual loss with symptoms of intraocular mass, optic nerve, or pre-chiasm.

a. *CT orbits with contrast* and choice (c) are equally the most appropriate.
b. CTA head and neck may be appropriate.
c. *MRI orbits* and choice (a) are equally the most appropriate.
d. MRA head and neck may be appropriate.

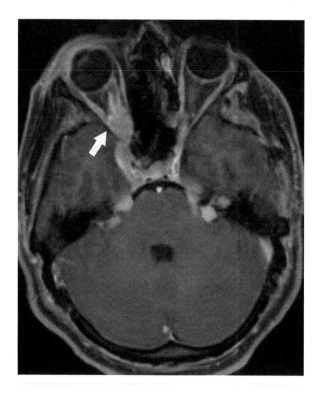

Fig. 11.44 Optic nerve meningioma. Head MR axial post-contrast image shows an enhancing mass (arrow) at the right orbital apex

Solution

Causes of monocular visual loss include intraocular mass, such as melanoma, and intra-orbital, intra-canalicular, or pre-chiasm optic nerve pathologies. MRI is the preferred exam for evaluating the soft tissue within and around the orbit, particularly for characterizing masses and evaluating the optic nerve. CT complements MRI by assessing for adjacent bone involvement not readily seen on MRI.

A 37-year-old woman presents with bilateral vision loss, suspected as originating at the level of the optic chiasm. Ischemic etiology is not suspected.

a. CT orbits with contrast
b. CT head with contrast
c. MRI head without and with contrast
d. MRI orbits without and with contrast
e. No ideal imaging exam

Nonischemic vision loss with chiasm or post-chiasm symptoms.

a. CT orbits with contrast is usually not appropriate.
b. CT head with contrast may be appropriate.
c. *MRI head without and with contrast* is the most appropriate.
d. MRI orbits without and with contrast is usually not appropriate.

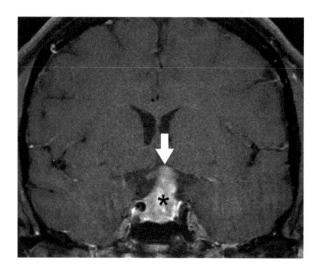

Fig. 11.45 Pituitary mass. Head MR coronal post-contrast image shows an enhancing mass centered in the pituitary fossa (star) that extends superiorly to displace and compress the optic chiasm (arrow)

Solution
Visual loss at the level of the optic chiasm suggests mass effect from a para-sellar lesion arising from the pituitary gland, hypothalamus, or adjacent dura. Post-chiasm visual loss suggests a lesion that involves the optic tracts, lateral geniculate nucleus, optic radiations, or primary visual cortex. MRI is the preferred imaging exam in both cases. Dedicated image acquisition for detailed assessment of the optic chiasm, and adjacent structures can be performed.

A 56-year-old man presents with ophthalmoplegia.

a. CT head with contrast
b. CTA head and neck
c. MRI head and/or orbits without and with contrast
d. MRA head and neck
e. No ideal imaging exam

Adult patient with ophthalmoplegia or diplopia.

a. CT head with contrast may be appropriate.
b. CTA head and neck may be appropriate.
c. *MRI head and/or orbits without and with contrast* is the most appropriate.
d. MRA head and neck may be appropriate.

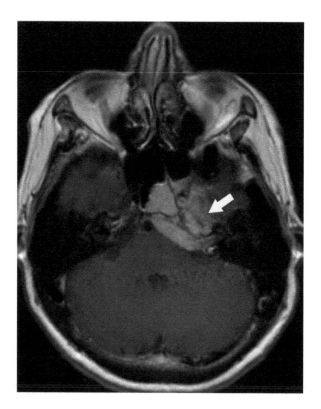

Fig. 11.46 Cavernous sinus meningioma. Head MR axial post-contrast image shows an enhancing suprasellar mass extending into the left cavernous sinus (arrow)

Solution
Ophthalmoplegia or diplopia may be caused by an intraorbital process affecting the extraocular muscles or by pathology involving the brain, brain stem, or cisternal segments of the cranial nerves. MRI is preferred for the evaluation of these sites and can be tailored for the dedicated evaluation of the orbits and/or cranial nerves.

11.10 Hearing Loss and Vertigo

A 61-year-old man presents with acquired conductive hearing loss. A middle ear mass is not clinically evident.

a. CT head without contrast
b. CT temporal bone without contrast
c. CT temporal bone with contrast
d. MRI head and internal auditory canal without and with contrast
e. No ideal imaging exam

Acquired conductive hearing loss in the absence of clinically evident mass in the middle ear.

a. CT head without contrast is usually not appropriate.
b. *CT temporal bone without contrast* is the most appropriate.
c. CT temporal bone with contrast is usually not appropriate.
d. MRI head and internal auditory canal without and with contrast is usually not appropriate.

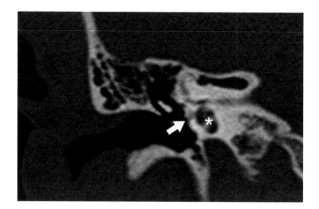

Fig. 11.47 Otosclerosis. Temporal bone CT coronal reconstruction image shows abnormal focal lucency (arrow) anteromedial to the cochlea (star)

Solution
Temporal bone CT is the preferred imaging exam and provides excellent visualization of the external auditory canal, ossicular chain, and bony inner ear structures. It can identify pathologies such as otosclerosis, ossicular erosion or fusion, round window occlusion, and dehiscence of the superior semicircular canal. Intravenous contrast is not useful for temporal bone assessment.

A 56-year-old woman with acquired conductive hearing loss from a cholesteatoma presents for imaging to guide surgical planning.

a. CT head without contrast
b. CT temporal bone without contrast
c. CT temporal bone with contrast
d. MRI head and internal auditory canal without and with contrast
e. No ideal imaging exam

Acquired conductive hearing loss secondary to cholesteatoma or to a neoplasm with suspected intracranial or inner ear extension. Imaging for surgical planning.

a. CT head without contrast may be appropriate.
b. *CT temporal bone without contrast* and choice (d) are equally the most appropriate.
c. CT temporal bone with contrast may be appropriate.
d. *MRI head and internal auditory canal without and with contrast* and choice (b) are equally the most appropriate.

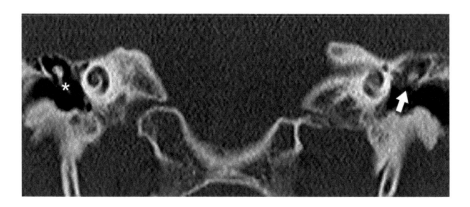

Fig. 11.48 Cholesteatoma. Temporal bone CT coronal reconstruction image shows abnormal soft tissue (arrow) in the left middle ear cavity with bony erosion, compared to a normal right middle ear cavity (star)

Solution
Temporal bone CT can demonstrate small inflammatory or neoplastic masses within the middle ear as well as the resulting erosions of ossicles and inner ear structures. MRI can help delineate the extent of a middle ear mass, and its superior soft tissue characterization complements the detailed evaluation of bony structures provided by CT.

A 57-year-old woman with acquired sensorineural hearing loss.

a. CT head without contrast
b. CT temporal bone without contrast
c. CT temporal bone with contrast
d. MRI head and internal auditory canal without and with contrast
e. No ideal imaging exam

Acquired sensorineural hearing loss.

a. CT head without contrast is usually not appropriate.
b. CT temporal bone without contrast may be appropriate.
c. CT temporal bone with contrast may be appropriate.
d. *MRI head and internal auditory canal without and with contrast* is the most appropriate.

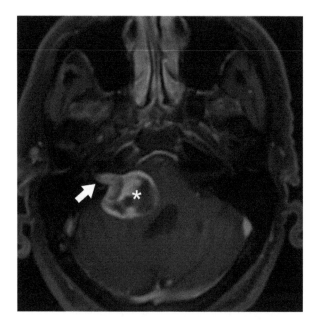

Fig. 11.49 Vestibular schwannoma. Head MR axial post-contrast image shows a mass (star) at the right cerebellopontine angle extending into the internal auditory canal (arrow)

Solution
Dedicated MRI protocols provide detailed evaluation of cochlear contents, the vestibulocochlear nerve, and auditory pathways. High-resolution MRI sequences with sub-millimeter spatial resolution are highly sensitive for etiologies of sensorineural hearing loss. Contrast use improves the detection of inflammation and neoplasm.

A 2-year-old boy with total deafness. He is undergoing surgical planning for cochlear implants.

a. CT head without contrast
b. CT temporal bone without contrast
c. CT temporal bone with contrast
d. MRI head and internal auditory canal without and with contrast
e. No ideal imaging exam

Congenital hearing loss, total deafness, or a cochlear implant candidate. Imaging for surgical planning.

a. CT head without contrast is usually not appropriate.
b. *CT temporal bone without contrast* and choice (d) are equally the most appropriate.
c. CT temporal bone with contrast is usually not appropriate.
d. *MRI head and internal auditory canal without and with contrast* and choice (b) are equally the most appropriate.

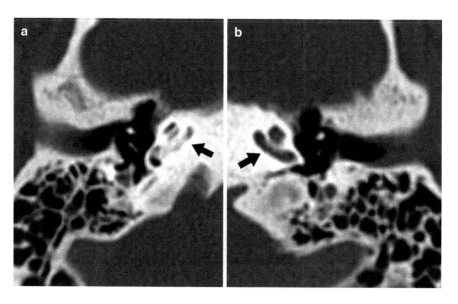

Fig. 11.50 Labyrinthitis ossificans. Temporal bone CT coronal reconstruction images show abnormal ossification of the right cochlea (**a**, arrow) compared to a normal left cochlea (**b**, arrow)

Solution
CT can identify the causes of hearing loss such as cochlear malformations and labyrinthitis ossificans and is valuable for surgical planning by accurately delineating relevant anatomic details such as the size of cochlear and vestibular aqueducts and variant anatomy. MRI is complementary by providing high-resolution assessment of inner ear structures.

A 52-year-old woman with episodic vertigo.

a. CT head without contrast
b. CT temporal bone without contrast
c. CT temporal bone with contrast
d. MRI head and internal auditory canal without and with contrast
e. No ideal imaging exam

Episodic vertigo with or without associated hearing loss or aural fullness (peripheral vertigo).

a. CT head without contrast is usually not appropriate.
b. *CT temporal bone without contrast* and choice (d) are equally the most appropriate.
c. CT temporal bone with contrast is usually not appropriate.
d. *MRI head and internal auditory canal without and with contrast* and choice (b) are equally the most appropriate.

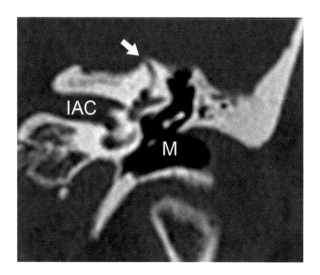

Fig. 11.51 Superior semicircular canal dehiscence. Temporal bone CT coronal reconstructed image shows a bony defect along the left superior semicircular canal (arrow). *IAC* internal auditory canal, *M* middle ear

Solution

A dedicated temporal bone CT can accurately evaluate the bony labyrinth to identify causes of peripheral vertigo including fractures, superior semicircular canal dehiscence, and bony erosions from inflammatory or iatrogenic causes. Potential etiologies that can be detected on MRI include labyrinthitis and neuritis.

A 61-year-old man presents with persistent central vertigo.

a. CT head without contrast
b. CT temporal bone without contrast
c. CT temporal bone with contrast
d. MRI head and internal auditory canal without and with contrast
e. No ideal imaging exam

Persistent vertigo with or without neurological symptoms (central vertigo).

a. CT head without contrast may be appropriate.
b. CT temporal bone without contrast is usually not appropriate.
c. CT temporal bone with contrast is usually not appropriate.
d. *MRI head and internal auditory canal without and with contrast* is the most appropriate.

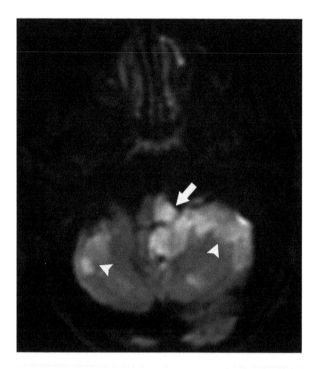

Fig. 11.52 Brainstem infarction. Head MR axial diffusion-weighted image shows restricted diffusion in the left lateral medulla (arrow) accounting for vertigo. Infarction of bilateral cerebellar hemispheres (arrowheads) are also present

Solution

MRI is the preferred imaging exam to detect causes of central vertigo including posterior fossa neoplasm and infarction, Chiari malformation, and demyelinating lesions. Of note, infarcts that cause isolated vestibular symptoms are usually small. Thus, a normal MRI does not exclude infarction as an etiology.

11.11 Tinnitus

A 51-year-old woman with pulsatile tinnitus. Exam reveals no myoclonus or Eustachian tube dysfunction.

a. US duplex Doppler carotid
b. CT temporal bone without contrast
c. CTA head and neck
d. MRA head without and with contrast
e. No ideal imaging exam

Subjective or objective pulsatile tinnitus (no myoclonus or Eustachian tube dysfunction).

a. US duplex Doppler carotid may be appropriate.
b. *CT temporal bone without contrast* and choice (c) are equally the most appropriate.
c. *CTA head and neck* and choice (b) are equally the most appropriate.
d. MRA head without and with contrast is usually appropriate, but there is a better choice here.

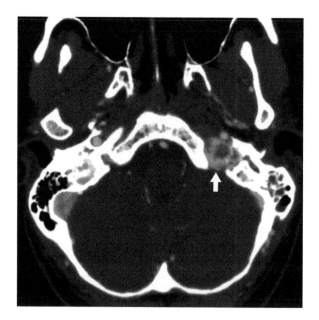

Fig. 11.53 Glomus jugulare paraganglioma. Head and neck CTA image shows an enhancing mass (arrow) expanding the left jugular foramen

Solution
Both temporal bone CT and CTA are recommended to assess pulsatile tinnitus. Causes include vascular masses such as paragangliomas, aberrant vascular anatomy, vascular malformations, and intracranial hypertension.

A 47-year-old man with unilateral subjective non-pulsatile tinnitus, without hearing loss, neurologic deficit, or recent trauma. Otoscopic exam is negative.

a. US duplex Doppler carotid
b. CT temporal bone without contrast
c. CTA head and neck
d. MRI head and internal auditory canal without and with contrast
e. No ideal imaging exam

Asymmetric or unilateral, subjective, non-pulsatile tinnitus. Negative otoscopic finding. No hearing loss, neurologic deficit, or recent trauma.

a. US duplex Doppler carotid is usually not appropriate.
b. CT temporal bone without contrast may be appropriate.
c. CTA head and neck is usually not appropriate.
d. *MRI head and internal auditory canal without and with contrast* is the most appropriate.

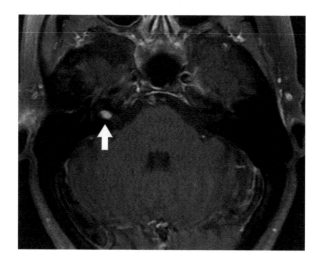

Fig. 11.54 Vestibular schwannoma. Head MR axial post-contrast image shows a mass (arrow) in the right internal auditory canal

Solution

MRI is the preferred imaging exam to identify causes of non-pulsatile unilateral tinnitus including retrocochlear lesions such as vestibular schwannoma, other cerebellopontine cistern angle lesions, or masses along the auditory pathway.

A 67-year-old man with bilateral subjective non-pulsatile tinnitus, without hearing loss, neurologic deficit, or trauma.

a. US duplex Doppler carotid
b. CT temporal bone without contrast
c. CTA head and neck
d. MRI head and internal auditory canal without and with contrast
e. No ideal imaging exam

Symmetric or bilateral, subjective, non-pulsatile tinnitus. No hearing loss, neuro-logic deficit, or trauma.

a. US duplex Doppler carotid is usually not appropriate.
b. CT temporal bone without contrast is usually not appropriate.
c. CTA head and neck is usually not appropriate.
d. MRI head and internal auditory canal without and with contrast is usually not appropriate.
e. *No ideal imaging exam* is the correct answer.

Solution
Imaging is usually unrevealing in this setting, where potential causes of tinnitus include medications, noise-induced hearing loss, presbycusis, or chronic bilateral hearing loss.

11.12 Sinonasal Disease

A 24-year-old man with 2 weeks of uncomplicated rhinosinusitis.

a. X-ray paranasal sinuses
b. CT paranasal sinuses without contrast
c. CT paranasal sinuses with contrast
d. MRI maxillofacial without and with contrast
e. No ideal imaging exam

Acute (<4 weeks) uncomplicated rhinosinusitis.

a. X-ray paranasal sinuses is usually not appropriate.
b. CT paranasal sinuses without contrast may be appropriate.
c. CT paranasal sinuses with contrast is usually not appropriate.
d. MRI maxillofacial without and with contrast is usually not appropriate.
e. *No ideal imaging exam* is the correct answer.

Solution
Acute bacterial rhinosinusitis is a clinical diagnosis for which imaging is not indicated in the absence of complications such as headache, facial swelling, orbital proptosis, or cranial nerve palsy.

A 31-year-old woman with 2 weeks of rhinosinusitis with orbital involvement now suspected.

a. CT cone beam paranasal sinuses
b. CT head without contrast
c. CT paranasal sinuses with contrast
d. MRI maxillofacial without and with contrast
e. No ideal imaging exam

Acute rhinosinusitis. Suspected orbital or intracranial complication.

a. CT cone beam paranasal sinuses is usually not appropriate.
b. CT head without contrast may be appropriate.
c. *CT paranasal sinuses with contrast* and choice (d) are equally the most appropriate.
d. *MRI maxillofacial without and with contrast* and choice (c) are equally the most appropriate.

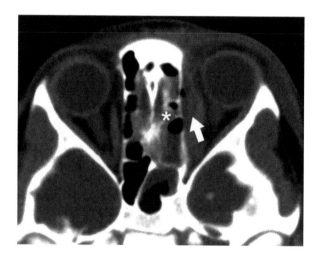

Fig. 11.55 Sinusitis with orbital complication. Sinus CT with contrast shows a subperiosteal abscess (arrow) in the left orbit and inflammation in the adjacent ethmoid sinus (star)

Solution

Infections from the ethmoid sinus can spread via perforations of the lamina papyracea and cribriform plate, veins that extend into the cavernous sinus, and direct extension through the bone. CT and MRI are complementary imaging exams to evaluate soft tissue structures, orbital contents, and the brain. CT is superior for determining bone integrity and erosion while MRI better depicts intraorbital and intracranial complications such as abscesses and cavernous sinus thrombosis.

A 52-year-old man with sinonasal obstruction. An underlying mass is suspected.

a. CT cone beam paranasal sinuses
b. CT head without contrast
c. CT paranasal sinuses without contrast
d. MRI maxillofacial without and with contrast
e. No ideal imaging exam

Sinonasal obstruction with suspected mass.

a. CT cone beam paranasal sinuses is usually not appropriate.
b. CT head without contrast is usually not appropriate.
c. *CT paranasal sinuses without contrast* and choice (d) are equally the most appropriate and complementary to each other.
d. *MRI maxillofacial without and with contrast* and choice (c) are equally the most appropriate and complementary to each other.

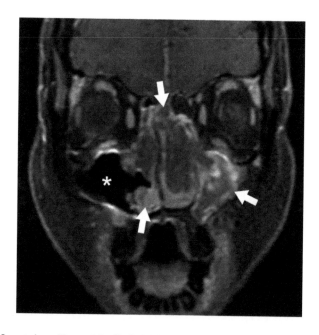

Fig. 11.56 Inverted papilloma. Maxillofacial MR coronal post-contrast image shows a mass (arrows) within the nasal cavity and paranasal sinuses with relative sparing of the right maxillary sinus (star)

Solution

Optimal evaluation of a suspected sinonasal mass usually requires both CT and MRI. Sinus CT characterizes bone erosion and destruction and evaluates for the presence of cartilaginous or bony matrix associated with the mass. MRI helps differentiate a mass from post-obstructive secretions and assesses orbital, skull base, or intracranial extension.

11.13 Thyroid Disease

A 55-year-old woman with a palpable thyroid nodule. She is euthyroid.

a. US thyroid
b. CT neck without contrast
c. MRI neck without contrast
d. I-123 radionuclide scan neck
e. No ideal imaging exam

Palpable thyroid nodule without goiter. Euthyroid.

a. *US thyroid* is the most appropriate.
b. CT neck without contrast may be appropriate.
c. MRI neck without contrast is usually not appropriate.
d. I-123 radionuclide scan neck is usually not appropriate.

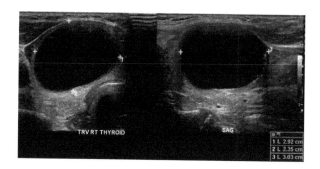

Fig. 11.57 Colloid cyst. Thyroid US shows a 3 cm cyst (calipers) in the right lobe of the thyroid gland

Solution

US is used to determine if the palpable abnormality corresponds to a thyroid nodule. Sonographic characteristics of thyroid nodules help estimate the risk for malignancy and helps guide the decision for biopsy.

A 42-year-old woman with a neck mass suspected to be goiter.

a. US thyroid
b. CT neck without contrast
c. MRI neck without contrast
d. I-123 radionuclide scan neck
e. No ideal imaging exam

Suspected goiter.

a. *US thyroid* and choice (b) are equally the most appropriate.
b. *CT neck without contrast* and choice (a) are equally the most appropriate.
c. MRI neck may be appropriate.
d. I-123 radionuclide scan neck may be appropriate.

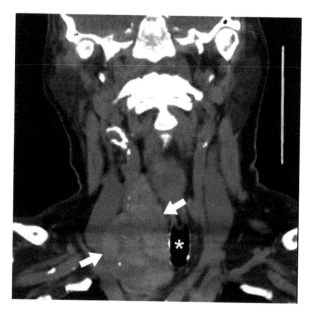

Fig. 11.58 Goiter. Neck CT coronal reconstruction image shows enlargement of the right lobe of the thyroid gland (arrows) with associated leftward deviation of the trachea (star)

Solution
US and CT are complementary in this setting. Sonographic evaluation helps confirm that the neck mass is arising from the thyroid and assesses its size and morphology. CT evaluates for substernal extension, deep extension into the retropharyngeal space, and tracheal compression. Contrast is not needed unless there is concern for an infiltrative neoplasm.

A 49-year-old woman with thyrotoxicosis.

a. US thyroid
b. CT neck without contrast
c. MRI neck without contrast
d. I-123 radionuclide scan neck
e. No ideal imaging exam

Thyrotoxicosis.

a. *US thyroid* and choice (d) are equally the most appropriate.
b. CT neck without contrast is usually not appropriate.
c. MRI neck without contrast is usually not appropriate.
d. *I-123 radionuclide scan neck* and choice (a) are equally the most appropriate.

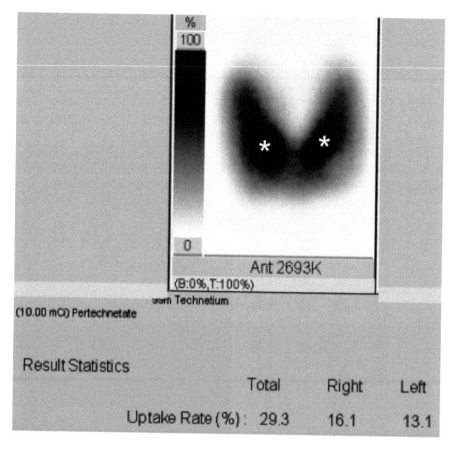

Fig. 11.59 Graves' disease. I-123 radionuclide scan of the neck shows diffusely increased tracer uptake in the thyroid gland (stars)

Solution

Radionuclide scans help distinguish between the causes of thyrotoxicosis with high uptake (i.e., Graves' disease, toxic adenoma, and toxic multinodular goiter) and low uptake (i.e., subacute thyroiditis and exogenous thyroid hormone). US can help confirm the presence of nodules suggested by the radionuclide scan.

A 32-year-old woman with primary hypothyroidism.

a. US thyroid
b. CT neck without contrast
c. MRI neck without contrast
d. I-123 radionuclide scan neck
e. No ideal imaging exam

Primary hypothyroidism.

a. US thyroid is usually not appropriate.
b. CT neck without contrast is usually not appropriate.
c. MRI neck without contrast is usually not appropriate.
d. I-123 radionuclide scan neck is usually not appropriate.
e. *No ideal imaging exam* is the correct answer.

Solution
Imaging does not play a role in the evaluation of hypothyroidism in adults. Neither evaluation of thyroid morphology nor radionuclide uptake differentiates among the causes of hypothyroidism.

11.14 Neck Mass and Adenopathy

A 67-year-old man with a non-pulsatile neck mass, not in the parotid or thyroid gland.

a. US neck
b. CT neck with contrast
c. CTA neck
d. MRI neck without and with contrast
e. No ideal imaging exam

Non-pulsatile neck mass(es), not in parotid or thyroid gland.

a. US neck may be appropriate.
b. *CT neck with contrast* and choice (d) are equally the most appropriate.
c. CTA neck is usually not appropriate.
d. *MRI neck without and with contrast* and choice (b) are equally the most appropriate.

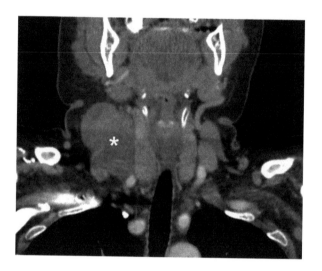

Fig. 11.60 Lymphoma. Neck CT with contrast coronal reconstruction image shows a right-sided neck mass (star)

Solution

CT and MRI allow precise localization of the palpable finding, and both can accurately evaluate for tumors and infections. Use of contrast helps detect abscesses, necrotic lymph nodes, and primary tumors and determines the relationship of neck masses to the vasculature.

A 49-year-old woman with a pulsatile neck mass, not in the parotid or thyroid gland.

a. US neck
b. CT neck with contrast
c. CTA neck
d. MRI neck without and with contrast
e. No ideal imaging exam

Pulsatile neck mass(es), not in the parotid or thyroid gland.

a. US neck may be appropriate.
b. *CT neck with contrast* and choices (c) and (d) are equally the most appropriate.
c. *CTA neck* and choices (b) and (d) are equally the most appropriate.
d. *MRI neck without and with contrast* and choice (b) and (c) are equally the most appropriate.

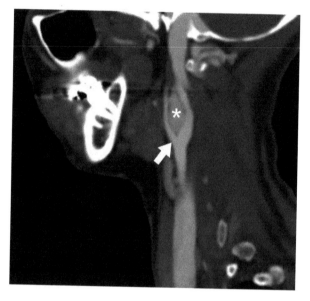

Fig. 11.61 Carotid body paraganglioma. Neck CTA sagittal reconstruction image shows an enhancing mass (star) located at the left carotid artery bifurcation (arrow)

Solution

A pulsatile neck mass may represent a tortuous artery, atypical lymphovascular malformation, arteriovenous fistula, pseudoaneurysm, paraganglioma, or a lymph node or tumor abutting an artery. These potential etiologies may be evaluated with either CT or MRI. Use of contrast helps differentiate vessels from lymph nodes.

A 64-year-old woman with bilateral parotid swelling.

a. US neck
b. CT neck with contrast
c. CTA neck
d. MRI neck without and with contrast
e. No ideal imaging exam

Parotid region mass(es).

a. *US neck* and choice (b) and (d) are equally the most appropriate.
b. *CT neck with contrast* and choices (a) and (d) are equally the most appropriate.
c. CTA neck is usually not appropriate.
d. *MRI neck without and with contrast* and choice (a) and (b) are equally the most appropriate.

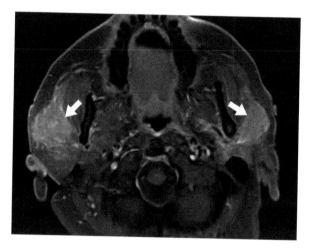

Fig. 11.62 Parotid tumors. Neck MR axial post-contrast image shows enhancing masses (arrows) in the parotid glands bilaterally. Surgical biopsy revealed metastatic melanoma

Solution
Imaging helps localize a mass as within or outside the parotid gland and allows a differential diagnosis. MRI provides the most complete evaluation and can assess for the extent of parotid involvement, local invasion, perineural tumor spread, and extension into the temporal bone. CT provides the evaluation of the adjacent bone and detects of sialoliths. US can accurately localize parotid masses and guide fine needle aspiration.

11.15 Low Back Pain

A 40-year-old man presents with 3 weeks of low back pain, for which he has not undergone any management. He is otherwise asymptomatic without any significant medical history.

a. X-ray lumbar spine
b. CT lumbar spine without contrast
c. MRI lumbar spine without contrast
d. CT myelography lumbar spine
e. No ideal imaging exam

Acute, subacute, or chronic uncomplicated low back pain or radiculopathy. No red flags. No prior management.

a. X-ray lumbar spine is usually not appropriate.
b. CT lumbar spine without contrast is usually not appropriate.
c. MRI lumbar spine without contrast is usually not appropriate.
d. CT myelography lumbar spine is usually not appropriate.
e. *No ideal imaging exam* is the correct answer.

Solution

Acute low back pain, lasting less than 6 weeks, is usually a benign, self-limited condition for which imaging is unlikely to be beneficial. However, imaging can be considered if there is little or no improvement in pain after 6 weeks of conservative management. Imaging is also indicated by red flags that raise suspicion for underlying conditions such as cauda equina syndrome, malignancy, fracture, or infection. For patients with chronic low back pain without red flags, the first-line treatment is likewise conservative management without routine imaging.

A 49-year-old man with low back pain and radiculopathy. His symptoms persisted over 6 weeks of conservative management, and now interventional treatment is being considered.

a. X-ray lumbar spine
b. CT lumbar spine without contrast
c. MRI lumbar spine without contrast
d. CT myelography lumbar spine
e. No ideal imaging exam

Acute, subacute, or chronic low back pain or radiculopathy with persistent or progressive symptoms during or following 6 weeks of conservative management. The individual is a candidate for surgery or intervention.

a. X-ray lumbar spine may be appropriate.
b. CT lumbar spine without contrast may be appropriate.
c. *MRI lumbar spine without contrast* is the most appropriate.
d. CT myelography lumbar spine may be appropriate.

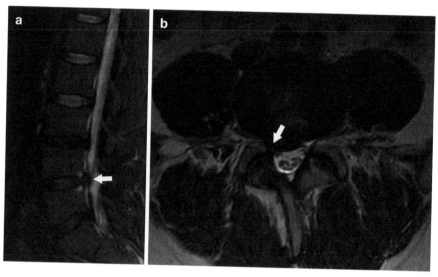

Fig. 11.63 Disc herniation with nerve root compression. Lumbar spine MR sagittal T2-weighted image (**a**) shows disc herniation at L4–L5 (arrow) which on axial T2-weighted image (**b**) is seen compressing the right L5 nerve root (arrow)

Solution

Imaging is indicated in patients who continue to be symptomatic after 4–6 weeks of conservative management, have signs of nerve root irritation, and are candidates for intervention. Imaging is also appropriate when the etiology of pain remains uncertain. MRI is preferred and can accurately demonstrate disc disease.

A 79-year-old woman with known osteoporosis and acute low back pain.

a. X-ray lumbar spine
b. CT lumbar spine without contrast
c. MRI lumbar spine without contrast
d. CT myelography lumbar spine
e. No ideal imaging exam

Acute, subacute, or chronic uncomplicated low back pain or radiculopathy with one or more of the following: low velocity trauma, osteoporosis, elderly, or chronic steroid use.

a. *X-ray lumbar spine* is the most appropriate.
b. CT lumbar spine without contrast is usually appropriate, but there is a better choice here.
c. MRI lumbar spine without contrast is usually appropriate, but there is a better choice here.
d. CT myelography lumbar spine is usually not appropriate.

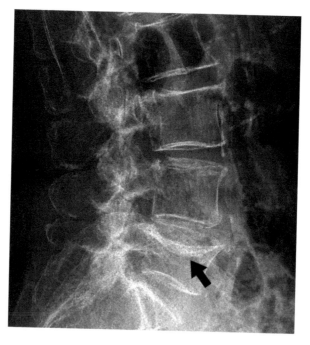

Fig. 11.64 Vertebral compression fracture. Lumbar spine X-ray lateral view shows lucent bones indicating diffuse osteopenia and a compression fracture of the L5 vertebral body superior end-plate (arrow)

Solution

Radiography is the preferred initial imaging exam in this setting to assess for vertebral body compression fracture. CT is used for fracture detection if there is concern for traumatic vertebral body injury. MRI is used to evaluate the spinal ligaments and canal and to assess for hemorrhage.

A 75-year-old man, chronically immunosuppressed, presents with acute low back pain.

a. X-ray lumbar spine
b. CT lumbar spine without contrast
c. MRI lumbar spine without and with contrast
d. CT myelography lumbar spine
e. No ideal imaging exam

Acute, subacute, or chronic low back pain or radiculopathy with one or more of the following: infection, immunosuppression, or suspicion for cancer.

a. X-ray lumbar spine may be appropriate.
b. CT lumbar without contrast spine may be appropriate.
c. *MRI lumbar spine without and with contrast* is the most appropriate.
d. CT myelography lumbar spine is usually not appropriate.

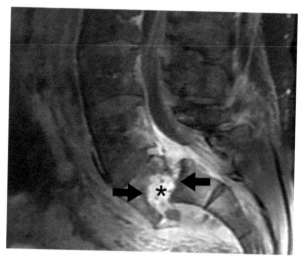

Fig. 11.65 Spondylodiscitis. Lumbar spine MR sagittal post-contrast image shows abnormal enhancement in the L5-S1 disc space (star) with the erosion of the adjacent vertebral body end-plates (arrows)

Solution

MRI is the preferred imaging exam to assess for spinal malignancy and infection. Intradural and spinal cord malignancies are better seen on MRI than CT. MRI is also highly sensitive and specific for infections and can make the diagnosis earlier in the course of disease than CT.

A 50-year-old man with prior lumbar spine surgery now with new low back pain.

a. X-ray lumbar spine
b. CT lumbar spine without contrast
c. MRI lumbar spine without and with contrast
d. CT myelography lumbar spine
e. No ideal imaging exam

Low back pain or radiculopathy. New or progressing symptoms or clinical signs and a history of prior lumbar surgery.

a. X-ray lumbar spine may be appropriate.
b. CT lumbar spine without contrast may be appropriate.
c. *MRI lumbar spine without and with contrast* is the most appropriate.
d. CT myelography lumbar spine may be appropriate.

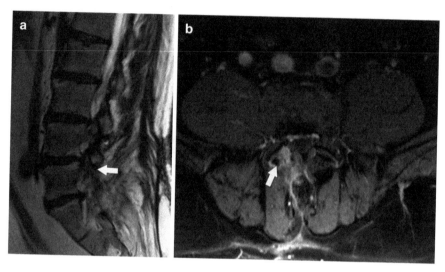

Fig. 11.66 Post-spine surgery scar with nerve root impingement. Lumbar spine MR sagittal T2-weighted (**a**) and axial post-contrast (**b**) images show soft tissue (arrows) encasing the right S1 nerve root

Solution

Causes for pain or radiculopathy that can be seen on MRI include free disc or bone fragments, postoperative scarring, bone graft failure, and recurrent disc protrusion or herniation. Use of contrast helps distinguish scars from recurrent disc protrusion or herniation. CT myelography may be used if MRI cannot be performed.

A 73-year-old woman presents with low back pain and cauda equina syndrome.

a. X-ray lumbar spine
b. CT lumbar spine without contrast
c. MRI lumbar spine without contrast
d. CT myelography lumbar spine
e. No ideal imaging exam

Low back pain and suspected cauda equina syndrome or rapidly progressing neurologic deficit.

a. X-ray lumbar spine is usually not appropriate.
b. CT lumbar spine without contrast may be appropriate.
c. *MRI lumbar spine without contrast* is the most appropriate.
d. CT myelography lumbar spine may be appropriate.

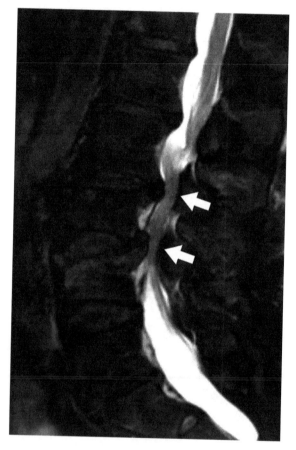

Fig. 11.67 Spinal stenosis. Lumbar spine MR sagittal T2-weighted image shows posterior disc
bulges at L2–L3 and L3–L4 (arrows), resulting in severe spinal canal stenosis and cauda equina
compression

Solution

Cauda equina syndrome results from the dysfunction of sacral and lumbar nerve
roots within the vertebral canal and is most commonly caused by disc herniation.
MRI is the preferred imaging exam as it depicts soft tissue pathology, evaluates the
vertebral marrow, and assesses spinal canal patency. Use of contrast is guided by the
specific clinical scenario and helps evaluate for infection, inflammation, and malignancy. CT myelography is an alternative if MRI cannot be performed.

Bibliography

Haydel MJ, et al. Indications for computed tomography in patients with minor head injury. New Engl J Med. 2000;343(2):100–5.
Mower WR, et al. Developing a decision instrument to guide computed tomographic imaging of blunt head injury patients. J Trauma. 2005;59(4):954–9.
Stiell IG, et al. The Canadian CT Head Rule for patients with minor head injury. Lancet. 2001;357(9266):1391–6.
Teasdale G, Jennett B. Assessment of coma and impaired consciousness. Lancet. 1974;2(7872):81–4.

Ingram Content Group UK Ltd.
Milton Keynes UK
UKHW021807230323
419040UK00002B/3